T0226791

Integrative Medicine

Editors

DEBORAH S. CLEMENTS
MELINDA RING

PRIMARY CARE:
CLINICS IN OFFICE PRACTICE

www.primarycare.theclinics.com

Consulting Editor
JOEL J. HEIDELBAUGH

June 2017 • Volume 44 • Number 2

ELSEVIER

1600 John F. Kennedy Boulevard • Suite 1800 • Philadelphia, Pennsylvania, 19103-2899

http://www.theclinics.com

PRIMARY CARE: CLINICS IN OFFICE PRACTICE Volume 44, Number 2
June 2017 ISSN 0095-4543, ISBN-13: 978-0-323-53027-9

Editor: Jessica McCool
Developmental Editor: Colleen Dietzler

Primary Care: Clinics in Office Practice (ISSN: 0095–4543) is published quarterly by Elsevier Inc., 360 Park Avenue South, New York, NY 10010-1710. Months of issue are March, June, September, and December. Periodicals postage paid at New York, NY and additional mailing offices. Subscription prices are $232.00 per year (US individuals), $451.00 (US institutions), $100.00 (US students), $283.00 (Canadian individuals), $511.00 (Canadian institutions), $175.00 (Canadian students), $355.00 (international individuals), $511.00 (international institutions), and $175.00 (international students). Foreign air speed delivery is included in all *Clinics* subscription prices. All prices are subject to change without notice. POSTMASTER: Send address changes to *Primary Care: Clinics in Office Practice*, Elsevier Periodicals Customer Service, 11830 Westline Industrial Drive, St. Louis, MO 63146. Customer Service Health Sciences Division, Subscription Customer Service, 3251 Riverport Lane, Maryland Heights, MO 63043. **Customer Service: 1-800-654-2452 (U.S. and Canada); 314-447-8871 (outside U.S. and Canada). Fax: 314-447-8029. E-mail: journalscustomerservice-usa@elsevier.com (for print support); journalsonlinesupport-usa@elsevier.com (for online support).**

Reprints. For copies of 100 or more, of articles in this publication, please contact the Commercial Reprints Department, Elsevier Inc., 360 Park Avenue South, New York, NY 10010-1710. Tel. 212-633-3874; Fax: 212-633-3820; E-mail: reprints@elsevier.com.

Primary Care: Clinics in Office Practice is covered in *MEDLINE/PubMed (Index Medicus)* and *EMBASE/ Excerpta Medica, Current Contents/Clinical Medicine,* and *ISI/BIOMED.*

Contributors

CONSULTING EDITOR

JOEL J. HEIDELBAUGH, MD, FAAFP, FACG
Clinical Professor, Departments of Family Medicine and Urology, University of Michigan
Medical School, Ann Arbor, Michigan; Ypsilanti Health Center, Ypsilanti, Michigan

EDITORS

DEBORAH S. CLEMENTS, MD, FAAFP
Nancy and Warren Furey Professor of Community Medicine, Professor of Medical
Education, Chair, Family and Community Medicine, Northwestern University Feinberg
School of Medicine, Chicago, Illinois

MELINDA RING, MD, FACP, ABOIM
Executive Director, Osher Center for Integrative Medicine, Drs Pat and Carl Greer
Distinguished Physician in Integrative Medicine, Clinical Associate Professor of Medicine
and Medical Social Sciences, Northwestern University Feinberg School of Medicine,
Chicago, Illinois

AUTHORS

ANNA BALABANOVA, MD
Family Medicine Chief Resident, Northwestern Medicine Lake Forest Hospital, Grayslake,
Illinois

ROMAN BECICKA, MD
Feinberg School of Medicine, Northwestern University, Chicago, Illinois

DAVID K. BECKER, MD, MPH, MA
Clinical Professor, Department of Pediatrics, Osher Center for Integrative Medicine,
University of California, San Francisco, San Francisco, California

DANNY BEGA, MD, MSCI
Assistant Professor, Department of Neurology, Northwestern University Feinberg School
of Medicine, Chicago, Illinois

KAREN L. CALDWELL, PhD
Professor, Department of Human Development and Psychological Counseling,
Appalachian State University, Boone, North Carolina

EZRA M. COHEN, MD
Fellow, Division of Immunology, Department of Rheumatology, Boston Children's
Hospital, Boston, Massachusetts

JONAH COHEN, MD
Fellow, Division of Gastroenterology and Hepatology, Beth Israel Deaconess Medical Center, Boston, Massachusetts

JUDITH CUNEO, MD
Osher Center for Integrative Medicine, University of California, San Francisco, San Francisco, California

MICHELLE L. DOSSETT, MD, PhD, MPH
Assistant Physician, Division of General Internal Medicine, Benson-Henry Institute for Mind Body Medicine, Massachusetts General Hospital, Instructor in Medicine, Harvard Medical School, Boston, Massachusetts

DEBORAH EDBERG, MD
Program Director, Northwestern Family Medicine Residency Program, Erie Family Health Center, Chicago, Illinois

ROY ELAM, MD
Associate Professor of Internal Medicine, Department of Physical Medicine and Rehabilitation, Osher Center for Integrative Medicine at Vanderbilt, Vanderbilt University Medical Center, Nashville, Tennessee

CHARLES C. FALZON, MD, MBA
Health System Clinician of Family and Community Medicine, Northwestern Memorial Hospital, Chicago, Illinois

JUDY A. FULOP, ND, MS, FABNO
Naturopathic Physician, Naturopathic Oncology, Osher Center for Integrative Medicine, Northwestern Memorial Hospital, Northwestern Medicine, Chicago, Illinois; Adjunct Faculty, Naturopathic Medicine, National University of Health Sciences, Lombard, Illinois

ANIA GRIMONE, MS, LAc
Acupuncturist, Herbalist, Health Coach, Osher Center for Integrative Medicine, Northwestern Memorial Hospital, Northwestern Medicine, Chicago, Illinois

MARNI G. HILLINGER, MD
Assistant Professor, Department of Physical Medicine and Rehabilitation, Director of Education, Osher Center for Integrative Medicine at Vanderbilt, Vanderbilt University Medical Center, Nashville, Tennessee

RUPA MAHADEVAN, MD
Osher Center for Integrative Medicine, Clinical Instructor of Pediatrics, Northwestern University Feinberg School of Medicine, Chicago, Illinois

LINDSEY C. McKERNAN, PhD
Assistant Clinical Professor, Departments of Psychiatry & Behavioral Sciences and Physical Medicine and Rehabilitation, Osher Center for Integrative Medicine at Vanderbilt, Vanderbilt University Medical Center, Nashville, Tennessee

DARSHAN MEHTA, MD, MPH
Associate Director of Education, Osher Center for Integrative Medicine, Brigham and Women's Hospital, Instructor in Medicine, Harvard Medical School, Medical Director, Director of Medical Education, Benson-Henry Institute for Mind-Body Medicine, Massachusetts General Hospital, Boston, Massachusetts

SREELA NAMBOODIRI, MD
Northwestern Fellow, Osher Center for Integrative Medicine and Family Medicine Residency Program, Erie Family Health Center, Chicago, Illinois

MELINDA RING, MD, FACP, ABOIM
Executive Director, Osher Center for Integrative Medicine, Drs Pat and Carl Greer
Distinguished Physician in Integrative Medicine, Clinical Associate Professor of Medicine
and Medical Social Sciences, Northwestern University Feinberg School of Medicine,
Chicago, Illinois

ANUJ K. SHAH, MD, MPH
Associate Program Director, Northwestern Family Medicine Residency Program,
Erie Family Health Center, Chicago, Illinois

MARY R. TALEN, PhD
Director, Primary Care Behavioral Health Education, Northwestern Family Medicine
Residency Program, Erie Family Health Center, Chicago, Illinois

DAVID VICTORSON, PhD
Associate Professor, Department of Medical Social Sciences, Northwestern University
Feinberg School of Medicine, Associate Director of Research, Osher Center for
Integrative Medicine, Northwestern Medicine, Chicago, Illinois

RUTH Q. WOLEVER, PhD
Associate Professor, Department of Physical Medicine and Rehabilitation, Director
of Vanderbilt Health Coaching: Education, Research, & Practice, Osher Center for
Integrative Medicine at Vanderbilt, Vanderbilt University Medical Center, Vanderbilt
University School of Nursing, Department of Psychiatry & Behavioral Sciences, Vanderbilt
University Medical Center, Nashville, Tennessee

Contents

> Integrative Medicine has been described as "healing oriented medicine that takes account of the whole person (body, mind, and spirit) including all aspects of lifestyle. It emphasizes therapeutic relationships and makes use of all appropriate therapies, both conventional and alternative." National surveys consistently report that approximately one-third of adults and 12% of children use complementary and integrative medicine approaches. Although there are barriers to primary care professionals engaging in discussions about lifestyle change and complementary and integrative medicine options, there is also great potential to impact patient well-being.

> Herbal medications are commonly used in all medical settings, making it essential for primary care providers to learn about the products being used and resources they can access for continuing education. Understanding how herbal medicines are sourced, processed, and standardized can help providers guide patients who are trying to choose the most clinically effective and affordable treatments. Multiple herbs are often combined and sold as proprietary blends, which can increase the risk of allergies, adverse reactions, or cross-reactivity with other pharmaceuticals and supplements. Several textbooks, online point-of-care resources, and conferences are available for primary care providers to expand their knowledge of herbal medicines.

> Until system reforms allow adequate time and reimbursement for primary care providers to focus on lifestyle change to prevent and mitigate chronic disease, primary care providers need a manageable, defined role to support lifestyle change. The authors suggest this role is to serve as a catalyst, priming the patient for change; educating and pointing the patient to appropriate, evidence-based resources for additional guidance and hands-on support; and providing ongoing encouragement throughout the long journey of change while patients work more intensely with health coaches or allied health providers.

Integrative health modalities can provide useful tools in the management of persistent pain in the primary care setting. These modalities, such as acupuncture, mind-body medicine, diet and herbs, and movement strategies can be safely used and may provide patients with hope and empowerment. It is highly recommended that the patient work alongside trained professionals for a given modality and/or an interprofessional team.

Gastrointestinal conditions are prevalent in the population and account for significant morbidity and health care costs. Patients with gastrointestinal conditions use integrative medicine. There is growing evidence that integrative medicine approaches can improve symptoms and affect physiology and disease course. This article reviews data on some common and well-studied approaches, including mind–body therapies, acupuncture, diet, probiotics, and dietary supplements and herbs. Although clear recommendations can be made for some conditions, in others there are challenges in translating these findings owing to small study size, lack of standardization, and trial heterogeneity.

An integrative approach to individuals with mood, emotional or mental health concerns involves a comprehensive model of care that is person-centered. Integrative medicine builds on a patient's personal meaning and goals (spiritual aspects) and includes herbal therapies, nutritional support, movement and physical manipulative therapies, mindfulness, relaxation strategies, and psychotherapies.

Chronic neurologic conditions are frequently managed in the primary care setting, and patients with these conditions are increasingly seeking nonconventional treatment options. This article provides a review and summary of the evidence for some of the most commonly studied and most frequently used complementary and integrative interventions for 3 conditions managed every day in primary care offices – diabetic neuropathy, migraine, and dementia.

Integrative Oncology incorporates conventional and western cancer treatment approaches with the best of ancient and traditional medicine including nutrition, supplements, Qigong, herbal medicine, mind-body practices, and more. This article offers a guiding conceptual paradigm from an integrative perspective based on the principles of balance and imbalance. An integrative approach is used to help improve quality of life, enhance lifestyle choices and mitigate symptoms and side effects from conventional treatments. By supporting the patient's mind, body and spirit throughout the cancer treatment journey, the primary care physician is in a key position to work with their patient's oncologist to provide supportive care and recommendations during cancer treatment.

Integrative Medicine

PRIMARY CARE:
CLINICS IN OFFICE PRACTICE

Foreword

"Too Much?"

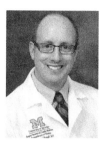

Joel J. Heidelbaugh, MD, FAAFP, FACG
Consulting Editor

A few years ago, I met a new patient to my practice, who walked in with a shopping bag, which she brought into the exam room. Covertly, she had it tucked behind her chair during the interview. We discussed the current state of her fibromyalgia, her polycystic ovarian syndrome and infertility, and her chronic pain. She felt very frustrated by the dozens of previous doctors who "didn't listen to her" and "told her that [her symptoms were] all in her head." At the end of our interview, she brought out the shopping bag and lined up 22 different bottles of supplements that she had ordered on the Internet to treat these conditions. She explained how she viewed the pharmaceutical companies as "unethical," and she only wanted to take "holistic and organic" supplements to treat her conditions. Honestly and sheepishly, I admitted that I would have to look up the majority of the supplements to find out their ingredients, their therapeutic purpose, as well as any evidence behind their efficacy. Then, she asked me if what she was taking was "just too much?"

Over the past decades, integrative medicine has exploded as a mainstream alternative to conventional medicine, marrying a holistic approach with directed attention toward the mind-body connection, nutrition, and biophysiologic medicine with a patient-centered approach. It's popular; it's in demand, and the demand often can't be adequately met in many areas of the country. Most US medical schools still eschew any codified curricula to provide adequate education in integrative medicine, nutrition, or any other form of alternative medicine. Fortunately, fellowship and additional training programs now provide the venue for practitioners across all medical fields to learn and incorporate such knowledge into their practices. Insurance companies still view most alternative therapies as nontraditional and rarely cover any therapeutic provisions or supplements. The landscape of health care in the coming years has the opportunity to embrace integrative medicine, but the story is yet to be told.

This issue of *Primary Care: Clinics in Office Practice* includes articles dedicated to phytotherapy, changing patient behavior, and centering patients within their health care. Additional articles highlight integrative approaches to cardiovascular,

Prim Care Clin Office Pract 44 (2017) xi–xii
http://dx.doi.org/10.1016/j.pop.2017.04.001
0095-4543/17/© 2017 Published by Elsevier Inc.

gastrointestinal, psychological, and neurologic disorders. Detailed reviews on an integrative approach to women's health and cancer topics are also presented.

I would like to thank Dr Clements and Dr Ring as well as their dedicated authors for their contributions to this very timely and important issue of articles on integrative medicine. My hope is that this knowledge will benefit primary care clinicians in their practices, and that these practical pearls can be used in advancing the medical care of your patients.

Joel J. Heidelbaugh, MD, FAAFP, FACG
Departments of Family Medicine and Urology
University of Michigan Medical School
Ann Arbor, MI 48109, USA

Ypsilanti Health Center
200 Arnet, Suite 200
Ypsilanti, MI 48198, USA

E-mail address:
jheidel@umich.edu

Preface

Integrative Medicine and Primary Care

 CrossMark

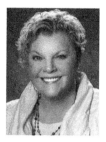 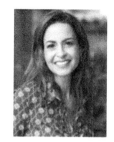

Deborah S. Clements, MD, FAAFP   Melinda Ring, MD, FACP, ABOIM
Editors

In primary care, we have become increasingly aware of our patients' interest in seeking alternatives to conventional approaches to treatment. This interest often arises from a patient's desire to have their care aligned with their values, beliefs, and philosophies about wellness. Patients understand they are more than the sum of their illnesses. Integrative medicine, the practice of medicine that focuses on caring for the whole person, using all available therapeutic choices from a variety of cultures, is a way to introduce additional healing tools into primary care practice.

The principles we associate with primary care—comprehensiveness, continuous, coordinated care in the context of the community—are reflected in the integrative medicine model as well. In caring for the whole person, we recognize that both physical and nonphysical factors impact health, well-being, and disease. This interrelatedness of the patient and their environment is at the heart of both primary care and integrative medicine.

Integrative medicine centers have opened across the country, with their numbers more than doubling in the past decade. Academic health centers and medical schools are increasingly incorporating principles of integrative medicine into medical education, including emerging integrative medicine postgraduate fellowships to prepare physicians for board certification and practice. And significant research is underway to provide the necessary evidence for the safe and effective practice of integrative modalities.

This issue of *Primary Care: Clinics in Office Practice* addressing "Integrative Medicine" brings recommendations from leading experts in integrative medicine to the point of care with practical, evidence-based recommendations for common concerns. We have organized the issue by condition, recognizing that many principles cross systems and are valuable to all patients, not the least of which are nutrition, exercise, and

Prim Care Clin Office Pract 44 (2017) xiii–xiv
http://dx.doi.org/10.1016/j.pop.2017.04.002
0095-4543/17/© 2017 Published by Elsevier Inc.
         primarycare.theclinics.com

mindfulness. Through the use of a patient-centered approach, our hope is that this resource will enhance both the care you provide and your own joy in practice.

Deborah S. Clements, MD, FAAFP
Family and Community Medicine
Northwestern University
Feinberg School of Medicine
710 North Lake Shore Drive
4th Floor Abbott Hall
Chicago, IL 60611, USA

Melinda Ring, MD, FACP, ABOIM
Northwestern Medicine
Osher Center for Integrative Medicine
Northwestern University
Feinberg School of Medicine
150 East Huron Avenue, Suite 1100
Chicago, IL 60611, USA

E-mail addresses:
dclements@northwestern.edu (D.S. Clements)
melinda.ring@nm.org (M. Ring)

Introduction to Integrative Medicine in the Primary Care Setting

Melinda Ring, MD, ABOIM*, Rupa Mahadevan, MD

KEYWORDS

• Integrative medicine • Complementary medicine • Alternative medicine • Philosophy

KEY POINTS

- Integrative medicine has been described as "healing oriented medicine that takes account of the whole person (body, mind, and spirit) including all aspects of lifestyle; it emphasizes therapeutic relationships and makes use of all appropriate therapies, both conventional and alternative."
- National surveys consistently report that approximately one-third of adults and 12% of children use complementary and integrative medicine approaches.
- Although there are barriers to primary care professionals engaging in discussions about lifestyle change and complementary and integrative medicine options, there is also great potential to impact patient well-being.
- Primary care providers can begin to incorporate integrative care into their current practice by engaging in education; collecting key tools and reliable resources; identifying local organizations or integrative medicine professionals to support care; considering new care models; and learning how to identify patients who will be most amenable to the information.
- Primary care professionals are in a strong position to advise patients in the safe use of integrative medicine and can collaborate with integrative medicine–trained physicians as well as complementary medicine providers to provide integrative team-based care.

INTEGRATIVE MEDICINE PHILOSOPHY AND PRACTICE

Sir William Osler said, "The good physician treats the disease; the great physician treats the patient who has the disease." Great health professionals differ from good ones because they understand the entire story. Each patient represents a story that includes their disease process, their environment, their social situation, and their belief

Departments of Medicine and Medical Social Sciences, Osher Center for Integrative Medicine, Northwestern University Feinberg School of Medicine, 150 East Huron Avenue, Suite 1100, Chicago, IL 60611, USA
* Corresponding author.
E-mail address: mring@nm.org

Prim Care Clin Office Pract 44 (2017) 203–215
http://dx.doi.org/10.1016/j.pop.2017.02.006
0095-4543/17/© 2017 Elsevier Inc. All rights reserved.
primarycare.theclinics.com

system. As the full story is explored, information is gained to guide appropriate diagnoses and management plans that are aligned with a patient's goals. This partnership between a health professional and a patient is at the heart of integrative medicine, and indeed, all of medicine. Integrative medicine changes the focus from disease and illness to health and healing and uses lifestyle approaches as the base of all subsequent care. An integrative approach additionally recognizes that many patients seek complementary and alternative modalities; primary care providers need to have at least basic comfort levels to guide patients in making safe and wise choices about their care.

The field of integrative medicine has been described as "healing oriented medicine that takes account of the whole person (body, mind, and spirit) including all aspects of lifestyle. It emphasizes therapeutic relationships and makes use of all appropriate therapies, both conventional and alternative."[1] Social, spiritual, behavioral, environmental, demographic, and cultural influences should always be taken into consideration when recommending lifestyle-based changes and treatment options. Recognizing external barriers, such as access issues, or internal barriers based on personal beliefs, is an important factor in the success of any therapeutic plan. In addition, a skillful integrative provider can provide the right level of advice by understanding where a patient is starting and how ready they are to change. Behavioral change in nutrition, physical activity, sleep, social relationships, exercise, and stress management often needs to be done in a stepwise fashion, with regular visits promoting long-term changes that will impact disease outcomes.[2,3] Unfortunately, conventional medical training does not adequately prepare physicians to counsel patients in these lifestyle behaviors. Studies have found that physicians held negative views regarding their ability to manage weight in primary care and cited a lack of time during routine primary care appointments, lack of reimbursement, and lack of knowledge and resources as barriers to this vehicle of weight management.[4,5] Fortunately, there is a growing number of high-quality continuing education resources as well as a network of health coaches, nutritionists, and integrative health professionals, available to work as a team to support patients in behavior change.

Integrative medicine has been criticized for promoting therapies unsupported by science.[6] Indeed, research on approaches, such as acupuncture, herbal supplements, and whole healing traditions, presents unique challenges and is not always best suited to a double-blind placebo controlled trial. Fortunately, a growing number of academic institutions have integrative medicine research departments. The biennial International Congress for Integrative Medicine and Health has blossomed since the inaugural meeting in 2004, attracting up to 1000 attendees worldwide. In those areas of integrative medicine where definitive evidence is lacking, the primary care provider should take into account the relative risks versus potential benefits, using available information and reliable resources as detailed in this journal.

THE ROLE OF INTEGRATIVE MEDICINE IN PRIMARY CARE

Integrative medicine encourages the collaboration of health and healing into the larger medical model and focuses on the least invasive methods to bring about change. Patients need effective prevention strategies to cope with the environmental influences that make achieving health a challenge. Empowering patients to learn how to take care of themselves, in order to be an active participant in the healing process, is a fundamental aspect of this approach. Although there are significant barriers to primary care professionals engaging in discussions about lifestyle change and complementary and integrative medicine options, there is also great potential to impact patient well-being, as well as provider career satisfaction.

In 2006, a report from the American College of Physicians stated that "Primary Care, the backbone of the nation's health care system, is at grave risk of collapse due to a dysfunctional financing and delivery system. Immediate and comprehensive reforms are required to replace systems that undermine and undervalue the relationship between patients and their personal physician."[7] Many patients turn to integrative medicine not because of a desire to abandon conventional medicine but rather because they are seeking "a strong therapeutic relationship with providers who listen and provide time and knowledgeable advice."[8] Primary care physicians report stress, burnout, and depression due to work conditions, including workflow and lack of autonomy, that prohibit them from providing the kind of care that would be more satisfying to them and their patients.[9] Although a system-level change that values provider time with patients would create the space for these therapeutic relationships, it is possible for providers on the frontline to succeed within the current care paradigm. This positive shift can be done through focused counseling using available tools in patient visits, through supplemental handouts, or by incorporating models such as group visits or team-based chronic care, which can improve access, education, and behavioral change.

For example, with growing evidence and public awareness of the benefit of mindfulness-based therapies for stress, and the relationship linking stress and disease, many patients are curious about how they can incorporate a mindfulness practice into their daily lives.[10] Practitioners should be aware of such therapies, the basic research that supports their use, and be able to suggest reliable resources for further education, or even better, guide the patient in a brief experience such as a breathing exercise or a guided meditation during the office visit.

In addition to having brief counseling tools and referral resources, choosing patients most likely to benefit from counseling also helps a provider be more effective without feeling burdened by extra responsibilities in office visits. Given that more than one-third of Americans are overweight or obese, or have related risk factors, lifestyle changes are included in most disease-based consensus statements as a first-line approach.[11] Many clinicians dealing with prediabetes or prehypertension will provide suggestions for diet and exercise to patients, but after 3 to 6 months, if there is no significant improvement, a prescription is provided for a salutary effect. However, it is important to note, when diet and lifestyle changes are recommended, data show that the time one spends on lifestyle as a remedy is often minimal and the emphasis on its importance is understated.[12] Given the limited resources available in the outpatient setting, the US Preventive Task Force recommendations of doing brief behavior change counseling for the general public has only a small potential impact; in order to identify which patients will benefit the most, providers must consider "risk factors for cardiovascular disease, patient readiness for change, social support and community resources that support behavioral change, and other health care and preventive service priorities."[13]

Primary care providers can thus begin to incorporate integrative care into their current practice by engaging in education, such as reading this journal issue, attending conferences, or watching Webinars; identifying key tools and reliable resources to be available during patient care; exploring local organizations or integrative medicine professionals to support care; considering care models that allow greater time on prevention like group visits; and learning how to identify patients who will be most amenable to the information.

THE INTEGRATIVE MEDICINE MOVEMENT

There is increased awareness of integrative medicine since the first major publication in the *New England Journal of Medicine* in 1993 detailing that 34% of Americans reported use of "unconventional" medicine within the past year, spending $13.7 billion, most of which was paid out of pocket.[14] Since then, the National Health Interview Survey conducted by the Centers for Disease Control and Prevention, in which tens of thousands of Americans are interviewed about health- and illness-related experiences, showed consistent use of complementary and integrative medicine approaches: 2002 (32.3% of adults), 2007 (35.5% adults, 12% children), and most recently, 2012 (33.2%, adults, 11.6% children).[15]

Terminology has changed over the past several decades, transitioning from "alternative medicine" to "complementary and alternative medicine or CAM" to the current more inclusive "integrative medicine" or "integrative health care" and "complementary and integrative medicine or CIM." Congress adopted a name change in 2014 for the National Institute of Health National Center for Complementary and Alternative Medicine to the National Center for Complementary and Integrative Health, with the rationale: "The change was made to more accurately reflect the Center's research commitment to studying promising health approaches that are already in use by the American public. Since the Center's inception, complementary approaches have grown in use to the point that Americans no longer consider them an alternative to medical care."[16]

Integrative medicine centers are a growing resource for patients, providers, and communities and are now embraced by many leading academic centers. Academic training in integrative medicine is also becoming a viable career option for trainees: as of 2016, there were 17 established integrative medicine fellowships, and the American Board of Physician Specialties offered the first American Board of Integrative Medicine in November 2014.

In addition to the growing number of physicians specializing in integrative medicine, either as integrative medicine specialty consultants or by incorporating it into their current practice, there are many other members of the integrative health care team. One of the core principles for integrative medicine is the role of collaborative treatment with other providers and familiarity with the variety of modalities available. A diverse group of providers, such as nutritionists, acupuncturists, massage therapists, chiropractic doctors, naturopathic doctors (NDs), health coaches, and behavioral health and mind-body specialists, can work together to create an optimal healing experience. Each discipline has unique training requirements, and licensure and certification standards vary from state to state. Ensuring the providers your patients see have met the highest standards for training and licensure is integral to maintaining the credibility of the field. Meeting local CIM providers and trying the therapies firsthand can be an optimal way to learn about a therapy and feel comfortable explaining the treatment to patients. In addition, working in transdisciplinary teams allows for greater insight into developing new creative ways to solve patient problems.[17]

BRANCHES OF INTEGRATIVE MEDICINE

Often chronic illnesses, such as depression, diabesity, and chronic pain, are best managed with a combination of pharmaceuticals, supplements, nutrition, preventive screening measures, healthy lifestyle behaviors, exercise, and relaxation therapies.[1] In addition to providing top conventional medical care, integrative medicine emphasizes the importance of lifestyle and prevention, treating the root cause of illness not just symptoms, and using all available evidence-informed approaches from around the world to promote health and healing. The following descriptions detail briefly some of the key disciplines incorporated into an integrative assessment and treatment plan, such as Mind Body Medicine, Manual Therapies, and Whole Healing Systems. This article also explores current movements in medicine that overlap significantly with integrative medicine, such as preventive medicine, lifestyle medicine, and functional medicine.

Lifestyle Medicine

Lifestyle medicine can be broadly defined as the nonpharmacologic and nonsurgical management of chronic disease with a focus on the 4 pillars of health: nutrition, physical activity, stress management, and sleep. Lifestyle is fundamental to health, wellness, and disease prevention, and comprehensive lifestyle interventions decrease illness burden and improve clinical outcomes.[17] Lifestyle medicine should be seen as a core competency for preventive and primary care medicine and is implicit in any integrative medicine care plan. (Please see Ruth Q. Wolever and colleagues article, "Integrative Medicine Strategies for Changing Health Behaviors: Support for Primary Care," in this issue).

Preventive Medicine

According to the American College of Preventive Medicine, preventive medicine focuses on the health of individuals, communities, and defined populations.[18] The goal of preventive medicine is to protect, promote, and maintain health and well-being and to prevent disease, disability, and death through education, high-quality research, service, and creative partnerships. Three specialty areas and competencies include aerospace medicine, occupational medicine, and public health and general preventive medicine. The concepts of being proactive in the prevention of disease is also a key tenet of integrative medicine and may range from an individual disease risk assessment and plan, to a more global assessment of the impact of environmental toxins on community health.

Mind-Body Medicine

Mind-body medicine uses the power of thoughts and emotions to influence physical health. Mind-body therapies activate the relaxation response to reduce stress and improve overall well-being. These therapies can include biofeedback, yoga, various forms of meditation, MBSR (mindfulness-based stress reduction), prayer, hypnosis, or guided imagery.[19] The basic elements for eliciting the relaxation response include a nonjudging receptive awareness, a mental focus, such as repetition of the word, phrase, prayer, or image. A comfortable position and a quiet environment are helpful, but not essential. The relaxation response counters the harmful effects of the physiologic and behavioral stress response, referred to as allostatic loading.[20]

Biofeedback is a self-regulation technique where patients learn to have voluntary control over aspects of their physiology, such as their heart rate, blood pressure, and respirations. Yoga is an ancient system of relaxation using movement exercise along with breathwork.[17] There are different forms of meditation, and 2 growing techniques include transcendental meditation, whereby the practice is to repeat a mantra (a single word or phrase), whereas in MBSR individuals focus their attention on their moment-by-moment thoughts and sensations. Hypnosis is an exercise that helps the body progressively relax while thought and emotions become more focused. In this state of deep concentration, some people are highly responsive to suggestions made by a hypnotherapist.[21] There is now considerable evidence that many mind-body therapies can be used for several common clinical conditions as effective adjuncts to conventional medical treatment.[22,23]

Energy Medicine

Energy medicine is based on the idea that living beings have energy fields, and that disruptions or imbalances to this field have a negative impact on well-being. A typical energy medicine session consists of a patient lying clothed on a table as a trained energy medicine healer places their hands in specific locations on the body or in the field around the body. Energy medicine therapies can be found in cultures throughout the world, such as therapeutic touch (TT) and healing touch (HT) in Western medicine, Reiki (ray-key) in Japan, and Qigong (chee-gong) in China.[17] Early studies in TT and HT demonstrated its efficacy in muscle relaxation, pain and stress, and anxiety reduction, along with a decrease in blood pressure and temperature.[24] Reiki claims to provide healing energy to recharge and rebalance the human energy fields, creating optimal conditions needed by the body's natural healing system.[25] These therapies are great first-line treatments because they are generally very low risk and can be used by children and adults.

Manual Therapies

Manual therapies include hands-on approaches, such as chiropractic medicine, osteopathic manipulative treatment (OMT), and massage therapy. The goal of manual therapies is to correct alignment, alleviate pain, and improve function to help support the body's innate ability to heal itself. Massage promotes well-being through application of pressure to manipulate muscles, connective tissue, tendons, and ligaments to enhance relaxation and reduce pain.[1] Many types of bodywork are available, ranging from the common Swedish or myofascial therapy to less known approaches, such as the Bowen technique or Core Structural Integration Therapy. Board certification from the National Certification Board for Therapeutic Massage and Bodywork indicates that a massage therapist has attained a higher level of achievement beyond entry level licensure.

Doctors of Chiropractic undergo 4 years of training, comparable in hours to medical school. Doctors of Osteopathy (DOs) generally complete a typical medical school training, with the addition of osteopathic manipulation. According to the American Osteopathic Association, with an advanced understanding of the interrelationships between the body's structure and function, and an understanding of how the body can be influenced by human's emotional or spiritual nature, the DO uses palpation and manipulation to provide patient-specific care that promotes health and treats disease.[26] Studies show that 15% to 20% of Americans experience low back pain and has become the second leading cause of primary care visits.[27,28] One clinical trial found that in comparison with usual care alone, usual care and OMT provided better 1-month outcomes in physical functioning, mental health, and back pain, whereas only the latter finding persisted more than 6 months.[29] OMT also resulted in the use of fewer cotreatments at 6 months and provided greater patient satisfaction overall. Several large reviews of chiropractic manipulation for back pain conclude that chiropractic care is potentially helpful and comparable to other recommended interventions for chronic and acute back pain.[30–32] Given the prevalence of chronic back pain, manual therapies can be a low-cost and beneficial treatment plan.

Whole Healing Systems

Whole healing systems in integrative medicine include Naturopathic Medicine, Functional Medicine, Homeopathy, Traditional Chinese Medicine (TCM), and Ayurvedic Medicine.

Naturopathic medicine

NDs are trained as primary care providers in a 4-year graduate level naturopathic medical school that includes both academic and clinical training. Their focus spans topics such as nutrition, homeopathy, botanical medicine, herbs, balneotherapy, and supplements.[33] The foundation of naturopathic medicine includes the following:

1. The healing power of nature: The recognition of an inherent self-healing process in people that is ordered and intelligent
2. Identifying and treating the cause: The removal of the underlying causes of illness rather than to merely eliminate or suppress symptoms
3. Avoid harming the patient: The minimization of the risk of harmful side effects using the least invasive techniques to diagnose and treat
4. Teaching: The education of the patients and encouragement of self-responsibility focusing on the doctor-patient relationship
5. Treating the whole person: Taking into account the physical, spiritual, mental, and social aspects of every individual
6. Prevention: Assessment of risk factors, heredity and susceptibility to disease, and appropriate interventions

Currently, 17 states, the District of Columbia, and the US territories of Puerto Rico and the Virgin Islands have licensing or regulation laws for NDs.[34] In some licensed states, NDs can function as primary care physicians, including performing examinations, ordering diagnostic tests, making clinical diagnoses, recommending interventions such as dietary supplements, and performing minor surgeries.[35] There are many integrative clinics nationwide that employ both NDs and MDs, and at least 20 hospitals that staff NDs. Some data support the benefit of a naturopathic whole-system approach: for example, a retrospective analysis of medical records at an academic naturopathic outpatient clinic as well as a prospective cohort study of adjunctive naturopathic medicine showed improvements in behavior change related to nutrition and physical activity, and better glycemic control in diabetic patients.[36,37] However, it is important for primary care providers to be aware of their patients' recommendations by NDs, particularly for dietary supplements.

In addition, interviews were conducted with 75 families of pediatric patients with cancer diagnosed with primary neoplasms identified from the Cancer Surveillance System of western Washington. The study found that 73% of patients used at least one alternative treatment, and 21% of patients consulted one alternative provider, either a ND, a homeopathic physician, or an acupuncturist, with insurance companies covering 75% of these costs.[38] Given the potential risks of dietary supplement interactions with pharmaceuticals and treatments such as radiation therapy, it is important that primary care providers remain informed about the therapies families are using in conjunction with conventional care.

Functional medicine

In 1990, Dr Bland founded the Institute for Functional Medicine (IFM) to encompass a systems biology approach to the prevention and management of disease. Training is available through the IFM and other functional medicine education programs, providing continuing medical education credits to physicians to learn this approach to care.[17] Other providers, including chiropractors, nutritionists, dentists, and pharmacists, can also complete certification in functional medicine. According to the IFM: "Functional Medicine is an approach to health care that conceptualizes health and illness as part of a continuum in which all components of the human biological system interact dynamically with the environment, producing patterns and effects that change over time. Functional Medicine helps clinicians identify and ameliorate dysfunctions in the physiology and biochemistry of the human body as a primary method of improving patient health.[39] This relatively new field is attracting many health care professionals who are seeking practical tools and algorithms for treating patients. Research in a functional medicine approach is scant, although recent affiliations with academic centers may lead to a stronger evidence base.[40]

Homeopathic medicine

Homeopathy is a system of medicine developed by Samuel Hahnemann in the early 1800s based on the law of similarity that "like cures like."[41] Core principles include those of using the minimum dose possible and the use of "potentization," whereby a substance is sequentially diluted and vigorously shaken between each dilution. Homeopathic products can be made from plants, minerals, and organic compounds. The extreme dilution of homeopathic medications, to a point where in some cases less than Avogadro's number of molecules are present, confounds many Western trained scientists in regards to the plausibility of having any effect. Despite this apparent contradiction, there is some evidence from randomized, controlled trials that homeopathy may be effective for the treatment of influenza, allergies, postoperative ileus, and childhood diarrhea.[42] Perhaps the most well-known homeopathic preparation, that of *Arnica montana* for reduction of bruising and swelling such as in the postoperative setting, has had mixed results in studies.[43–45] Homeopathic medicines have been considered to be drugs under the law since the inception of the Food, Drug, and Cosmetic Act in 1938 and are regulated by the Homeopathic Pharmacopoeia of the United States (HPUS). HPUS-regulated homeopathic drugs, when used in dilute preparations, are very unlikely to cause harm; however, more research is needed to verify its value and efficacy.

Traditional Chinese medicine

TCM has evolved over thousands of years from a system developed in ancient China. The TCM concept of health includes a harmonious balance between Yin and Yang, the 2 opposing but complementary forces of the body represented in the ancient Chinese philosophy; the flow of Qi (chee), a vital life force energy; and the interplay of 5 elements—fire, earth, wood, metal, and water—in nature and the body. TCM practice encompasses acupuncture (insertion of fine needles into specific body points), moxibustion (burning an herb above the skin to apply heat to acupuncture points), herbal medicine, tui na (Chinese therapeutic massage), dietary therapy, and Tai chi and Qigong (movements, postures, coordinated breathing, and mental focus).[17] Numerous clinical studies and systematic reviews have been done on acupuncture, herbal medicine, and Tai chi. However, lack of quality led to an inability to reach conclusions in 19 of 26 reviews on acupuncture for a variety of conditions and 22 of 42 reviews on Chinese herbal medicine.[46] The remaining reviews suggested possible benefits. Given the current public concern regarding the prevalence of chronic pain and the opioid epidemic, alternative options are desperately needed. A 2012 analysis of 29 studies of acupuncture for pain showed improved pain relief in patients who received acupuncture for back or neck pain, osteoarthritis, or chronic headache.[47] Tai chi is most well studied for improving balance and stability in people with Parkinson disease, although more recent data support reduced pain from knee osteoarthritis and fibromyalgia, and improved quality of life and mood in people with heart failure.[48] Traditional use of Chinese herbal medicine is based on complex formulation, and more research on the synergic effects of herbal combinations is required for a comprehensive understanding of the underlying effect on the disease process.[49]

Ayurvedic medicine

Ayurvedic medicine, as practiced in India, is one of the oldest systems of medicine in the world. The term "Ayurveda" combines the Sanskrit words *ayur* (life) and *veda* (science or knowledge). Many Ayurvedic therapies have been time tested and handed down by word of mouth and through the Vedas (ancient Indian scripture). Key philosophic underpinnings of Ayurvedic medicine include the belief in universal interconnectedness between people, health, and the universe; the role of the body's constitution (prakriti), and the concept of life forces (doshas). Ayurvedic physicians prescribe individualized treatments, including compounds of herbs or proprietary ingredients, and diet, exercise, and lifestyle recommendations.[50] According to Ayurvedic medicine, every living being is composed of 5 basic elements in the universe: space, air, earth, water, and fire. In the body, these elements form "doshas," which are energy forces that govern all biological processes. The 3 main doshas are vata (space and air), kapha (earth and water), and pitta (fire and water); optimal health is achieved when the structural elements as well as the 3 doshas are in a state of equilibrium.[17] Although many Ayurvedic herbs, such as curcumin (the active ingredient in turmeric), are being studied, there is minimal research on the whole system practice.

VISION FOR THE FUTURE

The Summit on Integrative Medicine and the Health of the Public held in 2009 was convened by the Institute of Medicine (IOM, now called the National Academy of Medicine) and The Bravewell Collaborative to examine emerging strategies to address major issues in the current health care system, and how to improve the prospects for integrative medicine's contributions to a better health care system.[51]

The themes and priorities for an idealized health care system included the following:

Vision of optimal health: Alignment of individuals and their health care for optimal health and healing across a full lifespan.

Conceptually inclusive: Seamless engagement of the full range of established health factor, physical, psychological, social, preventive, and therapeutic.

Lifespan horizon: Integration across the lifespan to include personal, predictive, preventive, and participatory care.

Person-centered: Integration around, and within, each person.

Prevention-oriented: Prevention and disease minimization as the foundation of integrative health care.

Team-based: Care as a team activity, with the patient as a central team member.

Care integration: Seamless integration of the care processes, across caregivers and institutions.

Caring integration: Person- and relationship-centered care.

Science Integration: Integration across scientific disciplines, and scientific processes that cross domains.

Integration of approach: Integration across approaches to care, for example, conventional, traditional, alternative, complementary, as the evidence supports.

Policy opportunities: Emphasis on outcomes, elevation of patient insights, consideration of family and social factors, inclusion of team care and supportive follow-up, and contributions.

Dr Harvey Feinberg, President of the IOM, stated that integrative medicine has 5 critical dimensions that show alignment with this health care vision:

Broad definition of health: Integrative medicine offers the possibility to fulfill the longstanding World Health Organization definition of health as more than the absence of disease. It should include physical, mental, emotional, and spiritual factors, enabling a comprehensive understanding of what makes a person healthy.

Wide range of interventions: Integrative medicine encompasses the whole spectrum of health interventions, from prevention to treatment to rehabilitation and recovery.

Coordination of care: Integrative medicine emphasizes coordination of care across an array of caregivers and institutions.

Patient-centered care: Integrative medicine integrates services around and within the individual patient, which is perhaps the most fundamental and the most neglected aspect of high-quality care.

Variety of modalities: Integrative medicine is open to multiple modalities of care, not just usual care, but also unconventional care that helps patients manage, maintain, and restore health.

As the evidence base grows for integrative medicine approaches, including efficacy, cost-effectiveness, and patient-provider satisfaction, the field will gain greater credibility. A shift in how this approach to care is perceived has already been seen: from alternative to complementary, then to integrative medicine, and it is hoped soon to just good medicine.

SUMMARY

The art of listening to a patient's story, seeing the way life's events impact disease presentation, and then going past superficial diagnoses to get to the root cause of illness has been lost as health professionals face their own struggles working in primary care. The US health care system spends more per capita on health care than other developed countries, yet falls short on outcomes, including shorter life expectancy and greater prevalence of chronic conditions.[52] The investment in expensive technology and pharmaceuticals rather than social services, prevention, and high-touch, low-cost interventions is proven a failure.[53]

Informed patients are seeking competent and empathic providers who can help them navigate the multiple therapeutic options available for conditions in which conventional therapies often fall short. Knowing about complementary and integrative approaches such as acupuncture, dietary supplements, and nutrition is helpful, as is developing a network of colleagues who can create an integrative medical home for your patient.

Oftentimes the answers are not always obvious in medicine; ultimately, the healing process begins not when one prescribes a medication or herb, but rather when patients suffering feel that their health care provider sees them for who they are, listens with intent, and is willing to be an active partner and health advocate in their journey to wellness. In the end, Sir William Osler got it right. Great clinicians understand the patient and the context of his/her illness; that is the basis of integrative medicine.

REFERENCES

1. Rakel D. Integrative medicine. Philadelphia: Elsevier Saunders; 2012.

2. Ring M, Brodsky M, Low Dog T, et al. Developing and implementing core competencies for integrative medicine fellowships. Acad Med 2014;89(3):421–8.

3. American Board of Physician Specialties. 2006. Available at: http://www.abpsus. org/. Accessed August 18, 2016.

4. Ruelaz AR, Diefenbach P, Simon B, et al. Perceived barriers to weight management in primary care—perspectives of patients and providers. J Gen Intern Med 2007;22(4):518–22.

5. Kolasa KM, Rickett K. Barriers to providing nutrition counseling cited by physicians a survey of primary care practitioners. Nutr Clin Pract 2010;25(5):502–9.

6. Fontanarosa PB, Lundberg GD. Alternative medicine meets science. JAMA 1998; 280(18):1618–9.

7. Bodenheimer T, Berenson RA, Rudolf Paul. The primary care–specialty income gap: why it matters. Ann Intern Med 2007;146(4):301–6.

8. McCaffrey AM, Pugh GF, O'Connor BB. Understanding patient preference for integrative medical care: results from patient focus groups. J Gen Intern Med 2007;22(11):1500–5.

9. Linzer M, Manwell LB, Williams ES, et al. Working conditions in primary care: physician reactions and care quality. Ann Intern Med 2009;151(1):28–36.

10. Cherkin DC, Sherman KJ, Balderson BH, et al. Effect of mindfulness-based stress reduction vs cognitive behavioral therapy or usual care on back pain and functional limitations in adults with chronic low back pain: a randomized clinical trial. JAMA 2016;315(12):1240–9.

11. Mitchell NS, Catenacci VA, Wyatt HR, et al. Obesity: overview of an epidemic. Psychiatr Clin North Am 2011;34(4):717.

12. Smith AW, Borowski LA, Liu B, et al. US primary care physicians' diet-, physical activity-, and weight-related care of adult patients. Am J Prev Med 2011;41(1): 33–42.

13. US Preventive Services Task Force. Behavioral counseling in primary care to promote a healthy diet: recommendations and rationale. Am J Nurs 2003;103(8): 81–92.

14. Eisenberg DM, Kessler RC, Foster C, et al. Unconventional medicine in the United States–prevalence, costs, and patterns of use. N Engl J Med 1993; 328(4):246–52.

15. 2012 National Health Interview Survey - National Center for Complementary and Integrative health. 2015. Available at: https://nccih.nih.gov/research/statistics/ NHIS/2012/key-findings. Accessed August 31, 2016.

16. Frequently Asked Questions: Name Change | NCCIH. 2015. Available at: https:// nccih.nih.gov/news/name-change-faq. Accessed August 31, 2016.

17. Mechanick JI, Kushner RF, editors. Lifestyle medicine: a manual for clinical practice. Cham (Switzerland): Springer; 2016.

18. American College of Preventive Medicine. Available at: http://www.acpm.org/. Accessed August 18, 2016.

19. Rakel D. Integrative medicine. Philadelphia: Saunders Elsevier; 2012.

20. Fricchione GL. The science of mind body medicine and the public health challenges. S Afr J Psychol 2014;44(4):404–15.

21. Maizes V, Rakel D, Niemiec C. Integrative medicine and patient-centered care. Explore (NY) 2009;5(5):277–89.

22. Astin JA, Shapiro SL, Eisenberg DM, et al. Mind-body medicine: state of the science, implications for practice. J Am Board Fam Pract 2003;16(2):131–47.

23. Gordon JS. Mind-body medicine. Complementary medicine in clinical practice 2006. p. 147–50.

24. Gagne D, Toye RC. The effects of therapeutic touch and relaxation therapy in reducing anxiety. Arch Psychiatr Nurs 1994;8(3):184–9.

25. vanderVaart S, Gijsen VM, de Wildt SN, et al. A systematic review of the therapeutic effects of Reiki. J Altern Complement Med 2009;15(11):1157–69.

26. American Osteopathic Association, Ward RC. Foundations for osteopathic medicine. Philadelphia: Lippincott Williams & Wilkins; 2003.
27. Gary HL, Deyo RA, Cherkin DC. Physician office visits for low back pain: frequency, clinical evaluation, and treatment patterns from a US national survey. Spine 1995;20(1):11–9.
28. Kent PM, Keating JL. The epidemiology of low back pain in primary care. Chiropr Osteopat 2005;13(1):1.
29. Licciardone JC, Stoll ST, Fulda KG, et al. Osteopathic manipulative treatment for chronic low back pain: a randomized controlled trial. Spine 2003;28(13):1355–62.
30. Bronfort G, Haas M, Evans R, et al. Effectiveness of manual therapies: the UK evidence report. Chiropr Osteopat 2010;18(1):1.
31. Dagenais S, Tricco AC, Haldeman S. Synthesis of recommendations for the assessment and management of low back pain from recent clinical practice guidelines. Spine J 2010;10(6):514–29.
32. Rubinstein SM, van Middelkoop M, Assendelft WJ, et al. Spinal manipulative therapy for chronic low-back pain: an update of a Cochrane review. Spine (Phila Pa 1976) 2011;36(13):E825–46.
33. House of Delegates Position Paper Definition of Naturopathic Medicine. 2012. Available at: http://www.naturopathic.org/files/Committees/HOD/Position%20Paper%20Docs/Definition%20Naturopathic%20Medicine.pdf. Accessed August 18, 2016.
34. Licensed States - AANP - American Association of Naturopathic Physicians. Available at: http://www.naturopathic.org/content.asp?contentid=57. Accessed August 31, 2016.
35. Fleming SA. Naturopathy and the Primary Care Practice. 2010. Available at: http://www.ncbi.nlm.nih.gov/pmc/articles/PMC2883816/. Accessed August 18, 2016.
36. Bradley R, Oberg EB. Naturopathic medicine and type 2 diabetes: a retrospective analysis from an academic clinic. Altern Med Rev 2006;11(1):30.
37. Bairy S, Kumar AM, Raju M, et al. Is adjunctive naturopathy associated with improved glycaemic control and a reduction in need for medications among type 2 diabetes patients? A prospective cohort study from India. BMC Complement Altern Med 2016;16(1):290.
38. Neuhouser ML, Patterson RE, Schwartz SM, et al. Use of alternative medicine by children with cancer in Washington state. Prev Med 2001;33(5):347–54.
39. Jones DS, Hofmann L, Quinn S. 21st century medicine: a new model for medical education and practice. Gig Harbor (WA): The Institute for Functional Medicine; 2009.
40. Center for Functional Medicine - Cleveland Clinic. 2014. Available at: http://my.clevelandclinic.org/services/center-for-functional-medicine. Accessed August 31, 2016.
41. Reilly D. The puzzle of homeopathy. J Altern Complement Med 2001;7(1):103–9.
42. Jonas WB, Kaptchuk TJ, Linde K. A critical overview of homeopathy. Ann Intern Med 2003;138(5):393–9.
43. Seeley BM, Denton AB, Ahn MS, et al. Effect of homeopathic Arnica montana on bruising in face-lifts: results of a randomized, double-blind, placebo-controlled clinical trial. Arch Facial Plast Surg 2006;8(1):54–9.
44. Stevinson C, Devaraj VS, Fountain-Barber A, et al. Homeopathic arnica for prevention of pain and bruising: randomized placebo-controlled trial in hand surgery. J R Soc Med 2003;96(2):60–5.
45. Brinkhaus B, Wilkens JM, Lüdtke R, et al. Homeopathic arnica therapy in patients receiving knee surgery: results of three randomised double-blind trials. Complement Ther Med 2006;14(4):237–46.

46. Manheimer E, Wieland S, Kimbrough E, et al. Evidence from the Cochrane Collaboration for traditional Chinese medicine therapies. J Altern Complement Med 2009;15(9):1001–14.
47. Vickers AJ, Cronin AM, Maschino AC, et al. Acupuncture for chronic pain: individual patient data meta-analysis. Arch Intern Med 2012;172(19):1444–53.
48. Birdee GS, Wayne PM, Davis RB, et al. T'ai chi and qigong for health: patterns of use in the United States. J Altern Complement Med 2009;15(9):969–73.
49. Li CG, Moyle K, Xue CC. Problems and challenges of Chinese herbal medicine. In: Leung P-C, Xue CC, Cheng Y-C, editors. A comprehensive guide to Chinese medicine. River Edge (NJ): World Scientific Publishing Co; 2003. p. 85–112.
50. Chopra A, Doiphode VV. Ayurvedic medicine: core concept, therapeutic principles, and current relevance. Med Clin North Am 2002;86(1):75–89.
51. Schultz AM, Samantha MC, Michael McGinnis J. Integrative medicine and the health of the public: a summary of the February 2009 Summit. Washington, DC: National Academies Press; 2009.
52. U.S. Health Care from a Global Perspective - The Commonwealth Fund. 2015. Available at: http://www.commonwealthfund.org/publications/issue-briefs/2015/oct/us-health-care-from-a-global-perspective. Accessed August 31, 2016.
53. Weil A. Health and healing: the philosophy of integrative medicine. Boston: Houghton Mifflin Harcourt; 2004.

Phytotherapy
An Introduction to Herbal Medicine

Charles C. Falzon, MD, MBA[a],*, Anna Balabanova, MD[b]

KEYWORDS

- Phytotherapy • Herbal medicine • Integrative medicine

KEY POINTS

- Herbal medications are commonly used in all medical settings, making it essential for primary care providers to learn about the products being used, and resources they can access for continuing education.
- Understanding how herbal medicines are sourced, processed, and standardized can help providers guide patients that are trying to choose the most clinically effective and affordable treatments.
- Multiple herbs are often combined and sold as proprietary blends, which can increase the risk of allergies, adverse reactions, or cross-reactivity with other pharmaceuticals and supplements.
- Several textbooks, online point-of-care resources, and conferences are available for primary care providers to expand their knowledge of herbal medicines.

BACKGROUND

This article is a primer for health care professionals who are interested in understanding the origins of phytotherapy, being introduced to some commonly used herbal medicines, learning about reputable resources that can help with point-of care decision-making and educational programs to build their knowledge-base, and knowing referral options for physicians and providers with expertise in phytotherapy.

Phytotherapy is a field of medicine that uses plants either to treat disease or as health-promoting agents. It is often referred to as herbalism in Western medicine. Traditional use of phytotherapies generally preserves the original composition and integrity of the source plant, so that either the whole plant, or a desired percentage of its minimally adulterated components, is used for medicinal purposes.

Several medical traditions use plant-based therapies, including anthroposophic medicine, naturopathic medicine, traditional Chinese medicine (TCM), Ayurvedic medicine,

[a] Northwestern University, Feinberg School of Medicine, Department of Family and Community Medicine, 710 N. Lake Shore Drive, Abbott Hall, 4th Floor, Chicago, IL 60611-3006, USA; [b] Northwestern University, Feinberg School of Medicine, McGaw Family Medicine Residency at Lake Forest, 1475 E. Belvidere Road, Suite 385, Grayslake, IL 60030-2012, USA
* Corresponding author.
E-mail address: charles.falzon@nm.org

Prim Care Clin Office Pract 44 (2017) 217–227
http://dx.doi.org/10.1016/j.pop.2017.02.001
primarycare.theclinics.com

and allopathic medicine. Physicians and providers may use either single-herb treatments, multiple herbs thought to have complementary properties, or mixtures with non-herbal substances such as minerals and vitamins. The more traditional use of phytotherapy often includes the whole part of the plant, such as a chamomile herb infusion (tea), whereas Western herbal medicine more commonly uses single herbs standardized to a component of the extract. In contrast, pharmaceutical medications derived from plants are typically single compounds isolated through the industrial separation and extraction of components identified as having therapeutic properties.

Manufacturing phytotherapies involves uniformly processing source plant materials so that the end-product contains a reference marker constituent at a verified concentration. Because plants contain multiple chemical constituents, the end-product is labeled as standardized to the marker constituent. The purpose of identifying a marker constituent is to generate an end-product that contains the desired concentration of the active constituent. In treatment, what matters most is delivering the active constituent at a therapeutically appropriate dose.

When health care professionals help patients choose phytotherapies from the marketplace, it is important to be aware that the active ingredient and the marker constituent of a phytotherapeutic agent are not always the same chemical. For example, many St. John's wort products are standardized to the chemical component hypericin, which was previously thought to be the active ingredient responsible for the antidepressive properties of the plant. However, it has since been determined that many of these effects are attributable to the hyperforin compound.[1,2]

Consumers should also be aware that a product's potency or therapeutic benefit may be overstated if the manufacturing process does not retain necessary concentrations of the active constituent's cofactors. Identifying the most reliable and effective product on the market becomes more complicated when an herbal medicine's active constituent has either not been identified, or is still the subject of debate.

Ultimately, the processes for determining source material selection, marker constituent standardization, active constituent and cofactor concentrations, and medication assembly can vary by both product and manufacturer. Because most herbal medicines are not covered by either government or commercial medical insurances, the variances identified increase the importance of being familiar with product quality and safety resources before recommending phytotherapeutic products for general use that are potentially costly and may have indeterminate efficacy.

COMMON HERBAL MEDICINES

The herbs presented here were chosen because they are representative of a range of common conditions seen in primary care, as well as their popularity in use among patients. For example, ginseng, garlic, and echinacea were among the 10 most common natural products used among adults in the most recent National Health Interview Survey.[3]

Butterbur

The perennial butterbur (*Petasites hybridus*) plant's clinical efficacy lies with migraines and allergy symptoms. Numerous well-controlled studies have been shown its efficacy in symptom management of intermittent allergic rhinitis. It should be considered as a treatment, especially in patients who cannot tolerate pharmacologic therapies due to drowsiness or other side effects.[4–7] Speculated to act through calcium channels and to influence the inflammatory cascade, butterbur is effective in migraine prophylaxis.[8,9] "The American Academy of Neurology and American Headache Society issued a guideline in 2012 recommending butterbur for migraine prophylaxis, but retracted the statement in 2015 due to potential product safety concerns."[10] The petasin compound that butterbur contains is speculated to work through the leukotriene pathway, making it perform favorably in comparison to antihistamines.[7] Although butterbur is generally well-tolerated, medication interactions should be taken into consideration: butterbur may amplify anticholinergic drug effects. In addition, a notable risk of certain preparations of butterbur is liver damage due to the pyrrolizidine alkaloid (PA) chemicals found in its raw, unprocessed state; recommended products should be certified as PA-free. Supplements or medications that induce cytochrome P450 3A4 should be avoided because these may increase conversion of PAs to toxic metabolites.[11,12]

Author recommendations
Butterbur has been used for migraine prophylaxis by adults, at a dose of 150 mg daily in a PA-free form, but is not universally endorsed as a preventive strategy by professional Medical organizations.

Chamomile, German

German chamomile (*Matricaria recutita*) is a commonly used herb for management of anxiety, depression, and insomnia. Although the specific mechanisms of action behind it is still unknown, chamomile flavonoids have demonstrated an ability to modulate several neurotransmitter pathways, including noradrenaline, dopamine, serotonin (5-hydroxytryptamine), and γ-aminobutyric acid (GABA), all of which have been identified as targets for conventional pharmacologic therapies.

German chamomile has been investigated in pilot studies for treatment of both behavioral and sleep disorders. In the Generalized Anxiety Disorder (GAD) study, chamomile (*M recutita,* 220 mg capsule, standardized to 1.2% apigenin) was administered in step-dose fashion, with a max daily dose of 1100 mg, over an 8-week period; the treatment group showed statistically significant superiority over placebo in reducing mean, total Hamilton Anxiety Rating scores.[13]

In a follow-up study, the same group evaluated subjects with anxiety and comorbid depression, anxiety and a history of depression, or anxiety-alone, and showed that chamomile (*M recutita*) was superior to placebo in lowering Hamilton Depression Ratings in all subjects but was not superior in treating anxiety with current comorbid depression.[14]

In a randomized, double-blind pilot study for treatment of chronic insomnia, subjects taking chamomile high-dose extract (*M recutita*, 270 mg 2 times per day for 4 weeks) experienced moderate improvement in daytime functioning, with small-to-moderate effects on sleep latency, nighttime awakenings, and fatigue severity; however, the study demonstrated no benefit over placebo with the dose or formulation used.[15]

Author recommendations
Chamomile is useful for generalized anxiety and insomnia in various forms: capsules, 300 to 400 mg taken 3 times per day; tincture (1:5, 45% alcohol), 30 to 60 drops of tincture, 3 times per day in hot water; and tea, pour 1 cup of boiling water over 2 to 3 heaping teaspoons (2–4 g) of dried herb, steep 10 to 15 minutes and drink 3 to 4 times per day between meals.

Echinacea

Echinacea is a plant primarily used to treat upper respiratory infections. A recent Cochrane review has shown that, in general, echinacea has some small preventive effects in terms of the common cold, though statistically significant reductions in illness occurrence are weak.[16] However, other meta-analyses of clinical trials have shown a positive, significant role in likelihood of experiencing a cold with echinacea use.[17,18] The mechanism of echinacea is immunomodulatory, including the enhancement of macrophage function, coming from its alkamides, oils, and other active chemical constituents.[19] Beliefs in treatments may affect these effects because those who believe echinacea to be effective experience shorter and less severe courses of illness even if given pills not containing echinacea.[20] Variations may also be attributable to the many preparations of echinacea that are available, all with varying bioavailability.[16] Overall echinacea is well-tolerated, with the most serious side effect seeming to be allergic reaction.[16,19] With this in mind, using echinacea for cold prevention may yield favorable results, as long as consumers and providers remain aware of the variation in preparations available. Multiple studies have evaluated the effect of echinacea on athletic performance, with conflicting conclusions as to the effect on maximal oxygen uptake (VO2 max) and running economy, meriting further research.[21–23]

Author recommendations
Certain extracts of echinacea may be useful for treatment of the common cold with an adult dose of 400 mg dried extract 3 times per day, 1 cup of tea (1 g root in 150 mL boiling water) 2 times per day, or 0.25 to 1 mL liquid alcohol extract 3 times daily until symptom improvement; however, not for more than 10 days.

Elderberry

Health benefits of the elderberry stem from its richness in flavonoids, which have antioxidant properties. It is thought that they play a role in the mechanism of its efficacy in the treatment of cold viruses and influenza. Numerous research findings show its contribution to significant symptom relief in cold and influenza patients, making it a safe and cost-effective treatment.[24–26] Most recently, a study has shown cold severity and duration to be reduced in air travelers.[27]

Small studies have shown elderberry to decrease triglycerides and cholesterol, as well as increase serum antioxidant capacity; however, further studies are needed to establish elderberry's effect on the lipid profile.[28,29] Only reliable elderberry sources should be used due to a risk of cyanide toxicity from uncooked berries or other plant parts.[30]

Author recommendations
1. "Cooked and/or reliably processed elderberry sources may be useful for the treatment of the common cold and influenza in adults for 3 to 5 days starting at symptom onset." 2. "Consider taking Elderberry syrup containing 3.8 g standardized liquid extract (2:1) per 10 ml, 2 teaspoons 1 to 3 times daily; or 2 lozenges (each containing 130 mg standardized extract) 1 to 3 times daily."

Feverfew

The feverfew (*Tanacetum parthenium*) herb, native to the Balkan area and now found worldwide, is used mostly for treatment of migraine headaches. A recent Cochrane review notes its statistical significance in effectively reducing migraine frequency, while encouraging further studies for confirmation. Duration, intensity, incidence, and severity were not found to be statistically significant in the reviewed studies.[31] Though a former human rheumatoid arthritis study yielded no apparent benefit,[32] feverfew continues to be promising in pain relief, including inflammatory and neuropathic pain.[33,34] The medicinal portions of the plant are the dried leaves, which are sold in various compositions.[31] Although the exact mechanism of feverfew's efficacy against migraines remains to be established, 3 main components of the plant are thought to contribute: the serotonin secretion inhibitor, parthenolide; the essential oil, chrysanthenyl acetate, with analgesic properties; and melatonin.[35] Studies have suggested patients have decreased melatonin excretion during migraine headaches, which feverfew may counteract.[36] The overall safety profile of feverfew is relatively favorable;

gastrointestinal complaints and other mild and transient side effects have been noted in migraine studies but no major safety concerns were found.[31]

Author recommendations
Feverfew may be useful for migraine prevention and treatment: 50 to 100 mg daily, standardized to contain 0.2% to 0.35% parthenolide.

Garlic

Garlic (*Allium sativum*) is associated in popular culture with its use as a treatment of the common cold and, although a trial does exist that suggests its efficacy in prevention of common cold occurrences, more evidence is necessary to confirm this.[37] Similarly, reviews of garlic's effect on hypertension and peripheral arterial disease have found positive effects on lowering blood pressure but there is a need for more studies before it can be claimed to improve cardiovascular health.[38,39] Garlic is speculated to possess antibiotic and antiviral properties, thought to come from allicin.[37] Also, an impact on cell proliferation and death have made it a promising target in cancer and benign prostatic hyperplasia research.[40–42] The most common side effects of garlic are rash and odor.[37] It should also be noted that garlic has been associated with prolonged bleeding time and the American Academy of Family Physicians recommends cessation of high doses of garlic 7 to 10 days before surgery.[43–45]

Author recommendations
Garlic may be useful against the common cold: 1000 mg (1.3% allicin) daily in supplement or fresh garlic equivalent form.

Ginseng

Popular in various forms from teas to powders to milks,[46] ginseng (*Panax ginseng*) has been shown to have a positive effect on cognition, memory, quality of life, and behavior, though further studies are warranted for confirmation.[47–58] Its positive effects on well-being, appetite, and sleep have made it a promising target for addressing quality of life, especially in patients with cancer, multiple sclerosis, and other chronic illnesses.[50,59] Ginseng seems to exert anti-inflammatory effects through its chemical ginsenosides.[48,60] No serious adverse side effects have been noted, though medication interactions should be noted.[47]

Author recommendations
Ginseng may be considered for psychological and immune function support: standardized extract 200 mg/d, or dry root (tea form or chewed) 0.5 to 2g per day. It is useful for cancer-related fatigue at 2000 mg daily.

MEDICATION INTERACTIONS

Physicians are generally knowledgeable that drug-drug interactions are a possibility and take them into consideration when prescribing. They are often concerned about dietary supplement-medication interactions but are not trained in how to assess the risk and may default to a recommendation to avoid supplements because they feel unprepared to counsel patients. Integrative medicine professionals who prescribe herbal medicines regularly have received training in possible medication-supplement interactions and available databases, and advise their patients accordingly.

Many herbal medicines and dietary supplements are packaged in proprietary combinations and can be purchased without a prescription. The popularity of multi-herb formulations can potentially increase the risk of herb-medicine interactions. To limit this risk, Drug-herb-supplement interaction checkers are available through point-of-care resources, like Natural Medicines:

- Banana
- Cucumber
- Melon, including cantaloupe, honeydew, watermelon
- Zucchini
- Echinacea
- Butterbur
- Honey
- Ragweed relatives (marsh elder, goldenrod, mugwort).

OFFICE-BASED RESOURCES

This section highlights educational materials that primary care providers can use to research phytotherapies in the clinic setting. Recommendations include free, 1-time purchase and subscription-based materials for providers with varying access to resources.

Building Herbal Vocabulary

Rakel's Integrative Medicine, 3rd edition, offers evidence-based recommendations to medical issues that are frequently encountered in the primary care setting, and provides succinct reviews of preventive and therapeutic options, including guidelines for recommending phytotherapy. This textbook is available from online retailers and medical bookstores, for download through Elsevier's Clinical Key, and for purchase directly through Elsevier's Web site.

A growing number of continuing-education conferences for clinicians are available through integrative health care organizations and academic institutions. The Academic Consortium for Integrative Medicine and Health convenes scientific conferences and maintains a list of conferences being hosted by its member academic health centers. The Academy of Integrative and Holistic Medicine (AIHM) sponsors an annual 4-day experience for clinicians interested in building their holistic medicine skills.

Researching Herbal Medicines

After identifying herbal medicines that may be useful for either treating diseases or improving overall health, the next step is understanding its indications for use, overall and comparative effectiveness, and potential side-effect profiles.

Natural Medicines is the combined product of two previously independent resources: *Natural Standard* and *Natural Medicines Comprehensive Database*. This resource has several helpful point-of-care resources for the clinic setting, including: "Herb-Supplement Interaction," "Medication Effectiveness," "Nutrient Depletion," and "Pregnancy-Lactation Checkers." The Clinical Management Series provides excellent diagnosis-based learning, and monograph-based courses provide in-depth overviews of individual herbal medicines. Access to this resource is subscription-based; it is frequently included in hospital and health system libraries. Information is available at: https://naturalmedicines.therapeuticresearch.com.

American Botanical Council (ABC) provides online access to the ABC's Clinical Guide to Herbs, The *Complete German Commission E Monographs* translated into English, commercial herbal product monographs, herbal product adulteration reports, and the ABC's electronic monthly newsletter, *Herbal EGram*. Certain online databases are only available to ABC Members, and individual memberships start at $50 per year. More information on ABC, and all of its educational resources, is available at http://abc.herbalgram.org.

Cochrane Complementary Medicine produces systematic reviews of complementary, alternative, and integrative medicine therapies that can be accessed for free. Under the "Evidence" heading and "Reviews by Type of Therapy" section, the "Natural Product-Based Therapies" subtopic lists nearly 100 analyses of herbal medicines, indexed by the specific medical conditions that have been investigated for treatment. The "Consumer Summaries" section contains subject-level explanations of study design, data analysis, and clinical impact. The "Plain-Language Summaries" section contains patient education-ready handouts in PDF format. For more information, see http://cam.cochrane.org/.

European Scientific Cooperative on Phytotherapy (ESCOP) represents several national herbal medicine and phytotherapy professional associations from across Europe, and has produced a collection of evidence-based and expert-reviewed monographs for more than 100 herbs. Monographs for more than 35 herbs can be purchased individually for €20. ESCOP's *Herb Reference* 2.0 app allows users to reference "Monograph Summaries" through its herb and condition directories, and can be downloaded to a mobile device for $1.99. Previous versions of the monographs have only been available in print, the last textbook edition was published in 2003, and a supplement was issued in 2009. For more information, please visit the organization's Web site: http://escop.com.

Free Point-Of-Care Resources

National Center for Complementary and Integrative Health (NCCIH) is a National Institute of Health initiative that supports research and education in this evolving field. Web site contains free online continuing medical education (CME) or continuing education unit (CEU), video casts of the annual Distinguished Lecture Series, and databases for both clinical guidelines and systematic reviews. For patients, "Understanding Drug-Supplement Interactions" is an online tutorial that describes the impact of herbal medicines on the effectiveness of Western pharmaceuticals, whereas "Herbs At-A-Glance" contains plain-language monographs of over 50 herbs, with information on general use, evidence-based recommendations, and potential side effects. The monographs are available for download in either PDF or eBook format, by visiting https://nccih.nih.gov/.

Longwood Herbal Task Force (LHTF) is a collaborative that started by evaluating the use of herbal medicines in the oncology setting. Educational resources include herbal monographs and clinician information summaries to guide clinical decision-making, and a "Patient Fact Sheets" section with clinic-ready patient education handouts in PDF format. The LHTF Web site is easy to navigate, the patient education materials are clear and thorough, and all of the online resources listed can be accessed for free. Of note, some educational materials are marked as last being revised in 1999 or 2000, and the Web site was last updated in 2003, so users should be aware that information from this site may not reference or incorporate more recent research. http://www.longwoodherbal.org/.

Federal Standards and Safety

Several national government agencies provide safety information to help patients and physicians educate themselves about the risks and benefits of starting herbal medicines.

The US Food and Drug Administration (FDA) maintains free, searchable databases of FDA-approved herbals and supplements, product recall press releases, generally regarded as safe ingredients, and current good manufacturing practices for dietary supplements. For more information, please visit the FDA Web site: http://www.fda.gov/.

Health Canada maintains an online *Licensed Natural Health Products Database* of natural health products that are sold in Canada, including herb and plant-based remedies, and have been found to be safe, effective, and of high quality under their recommended conditions of use. Data supporting product licensure is updated regularly. Please see Health Canada's Web site for more details: http://www.hc-sc.gc.ca/dhp-mps/prodnatur/applications/licen-prod/lnhpd-bdpsnh-eng.php.

Independent Quality-Control Agencies

In the United States, herbal medicines and dietary supplements are not subject to strict oversight by the FDA under the Dietary Supplement, Health, and Education Act (DSHEA) of 1994. In response to concerns about supplement quality, several third-party organizations now perform independent quality-control testing of actual products, providing information on whether supplements contain the stated ingredients and are free of contaminants. These organizations often have a seal or emblem that is applied to products that pass independent certification, meeting the internally generated quality-control standards.

A list of the most prominent and commonly encountered organizations includes

1. Consumer Lab: http://www.consumerlab.com, access to full reviews is available to consumers and clinicians for a reasonable annual fee
2. Natural Products Association: http://www.npainfo.org/
3. NSF International: http://www.nsf.org/services/by-industry/dietary-supplements
4. United States Pharmacopeia: http://www.usp.org/verification-services/usp-verified-dietary-supplements.

SUMMARY

It is essential for primary care health care professionals to have a foundational knowledge of dietary supplements and to become familiar with resources and professionals available for patients because herbal medicines are increasingly popular. When confronted with patients seeking more extensive guidance in the use of phytotherapy and other dietary supplements, referrals to trained integrative medicine physicians, naturopathic doctors, TCM providers, and herbalists can provide invaluable guidance in this area of medicine outside the scope of conventional training. It is also important to be aware that licensure and credentialing for naturopaths and TCM providers varies by state. In addition, although there are some extensively trained and experienced herbalists, this field has no formal oversight. It is the authors' hope that the information provided here in combination with the aforementioned resources can assist in making sure patients interested in using herbal medicine can do so with the support of their partnering health care provider to ensure safe and effective care.

REFERENCES

1. Chrea B, O'Connell JA, Silkstone-Carter O, et al. Nature's antidepressant for mild to moderate depression: isolation and spectral characterization of hyperforin from

a standardized extract of St. John's Wort (*Hypericum perforatum*). J Chem Educ 2014;91(3):440–2.

2. Lawvere S, Mahoney M. St. John's Wort. Am Fam Physician 2005;72(11):2249–54.

3. Clarke TC, Black LI, Stussman BJ, et al. Trends in the use of complementary health approaches among adults: United States, 2002–2012. National Health Statistics Reports. Hyattsville (MD): National Center for Health Statistics; 2015. Available at: https://nccih.nih.gov/research/statistics/NHIS/2012/natural-products.

4. Kaufeler R, Polasek W, Brattström A, et al. Efficacy and safety of butterbur herbal extract Ze 339 in seasonal allergic rhinitis: postmarketing surveillance study. Adv Ther 2006;23(2):373–84.

5. Schapowal A. Randomised controlled trial of butterbur and cetirizine for treating seasonal allergic rhinitis. BMJ 2002;324(7330):144–6.

6. Schapowal A. Butterbur Ze339 for the treatment of intermittent allergic rhinitis: dose-dependent efficacy in a prospective, randomized, double-blind, placebo-controlled study. Arch Otolaryngol Head Neck Surg 2004;130(12):1381–6.

7. Schapowal A. Treating intermittent allergic rhinitis: a prospective, randomized, placebo and antihistamine-controlled study of Butterbur extract Ze 339. Phytother Res 2005;19(6):530–7.

8. Diener H, Rahlfs VW, Danesch U, et al. The first placebo-controlled trial of a special butterbur root extract for the prevention of migraine: reanalysis of efficacy criteria. Eur Neurol 2004;51(2):89–97.

9. Lipton R, Göbel H, Einhäupl KM, et al. *Petasites hybridus* root (butterbur) is an effective preventive treatment for migraine. Neurology 2004;63(12):2240–4.

10. Holland S, Silberstein SD, Freitag F, et al. Evidence-based guideline update: NSAIDs and other complementary treatments for episodic migraine prevention in adults: report of the Quality Standards Subcommittee of the American Academy of Neurology and the American Headache Society. Neurology 2012;78(17):1346–53.

11. National Center for Complementary and Integrative Health. Butterbur. D464. 2016.

12. National Toxicology Program. Chemical information review document for butterbur. Research Triangle Park (NC): U.S Department of Health and Human Services; 2009. Available at: https://ntp.niehs.nih.gov/ntp/noms/support_docs/butterbur_nov2009.pdf.

13. Amsterdam JD, Li Y, Soeller I, et al. A randomized, double-blind, placebo-controlled trial of oral *Matricaria recutita* (chamomile) extract therapy for generalized anxiety disorder. J Clin Psychopharmacol 2009;29(4):378–82.

14. Amsterdam JD, Shults J, Soeller I, et al. Chamomile (*Matricaria recutita*) may provide antidepressant activity in anxious, depressed humans: an exploratory study. Altern Ther Health Med 2012;18(5):44–9.

15. Zick SM, Wright BD, Sen A, et al. Preliminary examination of the efficacy and safety of a standardized chamomile extract for chronic primary insomnia: a randomized placebo-controlled pilot study. BMC Complement Altern Med 2011;11:78.

16. Karsch-Völk M, Barrett B, Kiefer D, et al. Echinacea for preventing and treating the common cold. Cochrane Database Syst Rev 2014;(2):CD000530.

17. Schoop R, Klein P, Suter A, et al. Echinacea in the prevention of induced rhinovirus colds: a meta-analysis. Clin Ther 2006;28:174–83.

18. Shah S, Sander S, White CM, et al. Evaluation of echinacea for the prevention and treatment of the common cold: a meta-analysis. Lancet Infect Dis 2007;7:473–80.

19. Barnes J, Anderson LA, Gibbons S, et al. Echinacea species (*Echinacea angustifolia* (DC.) Hell., *Echinacea pallida* (Nutt.) Nutt., *Echinacea purpurea* (L.) Moench): a review of their chemistry, pharmacology and clinical properties. J Pharm Pharmacol 2005;57(8):929–54.

20. Barrett B, Brown R, Rakel D, et al. Placebo effects and the common cold: a randomized controlled trial. Ann Fam Med 2011;9(4):312–22.
21. Baumann C, Bond KL, Rupp JC, et al. *Echinacea purpurea* supplementation does not enhance VO2max in distance runners. J Strength Cond Res 2014; 28(5):1367–72.
22. Senchina D, Shah NB, Doty DM, et al. Herbal supplements and athlete immune function–what's proven, disproven, and unproven? Exerc Immunol Rev 2009; 15:66–106.
23. Whitehead M, Martin TD, Scheett TP, et al. Running economy and maximal oxygen consumption after 4 weeks of oral Echinacea supplementation. J Strength Cond Res 2012;26(7):1928–33.
24. Krawitz C, Mraheil MA, Stein M, et al. Inhibitory activity of a standardized elderberry liquid extract against clinically-relevant human respiratory bacterial pathogens and influenza A and B viruses. BMC Complement Altern Med 2011;11:16.
25. Roschek B, Fink RC, McMichael MD, et al. Elderberry flavonoids bind to and prevent H1N1 infection in vitro. Phytochemistry 2009;70(10):1255–61.
26. Zakay-Rones Z, Thom E, Wollan T, et al. Randomized study of the efficacy and safety of oral elderberry extract in the treatment of influenza A and B virus infections. J Int Med Res 2004;32(2):132–40.
27. Tiralongo E, Wee SS, Lea RA, et al. Elderberry supplementation reduces cold duration and symptoms in air-travellers: a randomized, double-blind placebo-controlled clinical trial. Nutrients 2016;8(4):182.
28. Ivanova D, Tasinov O, Kiselova-Kaneva Y, et al. Improved lipid profile and increased serum antioxidant capacity in healthy volunteers after *Sambucus ebulus L.* fruit infusion consumption. Int J Food Sci Nutr 2014;65(6):760–4.
29. Murkovic M, Abuja PM, Bergmann AR, et al. Effects of elderberry juice on fasting and postprandial serum lipids and low-density lipoprotein oxidation in healthy volunteers: a randomized, double-blind, placebo-controlled study. Eur J Clin Nutr 2004;58(2):244–9.
30. Ulbricht C, Basch E, Cheung L, et al. An evidence-based systematic review of elderberry and elderflower (*Sambucus nigra*) by the Natural Standard Research Collaboration. J Dietary Supplements 2014;11(1):80–120.
31. Wider B, Pittler MH, Ernst E, et al. Feverfew for preventing migraine. Cochrane Database Syst Rev 2015;(4):CD002286.
32. Pattrick M, Heptinstall S, Doherty M, et al. Feverfew in rheumatoid arthritis: a double blind, placebo controlled study. Ann Rheum Dis 1989;48(7):547–9.
33. Di Cesare Mannelli L, Tenci B, Zanardelli M, et al. Widespread pain reliever profile of a flower extract of *Tanacetum parthenium*. Phytomedicine 2015;22(7–8):752–8.
34. Galeotti N, Maidecchi A, Mattoli L, et al. St. John's Wort seed and feverfew flower extracts relieve painful diabetic neuropathy in a rat model of diabetes. Phytotherapy 2014;92:22–3.
35. Murch S, Simmons CB, Saxena PK. Melatonin in feverfew and other medicinal plants. Lancet 1997;350(9091):1598–9.
36. Brun J, Claustrat B, Saddier P, et al. Nocturnal melatonin excretion is decreased in patients with migraine without aura attacks associated with menses. Cephololgia 1995;15(2):136–9.
37. Lissiman E, Bhasale AL, Cohen M. Garlic for the common cold. Cochrane Database Syst Rev 2014;(11):CD006206.
38. Jepson R, Kleijnen J, Leng GC. Garlic for peripheral arterial occlusive disease. Cochrane Database Syst Rev 2013;(4):CD000095.

39. Stabler SN, Tejani AM, Huynh F, et al. Garlic for the prevention of cardiovascular morbidity and mortality in hypertensive patients. Cochrane Database Syst Rev 2012;(8):CD007653.
40. Chung K, Shin SJ, Lee NY, et al. Anti-proliferation effects of garlic (*Allium sativum L.*) on the progression of benign prostatic hyperplasia. Phytother Res 2016;30(7): 1197–203.
41. De Giorgio A, Stebbing J. Garlic: a stake through the heart of cancer? Lancet Oncol 2016;17(7):879–80.
42. Zhou Y, Li Y, Zhou T, et al. Dietary natural products for prevention and treatment of liver cancer. Nutrients 2016;8(3):156.
43. Ackermann RT, Mulrow CD, Ramirez G, et al. Garlic shows promise for improving some cardiovascular risk factors. Arch Intern Med 2001;161:813–24.
44. Burnham BE. Garlic as a possible risk for postoperative bleeding. Plast Reconstr Surg 1995;95:213.
45. Tattelman E. Health effects of garlic. Am Fam Physician 2005;72(01):103–6.
46. Tarrega A, Salvador A, Meyer M, et al. Active compounds and distinctive sensory features provided by American ginseng (*Panax quinquefolius L.*) extract in a new functional milk beverage. J Dairy Sci 2012;95(8):4246–55.
47. Geng J, Dong J, Ni H, et al. No convincing evidence of a cognitive enhancing effect of *Panax ginseng*. Cochrane Database Syst Rev 2010;(12):CD007769.
48. Geng J, Dong J, Ni H, et al. Ginseng for cognition. Cochrane Database Syst Rev 2010;(12):CD007769.
49. Ossoukhova A, Owen L, Savage K, et al. Improved working memory performance following administration of a single dose of American ginseng (*Panax quinquefolius L.*) to healthy middle-age adults. Hum Psychopharmacol 2015;30(2):108–22.
50. Yennurajalingam S, Reddy A, Tannir NM, et al. High-dose Asian ginseng (*Panax ginseng*) for cancer-related fatigue: a preliminary report. Integr Cancer Ther 2015;14(5):419–27.
51. Asero R, Mistrello G, Amato S. The nature of melon allergy in ragweed-allergic subjects: A study of 1000 patients. Allergy Asthma Proc 2011;32(1):64–7.
52. Choi J, Jang YS, Oh JW, et al. Bee pollen-induced anaphylaxis: a case report and literature review. Allergy Asthma Immunol Res 2015;7(5):513–7.
53. Egger M, Mutschlechner S, Wopfner N, et al. Pollen-food syndromes associated with weed pollinosis: an update from the molecular point of view. Allergy 2006; 61(4):461–76.
54. Enberg R, Leickly FE, McCullough J, et al. Watermelon and ragweed share allergens. J Allergy Clin Immunol 1987;79(6):867–75.
55. Anderson LB Jr, Dreyfuss EM, Logan J, et al. Melon and banana sensitivity coincident with ragweed pollinosis. J Allergy 1970;45(3):310–9.
56. Popescu F. Cross-reactivity between aeroallergens and food allergens. World J Methodol 2015;5(2):31–50.
57. Reindl J, Anliker MD, Karamloo F, et al. Allergy caused by ingestion of zucchini (*Cucurbita pepo*): Characterization of allergens and cross-reactivity to pollen and other foods. J Allergy Clin Immunol 2000;106(2):379–85.
58. Don't take echinacea if you're allergic to ragweed. Consum Rep 2012;77:12.
59. Etemadifar M, Sayahi F, Abtahi SH, et al. Ginseng in the treatment of fatigue in multiple sclerosis: a randomized, placebo-controlled, double-blind pilot study. Int J Neurosci 2013;123(7):480–6.
60. Lee D, Yang CL, Chik SC, et al. Bioactivity-guided identification and cell signaling technology to delineate the immunomodulatory effects of *Panax ginseng* on human promonocytic U937 cells. J Transl Med 2009;7:34.

Integrative Medicine Strategies for Changing Health Behaviors
Support for Primary Care

Ruth Q. Wolever, PhD[a,b,*], Karen L. Caldwell, PhD[c],
Lindsey C. McKernan, PhD[b,d], Marni G. Hillinger, MD[d]

KEYWORDS

- Primary care • Lifestyle • Behavior change • Health coach • Integrative medicine

KEY POINTS

- Integrative Medicine approaches are particularly useful to support lifestyle change.
- Addressing behavior change from a holistic perspective allows for success in an area in which the patient has intrinsic motivation. Success breeds further success.
- Sustainable behavior change is quite complex and lengthy; it requires much more than education and advice. Neither the primary care provider nor the individual patient should expect to carry the full burden alone.
- The primary care provider has a key role in health behavior change, namely catalyzing change, educating and linking to available resources, and supporting the patient in the background while health coaches or others guide the change process in the foreground.
- Stress undermines behavior change; stress must be addressed first or at least simultaneously to enact sustainable behavior change.

NEED FOR LIFESTYLE CHANGE

An estimated 86% of US health care expenses are related to chronic diseases: type II diabetes, heart disease, stroke, and obesity, driven by unhealthy lifestyles.[1,2] Prevention and mitigation of these diseases involve cultivation of health through daily lifestyle

Disclosure: See last page of article.
[a] Department of Physical Medicine and Rehabilitation, Osher Center for Integrative Medicine at Vanderbilt, Vanderbilt University Medical Center, Vanderbilt University School of Nursing, 3401 West End Avenue, Suite 380, Nashville, TN 37203, USA; [b] Department of Psychiatry & Behavioral Sciences, Vanderbilt University Medical Center, Nashville, TN, USA; [c] Department of Human Development and Psychological Counseling, Appalachian State University, 151 College Street, Boone, NC 28608, USA; [d] Department of Physical Medicine and Rehabilitation, Osher Center for Integrative Medicine at Vanderbilt, Vanderbilt University Medical Center, 3401 West End Avenue, Suite 380, Nashville, TN 37203, USA
* Corresponding author. 12 Hopewell Drive, Durham, NC 27705.
E-mail address: ruth.wolever@vanderbilt.edu

behaviors, including adequate intake of fruits, vegetables, and healthy dietary fat sources, regular exercise, moderate (if any) alcohol use, and no use of tobacco. Unfortunately, less than 10% of US adults consistently engage in these behaviors.[3] In addition, the rising burden of stress complicates and undermines attempts to change lifestyle.[4] Because the need to manage stress is so central to successful behavior change, stress should also be considered a key target in lifestyle change, along with nutrition, physical activity, substance management, and sleep. Although most providers are fully aware of both the scientific and the fiscal case for promoting health behaviors, they are typically not trained in behavior change beyond the provision of education and recommendations. In addition, the burgeoning requirements for primary care practice make it unrealistic to expect primary care providers to manage the complexities of behavior change without team-based approaches.

ROLE OF PRIMARY CARE IN LIFESTYLE CHANGE

Given the burgeoning need to improve health behaviors, federal initiatives to promote healthy lifestyle and disease prevention have enacted the Patient Protection and Affordable Care Act (2010), and new prevention models are slowly emerging.[5] Primary care must take a vital role in supporting health behaviors. Patients expect to receive behavioral counseling from their primary care providers,[6] and they respect and value their guidance.[7] In addition, primary care is built on a relationship over time, and relationship-based care provides the strongest motivator for sustainable behavior change.[8] Nonetheless, although the focus on prevention is growing, acute care still drives health care reimbursement, and hence, delivery.[9] Until system reforms allow adequate time and reimbursement for primary care providers to move the focus to prevention, primary care providers need a manageable, defined role in lifestyle change, easy-to-implement strategies, and evidence-based resources to provide patients.

Primary care providers play an enormously important role in the health behavior change process, but it is not fair or realistic to expect them to hold the whole process. Providers would do well to shift their expectations to a more realistic stance by identifying a patient's current stage in the change process for a specific behavior and targeting a single step forward rather than a total overhaul in patient behavior: "the goal for a single encounter is a shift from the grandiose to the realistic."[10] Given the enormity of the need for behavior change, and the lack of time and expertise on the part of most primary care providers, the authors suggest a particular role for primary care providers that is seminal: (1) to serve as a catalyst, priming the patient for change[11,12]; (2) to educate and point the patient to appropriate resources for additional guidance and hands-on support; and (3) to provide an umbrella of ongoing encouragement throughout the long journey of change while patients work more intensely with health coaches or allied health providers. In order to provide ongoing encouragement, clinicians must understand that behavior change is highly complex and not understood by many in the medical system. Patients become overwhelmed when presented with the end goal (eg, "you need to lose 40 pounds," "you need to exercise aerobically for 30 minutes at least 5 times per week). The primary care provider would do well to get patients headed in the right direction, taking small steps with *any* lifestyle goal that interests them (often stress management is first) and experiencing small successes to build self-efficacy. Sample open-ended questions to introduce lifestyle concepts and catalyze change are provided in **Box 1**. Providers can then refer to well-trained health coaches to support/guide the entire process of behavior change and to

> **Box 1**
> **Sample open-ended questions to catalyze exploration and change in lifestyle domains**
>
> - Lowered stress: What would your life be like if you actively worked on lowering your stress?
> - Increased physical activity and exercise: What type of physical movement do you enjoy or have you enjoyed in the past?
> - Increased fruit and vegetable intake: How would you know if you were getting enough vegetables (or fruit)?
> - Increased sources of healthy fat: What have you learned about healthy sources of fat?
> - Reduced sugar consumption: How would you physically feel if you ate less sugar?
> - Limited caffeine: What would your average day be like if you only drank 2 cups of coffee (stop drinking coffee at noon, etc)?
> - No more than moderate alcohol intake: What is at stake for you if you decide not to drink less?
> - No tobacco use or other recreational substance use: How will you know when it is time to quit smoking?
> - Adequate, restful sleep: What possibilities might open up for you if you had adequate, restful sleep?

specialists for specific skills training and more time-intensive education. Integrative Medicine (IM) strategies can aid the primary care provider in these crucial roles.

WHY USE INTEGRATIVE MEDICINE AS AN APPROACH FOR LIFESTYLE CHANGE?

IM aligns well with optimization of health and health behavior change. First, IM is holistic, allowing the patient ample choice of where to initiate change. Because self-determined goals predict sustainability of behavior change,[13,14] it is best for patients to choose where they want to begin to improve lifestyle, and subsequently, where they want to go next (**Fig. 1**). Second, IM is an excellent choice for supporting behavior change because IM uses lifestyle medicine as a foundation.[15] Specifically, IM strives to recruit and enhance the body's natural ability to heal; healthy lifestyle behaviors (eg, nutritious food, adequate physical activity, stress management, adequate sleep) are the primary mechanisms for optimizing functioning of the body.[15] Third, IM works for behavior change because it is aligned with a paradigm of growth rather than abnormality.[16] Behavior change requires sustained motivation as well as environmental supports that are best implemented through development and learning paradigms.[13,17] Few people sustain health behavior change when the motivation is grounded in fear or is avoidance based (that is, "I want to avoid this illness [often in the far future]"). On the other hand, approach-based motivation, founded on mastery and excitement, is both easier to access and more reliable (ie, "I want to create or to learn that skill"). Finally, health promotion is actually the primary reason that patients seek IM.[18] In addition, IM patient cohorts have healthier behaviors compared with the average US adult, further supporting the association of IM and preventive health.[18]

MIND-BODY TECHNIQUES FOR BEHAVIOR CHANGE

Listed in later discussion are key findings on IM approaches for lifestyle change. One caveat about research methodology used for IM merits mention, and in particular, those studies on mind-body programs. By definition, mind-body practices, such as

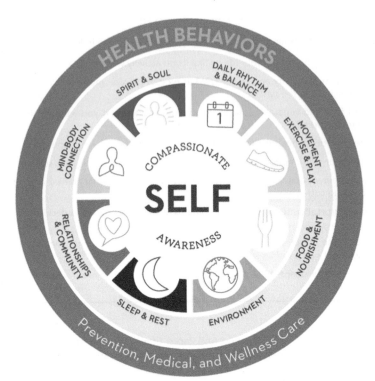

Fig. 1. Wheel of Health: Holistic model that allows patients to identify an area where they would like to begin to improve their lifestyle. (*Courtesy of* Osher Center for Integrative Medicine, Vanderbilt University Medical Center, Nashville, TN, 2015; with permission.)

meditation, tai chi, and yoga, focus on the complex interactions between the mind, body (including brain), and behavior. They specifically attend to the role of the mind in affecting physical functioning and health promotion.[19] Mind-body approaches depend on patients' active participation, perspectives, preferences, and beliefs. Hence, the very fabric of mind-body programs relies on internal factors that are difficult or even inappropriate to control as typically done in conventional medical research. To evaluate such interventions, one must consider the complexity of such approaches, along with the context in which they have arisen. Clinically, patient strengths and contextual factors are leveraged in these IM interventions to enhance the outcomes of mind-body interventions. For example, the patient-provider relationship is known to be central to the outcomes of such interventions. Thus, the actual cause-effect relationship of the intervention and the outcome does not occur in isolation from extraneous factors, but in synergy with them. In short, the extraneous factors that are considered "noise" that needs to be controlled in efficacy research in conventional medicine are the same factors that need to be *understood* and *leveraged* in mind-body interventions. Hence, investigation of the program's outcomes typically involves assessment of the program as a synergistic bundle that includes the context of the treatment, philosophy underlying the paradigm, the treatment components taken together, and their synergistic impact. Investigators do not attempt to dissect the program components, and there is less methodological control. For most of IM, it makes more sense to evaluate effectiveness first rather than efficacy first, as done in conventional medicine.[20] In sum, the gold standard is methodologically rigorous effectiveness trials, and hence, most of the trials noted in later discussion are effectiveness trials. The authors have attempted to provide a snapshot of the current state of effectiveness known about the approaches.

Given the extremely high burden on primary care practitioners to carry out their responsibilities, the authors present approaches that, once-learned, can be self-administered and sustained by patients without ongoing support from outside clinicians. Highly trained practitioners are important to initially teach patients these mind-body skills and support ongoing practices through difficult periods, but patients are able to sustain the practices with minimal support. Mind-body practices are also low risk, require very minor safety surveillance, and with few exceptions, do not have negative side effects. Furthermore, they require little or no equipment and can be taught to individuals or groups, allowing for more cost-effective implementation. Moreover, the techniques are portable, so can be demonstrated, taught, and used in multiple settings from primary care offices to the workplace. As an example, consider techniques that focus on using the breath; these can be practiced anywhere, anytime, without equipment, and without anyone else even knowing the person is practicing. Some of the IM approaches are simple and require such little time that the primary care provider with appropriate training can teach the patient during an encounter. For most, though, clinicians can direct the patient toward appropriate resources. Others require referral to a clinician with considerable training and credentials with the time to lead the patient carefully through the approach. Helpful IM resources are provided in **Box 2**.

EVIDENCE FOR SPECIFIC TECHNIQUES FOR LIFESTYLE CHANGE

A variety of techniques can empower patients in their lifestyle change process. Cognitive techniques include mindfulness meditation, hypnosis, and/or imagery/visualization. Behavioral techniques range from a simple listing of coping strategies to

---

Box 2
Resources for integrative medicine

- Natural Medicines (formerly Natural Standard and Natural Medicines Comprehensive Database) maintains a set of databases providing evidence ratings for dietary supplements, natural medicines, and complementary, alternative and integrative therapies (https://naturalmedicines.therapeuticresearch.com/).

- *Integrative Medicine*, 3rd edition. Philadelphia: Elsevier Saunders: 2012 is a definitive text on integrative medicine edited by family medicine physician Dave Rakel, MD (http://www.us.elsevierhealth.com/integrative-medicine-9781437717938.html).

- National Center for Complementary and Integrative Health at the National Institutes of Health provides many useful references for patients (https://nccih.nih.gov/).

- Health Coaching: See ichwc.org for updates on national certification standards and strategies for finding a qualified coach.

- Meditation: Individuals can find free recorded meditations at https://contemplativemind.wordpress.com/how-to-meditate-links-for-guided-meditation-practice/. Individuals can find live, in-person mindfulness classes at many local universities and live, on-line mindfulness courses through eMindful.com. Providers can find peer-reviewed literature on meditation and various mind-body approaches at https://contemplativemind.wordpress.com/peer-reviewed-research-mindfulness-meditation-contemplative-practice/. This site also has excellent explanations of the mechanisms of various practices.

- Hypnosis: For the latest research on hypnosis and strategies to find a qualified hypnotherapist, see the American Society of Clinical Hypnosis at http://www.asch.net.

complex skills training. Somatic relaxation techniques can include progressive muscle relaxation, diaphragmatic breathing, biofeedback, self-hypnosis, and guided imagery.[21] Many of these approaches, as well as some of the venues through which they are typically enacted, combine cognitive, behavioral, and somatic techniques. These combinations are particularly true of health coaching, psychotherapy, sleep therapy, self-monitoring exercises, meditation training, hypnosis, and meditative movement.

Health Coaching

Historically, many people have equated "coaching" with educating and advising, but neither are the primary tasks of health and wellness coaching (HWC). The role of an HWC was recently delineated by a job task analysis and validated by large surveys of practicing HWCs.[22] Coaching is a relationship-based approach that uses methodology from health psychology, positive psychology, and growth paradigms rather than working from a pathology paradigm of what is wrong.

- Coaches first elicit from the client a vision of their optimal health, self, or future through visioning and the use of the perceptual information processing system rather than solely relying on the conceptual information-processing system.[23] The visioning process appears to link to deeper sources of motivation, but takes time to cultivate and use well. As the vision percolates, patients are led through a gap analysis wherein they compare where they are now with where they want to be, in multiple domains of their lives.
- Patients are often not ready to take on something that the provider would prioritize from a medical perspective. However, by starting in one area where the patient has intrinsic interest and motivation to change, the chances of success are great. Success (in any behavior change) breeds success as patients become activated in self-care and gain self-efficacy.
- For the most part, effective health coaches avoid teaching, advising, or telling clients what to do but facilitate client learning and discovery.[22]
- Reviews strongly suggest the effectiveness of HWC in improving motivational processes, psychosocial outcomes, behavioral outcomes, and to a lesser degree, immediate biological indices of chronic illness.[24–28]
- The International Consortium for Health and Wellness Coaching (ICHWC) is implementing the first national examination in 2017, in partnership with the National Board of Medical Examiners.[22,29] Referral to National Board Certified Health and Wellness Coaches (NBC-HWC) will ensure that patients receive coaching from those that have at least a minimal standard of competencies in supporting behavior change. See ichwc.org for updates and strategies for finding a qualified coach.

Psychotherapy and Counseling

Counselors and psychotherapists use a range of techniques based on experiential relationship building, dialogue, communication, and enacting behavior change strategies designed to improve the mental health of a client or patient. There is strong evidence for its effectiveness for many different targets, including several lifestyle-related targets.[30]

Sleep therapy
Insomnia is a widespread condition characterized by a difficulty in falling asleep, staying asleep, or getting restful sleep.

- Cognitive-behavioral therapy for insomnia (CBT-I) is a multicomponent behavioral intervention providing sleep education, strategies for strengthening the associations between bed and sleep, and therapy for beliefs that can increase arousal mechanisms.[31] When compared with medications, CBT-I is as effective, and its effects may be more durable than medications.[31]

- For mild to moderate cases of insomnia, CBT-I can be self-administered through online programs such as Shut-i.[32] More severe cases should be referred to a therapist trained in the approach.
- There are considerable data to support use of 0.3 to 5.0 mg of melatonin at bedtime, particularly if the patient has an associated circadian rhythm disorder.[21,33]

Self-monitoring

Self-monitoring is a crucial aspect of healthy behavior change, and the strongest predictor of success in adoption of physical activity and dietary behaviors.[34] In addition to traditional paper-based methods of self-monitoring, technology-based methods are growing in use.

- Smartphone applications (apps) can help monitor and manage exercise, diet, weight, and sleep, providing rapid feedback with reminders of minimum goals.[35]
- Eighty percent of studies on mobile phones for weight loss reported positive effects. Important contributors to successful weight loss were (a) frequent self-recording of weight, (b) personalization of the intervention, and (c) participants' engagement in a proactive approach to everyday problems.[36]
- Text messaging interventions have increased adherence to antiretroviral treatment and smoking cessation.[37]

Hypnosis

Hypnosis is a state of inner absorption, concentration, and focused attention. It can help to modify automatic behavior patterns, such as addictions, habits, and ingrained reactive responses.[38]

- Hypnosis has a long history of success as a stress reduction technique.[39]
- Increased weight loss with hypnosis is fairly small and of arguable clinical significance.[40]
- Hypnotherapy may be effective for smoking cessation, but more rigorous evidence is needed to be certain.[41,42] One randomized contolled trial (RCT) found hypnotherapy to be more effective than nicotine replacement therapy for smoking cessation.[43]
- Strong evidence supports the use of clinical hypnosis in the treatment of both chronic and acute pain. Hence, when pain is the obstacle to lifestyle change, hypnosis is an excellent recommendation.[44]
- The primary contraindications to hypnosis are poor diagnostic and therapeutic skills of the therapist.[38] For the latest research on hypnosis and strategies to find a qualified hypnotherapist, see the American Society of Clinical Hypnosis at http://www.asch.net/.

Meditation training

Meditation practices are widely variable but typically involve training the mind to focus attention. Mindfulness meditation involves bringing attention to the present moment with openness and a nonjudgmental attitude.[45]

- For those who engage in binge eating and emotional eating, mindfulness meditation can decrease these behaviors, although the evidence for meditations' effect on weight change is mixed.[46]
- Meta-analyses show that mindfulness-based treatment is associated with reductions in stress and improvements in anxiety, depression, and pain.[47,48]

- Participants in a mindfulness-based course and a relapse-prevention treatment showed decreases in alcohol-related problems and reductions in substance use.[49,50]
- A few reports of negative psychological effects of meditation have been published. Caution is encouraged before recommending meditation to individuals with severe personality disorders, psychotic disorders, or severe depression without ongoing concurrent psychotherapy or medical treatment.[51]

Meditative Movement

The evidence base for the importance of physical exercise is substantial.[52] Meditative movement practices involve physical movement with a meditative mindset and include tai chi, qigong, and yoga. Tai chi and qigong practices come from traditional Chinese medicine and coordinate breath and mental focus with specific movements or postures. Yoga, with origins in Indian philosophy, typically includes various *asanas* (postures), breathing, and meditation or relaxation, although there is great variety between schools of yoga.

- Comprehensive reviews of qigong and tai chi found consistent results for several health benefits in RCTs, including improvement in physical function, quality of life, stress, and psychological symptoms.[53,54]
- Meditative movement has demonstrated beneficial effects on sleep, but the current research has significant methodological limitations.[55]
- More high-quality evidence is needed to determine the usefulness of yoga in substance use treatment,[56] although some evidence shows that yoga is useful in smoking cessation.[57]
- Tai chi is generally considered a safe exercise for all ages, even the elderly.[58] A systematic review found that yoga appears as safe as usual care and exercise.[59]
- There is no national standard for certification of yoga, tai chi, or qigong instructors. The National Qigong Association does have a certification process (http://nqa.org/membership/certification/).

Nutrition

A burgeoning body of evidence shows the impact of eating habits on chronic diseases. A Mediterranean diet reduces all-cause mortality in addition to disease-specific mortality, most notably, coronary heart disease.[60,61] In addition, lifestyle strategies improve blood glucose control,[62] and increased vegetable consumption is associated with lower dementia risk.[63,64]

The number and types of diets can be overwhelming to patients and providers alike and may be a barrier to initiating dietary changes. Nonetheless, many evidence-based diets share certain recommendations, such as the inclusion of nuts, seeds, fruits, vegetables, and olive oil[65] (**Table 1**, reprinted from Katz and Meller [2014]; their review provides a stellar comparison and summary of diets).[65] In short, no rigorous long-term studies comparing diets are without significant bias or confounders. At the same time, significant evidence supports the importance of healthful eating, namely, adopting a largely whole food, plant-based diet, with room for variation.[65–70] In other words, as Pollan[71] so succinctly states, "Eat food, not too much, mostly plants."

Listed in **Box 3** are evidence-based, easy-to-follow recommendations that can be used over multiple visits to move patients in the right direction. Developing healthy eating habits is complex and involves the intersection of many different factors, including family, culture, religion, economics, politics, marketing, wellness, addiction, and environment. Importantly, a discussion of eating habits often evokes an emotional response.[72] Use of a holistic model (see **Fig. 1**) can open discussion

Table 1
The theme of optimal eating

	Low-Carbohydrate	Low-Fat/ Vegetarian/Vegan	Low-Glycemic	Mediterranean	Mixed/Balance	Paleolithic
Health benefits relate to:	Emphasis on restriction of refined starches and added sugars in particular	Emphasis on plant foods direct from nature; avoidance of harmful fats	Restriction of starches, added sugars; high fiber intake	Foods direct from nature; mostly plants; emphasis on healthful oils, notably monounsaturates	Minimization of highly processed, energy-dense foods; emphasis on wholesome foods in moderate quantities	Minimization of processed foods; emphasis on natural plant foods and lean meats
Compatible elements:	Limited refined starches, added sugars, processed foods, limited intake of certain fats; emphasis on whole plant foods, with or without lean meats, fish, poultry, seafood					
And all potentially consistent with:	Food, not too much, mostly plants[a,b,c]					

Diverse diets making competing claims actually emphasize key elements that are generally compatible, complementary, or even duplicative. Competition for public attention and a share of weight-loss/health-promotion markets results in exaggerated claims and an emphasis on mutually exclusive rather than shared elements.

[a] From Pollan M. 2007. Unhappy meals. New York Times, Jan. 28. http://www.nytimes.com/2007/01/28magazine/28nutritionism.t.html?pagewanted=all.
[b] Portion control may be facilitated by choosing better-quality foods, which have the tendency to promote satiety with fewer calories.
[c] Although neither the low-carbohydrate nor Paleolithic diet need be "mostly plants," both can be.
From Katz D, Meller S. Can we say what diet is best for health? Annu Rev Public Health 2014;35:95; with permission.

Box 3
Evidence-based nutrition recommendations

- Focus on eating whole foods rather than individual micronutrients. Whole foods tend to naturally be lower in salt, sugar, and saturated fats while being high in fiber and phytonutrients.
- Build a balanced plate made up of at least ½ vegetables and fruit, ¼ unprocessed whole grains and ¼ plant protein, sustainable fish or grass-fed animal protein. Adding more of these foods to your plate will leave less room for other foods.
- Eat abundant amounts of vegetables and fruits (minimum 5 servings such as one cup of leafy greens, one medium-sized piece of fruit, or ½ cup of fruits or vegetables). Choose at least 2 to 3 colors to add to the plate, one of which should be green leafy vegetables.
- Choose healthy nonhydrogenated fats, such as olive oil, avocado, nuts, and seeds.
- Replace sugar-sweetened beverages with water.
- "Add" to the diet before "taking away" (eg, add more fruits and vegetables rather than remove ice cream or sweets).
- Set your kitchen up for success: place fruits and vegetables on the countertop and put prepped fruits and vegetables in see-through containers at eye level in the front of the refrigerator or pantry.
- Learn mindful eating techniques to manage stress; learn more about behavioral drivers; and increase connection with innate appetite regulation systems. The Mindful Diet has several tools to help patients change food-related patterns. In addition, guided eating-related mindfulness exercises are available at no charge at https://www.vanderbilthealth.com/osher/50336.
- Just like with other behavioral changes, small shifts that build on each other are much more likely to be successful.

Data from Refs.[64–69]

---

about the role of food in patients' lives. Once the provider catalyzes change in nutrition habits, ongoing change may be supported by referral to an interprofessional team member. Health coaching, dietician consultation, and psychotherapy can all facilitate behavior change related to dietary habits; the more rigid or compulsive the eating pattern (whether overly restrictive or seemingly devoid of guidelines), the more likely that psychotherapy should be a treatment component.

Other Interventions for Tobacco Cessation

- Current treatment guidelines recommend screening for tobacco use in health care settings and provision of behavioral counseling (individual, group, or telephone) and/or pharmacotherapy.[73,74]
- Internet tobacco cessation interventions are sustainable, cost-efficient, and acceptable and widely available to patients. Interactive internet cessation interventions may be equivalent to other currently recommended treatment modalities (ie, telephone, in-person counseling).[75] Several mobile phone apps for tobacco cessation are available, but there is a lack of scientific evidence for their efficacy.[76]

CASE STUDY
Introduction

The following case has been written with consent and permission of the patient treated. All personally identifying information has been removed or disguised to maintain patient confidentiality.

Background

Jody is a 28-year-old Asian-American woman referred to IM for unexplained weakness in both legs, fatigue, migraines, and bouts of extreme joint stiffness and pain. In a wheelchair, Jody came to the initial evaluation with the nurse practitioner. She reported being "bedridden" for 2 years because of highly unpredictable episodes of weakness in her legs, arms, face, and neck and "crushing" pain in her legs throughout the day. Her symptoms began with rapid onset, at age 17, when she experienced flulike symptoms and was "never the same." She discontinued college in her second year, stopped working as a dog trainer, and stopped driving. Social connections were limited to family. Her mood was extremely low with flat affect. Emotionally, she presented as defeated and despondent. Although she could not identify specific triggers for her symptoms, she stated that stress often worsened them. Jody had previously undergone extensive negative workups by Neurology, Rheumatology, and Interventional Pain. In addition, she had been evaluated twice at specialty hospitals with no conclusive diagnosis. During the initial interview, Jody denied anxiety/depression, but reported a significant disconnection from life goals. She noted that her life had been placed on hold by her symptoms, and she expressed a desire to progress in her life.

Using a whole-person perspective, the treatment team found that Jody had broad needs in understanding/managing her symptoms, increasing activity levels, reconnecting with life goals, establishing connection with others, and improving dietary intake. Jody's self-assessed primary needs were quite similar and included improving the mind-body connection, daily rhythm and balance, physical activity, developing community, and sleep. As such, the treatment plan codeveloped with her nurse practitioner involved the following: participation in mind-body therapy groups that included yoga, individual psychotherapy with a health psychologist, and a re-evaluation of her medication regimen to assess potential side effects that might contribute to symptom presentation.

Course of Treatment

Jody's treatment occurred over a 15-month period and included the synergistic components noted in **Fig. 2**. With a health psychologist, Jody completed a structured

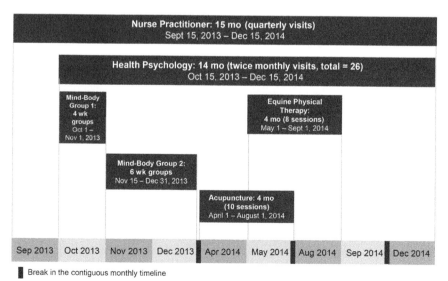

Fig. 2. Timeline for integrative treatment provided in case study.

goals and values assessment, which used principles of behavioral activation.[77,78] In this exercise, patients review specific life areas (eg, family, health, social relationships, hobbies) and identify satisfaction with each life area, past behaviors, desires for change, and specific needs. Jody constructed an activity hierarchy[79] from easiest to hardest to complete and systematically progressed through these activities over the next 10 months.[80] For Jody, key life areas involved improving family relationships/communication, establishing a hobby related to her love for animals, increasing independence, and reconnecting with music. One notable activity she undertook, using her gift with animals, was training her dog to become a service animal. Because she had to get her dog accustomed to novel environments as a part of training, this activity served a dual purpose: Jody began pursuing value-congruent goals and also left the house more often, increasing her independence through driving again.

Synergistic with psychotherapy, Jody participated in 2 mind-body groups that provided training in mind-body practices (specifically, mindfulness, yoga, and visualization), coping strategies for pain, and identity exploration using elements of Acceptance and Commitment Therapy.[81] She established a daily mindfulness practice and noted particular help from focused-awareness meditation (from mindfulness-based stress reduction[45]) and the use of comforting imagery to ward off paniclike symptoms and reduce catastrophic thinking when encountering pain. These strategies were important because catastrophic thought processes are known to lead to avoidance, increased pain intensity, and functional disability.[82]

Seven months into treatment, at quarterly follow-up with her nurse practitioner, Jody demonstrated symptom improvement but continued pain/weakness. She was referred for acupuncture and learned hypnosis in psychotherapy to overcome her fear of needles. Jody reported significant improvement in her pain through acupuncture and sought out hippotherapy (equine physical therapy) in the community halfway through her 10 sessions of acupuncture. At the urging of her integrative team, she also agreed to begin walking each day to prevent further atrophy in her legs and increase muscle strength. She began walking by merely standing, then walking short distances, and gradually moved to 10, 15, and then 30 minutes of walking per day. The physical activity led to increased strength and reduced her reliance on the wheelchair, and subsequently crutches, and then a cane until she walked independently again with the assistance of her service animal.

Thirteen months into treatment, Jody received a formal diagnosis: hypokalemic periodic paralysis. This condition is characterized by "attacks" of weakness resulting from low potassium concentration in the body.[83] She was prescribed acetazolamide to control episodes of weakness. In addition, through researching and understanding the condition further, Jody was able to identify numerous triggers for symptoms, many of which were dietary. She adopted a gluten-free diet with low sodium intake, as recommended by experts,[84] and reported almost immediate energy increase.

Outcomes

By participating in an integrative health treatment program, Jody's functioning significantly improved in multiple lifestyle domains. At the conclusion of her treatment, she no longer used a wheelchair, was walking independently, and driving regularly. Through values-congruent activity engagement, her former desire to work with animals resurfaced. Jody even set a long-term goal of developing a community organization to train service animals for those in need of medical and/or emotional support. Jody felt increasingly confident in her ability to manage symptoms through skills application and awareness/monitoring of triggers, and her symptoms no longer felt "unpredictable."

Follow-Up

Jody was seen for follow-up 4 months after treatment. She was working full time at a local animal shelter, which involved walking dogs throughout the day. Although she acknowledged a period of time where her body had to adapt to her increased pace, she had lost 30 pounds and reported feeling much stronger. She had learned to take regular breaks throughout the day, and she communicated her needs at the outset of her job to ensure that her employer would be flexible with her health needs. Jody reported feeling happy and fulfilled, stating she was working toward developing dog-training classes at her rescue organization.

Summary

Jody followed an integrative treatment program that collectively improved her quality of life and functioning in multiple lifestyle domains. No one aspect of this program was responsible for these changes alone; instead, the combination of services facilitated change. For example, Jody likely would have not pursued acupuncture without the assistance of Health Psychology and coping strategies to manage anxiety related to needles. Furthermore, acupuncture served as the impetus to her beginning to stand/walk, because she was in less pain and more able to use her legs. The coordination of a treatment plan by a nurse practitioner with quarterly follow-up serves as a useful model for how primary care providers can facilitate treatment in multiple lifestyle domains. In addition, the patient's ability to engage in physical activity and change her dietary intake came after she became meaningfully engaged in life again, and as a function of pursuing what she most cared about (ie, walking the animals she loved). Psychotherapy and mind-body groups, augmented by mindfulness training and acupuncture, formed a crucial foundation for her treatment. Jody's motivation for change clearly facilitated her treatment progression, and simultaneously, the cultivation of values-congruent activities iteratively led to greater motivation for subsequent lifestyle changes.

DISCLOSURES

R.Q. Wolever serves as the Chief Science Officer to eMindful, Inc, is on the Executive Committee for the nonprofit International Consortium for Health and Wellness Coaching, holds a contract with Nokia and grants from the US Air Force (FA8650-13-2-6374) and the National Heart, Lung, and Blood Institute (HL123500) for research that entails health coaching and mindfulness, respectively. She is also the coauthor of *The Mindful Diet*. Additional funding relevant to health coaching and mindfulness in the 3 years before the submission of this article includes grants from the National Institute of Deafness and Communication Disorders (DC011643), the Bravewell Philanthropic Collaborative, and the Duke Center for Personalized and Precision Medicine. K.L. Caldwell received funding from National Center for Complementary and Integrative Health (AT006795) for a grant evaluating the effects of Tai Chi in young adults. None (L.C. McKernan and M. Hillinger).

REFERENCES

1. Centers for Disease Control and Prevention (CDC). Chronic disease overview. Available at: http://www.cdc.gov/chronicdisease/overview/. Accessed February 23, 2016.

2. Yach D, Hawkes C, Gould CL, et al. The global burden of chronic diseases: overcoming impediments to prevention and control. JAMA 2004;291(21):2616–22.
3. Berrigan D, Dodd K, Troiano RP, et al. Patterns of health behavior in U.S. adults. Prev Med 2003;36(5):615–23.
4. Umberson D, Crosnoe R, Reczek C. Social relationships and health behavior across the life course. Annu Rev Sociol 2010;36(1):139–57.
5. Simmons LA, Wolever RQ, Bechard EM, et al. Patient engagement as a risk factor in personalized health care: a systematic review of the literature on chronic disease. Genome Med 2014;6(2):16.
6. Whitlock EP, Orleans CT, Pender N, et al. Evaluating primary care behavioral counseling interventions: an evidence-based approach. Am J Prev Med 2002;22(4):267–84.
7. Simpson V, Pedigo L. Nurse and physician involvement in health risk appraisals: an integrative review. West J Nurs Res 2016;1–22.
8. Deci EL, Ryan RM. Facilitating optimal motivation and psychological well-being across life's domains. Canadian Psychology/Psychologie canadienne 2008;49(1):14–23.
9. Nagykaldi ZJ, Voncken-Brewster V, Aspy CB, et al. Novel computerized health risk appraisal may improve longitudinal health and wellness in primary care: a pilot study. Appl Clin Inform 2013;4(1):75–87.
10. Zimmerman GL, Olsen CG, Bosworth MF. A 'stages of change' approach to helping patients change behavior. Am Fam Physician 2000;61(5):1409–16.
11. Kreuter MW, Chheda SG, Bull FC. How does physician advice influence patient behavior? Evidence for a priming effect. Arch Fam Med 2000;9(5):426–33.
12. Petrella RJ, Lattanzio CN. Does counseling help patients get active? Systematic review of the literature. Can Fam Physician 2002;48:72–80.
13. Deci EL, Ryan RM. Self-determination theory: a macrotheory of human motivation, development, and health. Canadian Psychology/Psychologie Canadienne 2008;49(3):182.
14. Sheldon KM. 3: The self-concordance model of healthy goal striving: when personal goals correctly represent the person. New York: Handbook Self Determination Res; 2004. p. 65.
15. Rakel D, Weil A. Philosophy of integrative medicine. In: Rakel D, editor. Integrative medicine. 3rd edition. Philadelphia: Elsevier, Inc.; 2012. p. 2–11.
16. Wolever RQ, Caldwell KL, Wakefield JP, et al. Integrative health coaching: an organizational case study. Explore (NY) 2011;7(1):30–6.
17. Wolever RQ, Simmons LA, Sforzo GA, et al. A systematic review of the literature on health and wellness coaching: defining a key behavioral intervention in healthcare. Glob Adv Health Med 2013;2(4):34–58.
18. Wolever RQ, Abrams DI, Kligler B, et al. Patients seek integrative medicine for preventive approach to optimize health. Explore (NY) 2012;8(6):348–52.
19. NCCIH. The science of mind-body therapies. Available at: https://nccih.nih.gov/video/series/mindbody. Accessed February 27, 2017.
20. Smith K, Firth K, Smeeding S, et al. Guidelines for creating, implementing, and evaluating mind–body programs in a military healthcare setting. Explore (NY) 2016;12(1):18–33.
21. Rakel D. Integrative medicine. 3rd edition. Philadelphia: Elsevier Saunders; 2012.
22. Jordan M, Wolever RQ, Lawson KL, et al. National training and education standards for health and wellness coaching: the path to national certification. Glob Adv Health Med 2015;4(3):46–56.

23. Pashko S. Implications of the differences between our perceptual and conceptual views. Psychol Neurosci 2016;9(2):267–81.
24. Ammentorp J, Uhrenfeldt L, Angel F, et al. Can life coaching improve outcomes? A systematic review of intervention studies. BMC Health Serv Res 2013;13:428.
25. Hill B, Richardson B, Skouteris H. Do we know how to design effective health coaching interventions: a systematic review of the state of the literature. Am J Health Promot 2015;29(5):e158–68.
26. Kivelä K, Elo S, Kyngäs H, et al. The effects of health coaching on adult patients with chronic diseases: a systematic review. Patient Educ Couns 2014;97(2): 147–57.
27. Lindner H, Menzies D, Kelly J, et al. Coaching for behaviour change in chronic disease: a review of the literature and the implications for coaching as a self-management intervention. Aust J Prim Health 2003;9(2/3):177–85.
28. Olsen JM, Nesbitt BJ. Health coaching to improve healthy lifestyle behaviors: an integrative review. Am J Health Promot 2010;25(1):e1–12.
29. Wolever RQ, Jordan M, Lawson K, et al. Advancing a new evidence-based professional in health care: job task analysis for health and wellness coaches. BMC Health Serv Res 2016;16(1):1.
30. American Psychological Association. Recognition of psychotherapy effectiveness. http://www.apa.org/about/policy/resolution-psychotherapy.aspx. Accessed February 27, 2017.
31. Mitchell MD, Gehrman P, Perlis M, et al. Comparative effectiveness of cognitive behavioral therapy for insomnia: a systematic review. BMC Fam Pract 2012; 13(1):1–11.
32. BeHealth Solutions L, University of Virginia, Behavioral Health & Technology. Shut-i. Available at: http://www.myshuti.com/. Accessed February 27, 2017.
33. Natural Medicines Data Base (2017). Available at: https://naturalmedicines. therapeuticresearch.com/databases/food,-herbs-supplements/professional.aspx? productid=940#dosing. Accessed February 27, 2017.
34. Michie S, Abraham C, Whittington C, et al. Effective techniques in healthy eating and physical activity interventions: a meta-regression. Health Psychol 2009;28(6): 690–701.
35. Higgins JP. Smartphone applications for patients' health and fitness. Am J Med 2016;129(1):11–9.
36. Aguilar-Martinez A, Sole-Sedeno JM, Mancebo-Moreno G, et al. Use of mobile phones as a tool for weight loss: a systematic review. J Telemed Telecare 2014;20(6):339–49.
37. Free C, Phillips G, Galli L, et al. The effectiveness of mobile-health technology-based health behaviour change or disease management interventions for health care consumers: a systematic review. PLoS Med 2013;10(1):e1–45.
38. Wickramsekera I. Hypnotherapy. In: Jonas WB, Levin JS, editors. Essentials of complementary and alternative medicine. Philadelphia: Lippincott Williams and Wilkins; 1999. p. 426–43.
39. Gruzelier JH. A review of the impact of hypnosis, relaxation, guided imagery and individual differences on aspects of immunity and health. Stress 2002;5(2):147–63.
40. Lovejoy JC. Integrative approaches to obesity treatment. Integr Med 2013;12(2): 30–6.
41. Tahiri M, Mottillo S, Joseph L, et al. Alternative smoking cessation aids: a meta-analysis of randomized controlled trials. Am J Med 2012;125(6):576–84.
42. Barnes J, Dong CY, McRobbie H, et al. Hypnotherapy for smoking cessation. Cochrane Database Syst Rev 2010;(10):CD001008.

43. Hasan FM, Zagarins SE, Pischke KM, et al. Hypnotherapy is more effective than nicotine replacement therapy for smoking cessation: results of a randomized controlled trial. Complement Ther Med 2014;22:1–8.

44. Patterson DR. Clinical hypnosis for pain control. Washington, DC: American Psychological Association; 2010.

45. Kabat-Zinn J. Full catastrophe living: using the wisdom of your body and mind to face stress, pain, and illness. New York: Delacorte Press; 1990.

46. Katterman SN, Kleinman BM, Hood MM, et al. Mindfulness meditation as an intervention for binge eating, emotional eating, and weight loss: a systematic review. Eat Behav 2014;15(2):197–204.

47. Carmody J, Baer RA. Relationships between mindfulness practice and levels of mindfulness, medical and psychological symptoms and well-being in a mindfulness-based stress reduction program. J Behav Med 2008;31(1):23–33.

48. Goyal M, Singh S, Sibinga EM, et al. Meditation programs for psychological stress and well-being: a systematic review and meta-analysis. JAMA Intern Med 2014;174(3):357–68.

49. Bowen S, Witkiewitz K, Dillworth TM, et al. Mindfulness meditation and substance use in an incarcerated population. Psychol Addict Behav 2006;20(3):343–7.

50. Bowen S, Witkiewitz K, Clifasefi SL, et al. Relative efficacy of mindfulness-based relapse prevention, standard relapse prevention, and treatment as usual for substance use disorders: a randomized clinical trial. JAMA Psychiatry 2014;71(5): 547–56.

51. Baime MJ. Meditation and mindfulness. In: Jonas WB, Levin JS, editors. Essentials of complementary and alternative medicine. Philadelphia: Lippincott Williams & Wilkins; 1999. p. 522–36.

52. Reiner M, Niermann C, Jekauc D, et al. Long-term health benefits of physical activity: a systematic review of longitudinal studies. BMC Public Health 2013;13(1): 1–9.

53. Jahnke R, Larkey L, Rogers C, et al. A comprehensive review of health benefits of qigong and tai chi. Am J Health Promot 2010;24(6):e1–25.

54. Wang C, Bannuru R, Ramel J, et al. Tai chi on psychological well-being: systematic review and meta-analysis. BMC Complement Altern Med 2010;10(1):1–16.

55. Wang F, Eun-Kyoung Lee O, Feng F, et al. The effect of meditative movement on sleep quality: a systematic review. Sleep Med Rev 2016;30:43–52.

56. Posadzki P, Choi J, Lee MS, et al. Yoga for addictions: a systematic review of randomised clinical trials. Focus Altern Complement Therapies 2014;19(1):1–8.

57. Carim-Todd L, Mitchell SH, Oken BS. Mind-body practices: an alternative, drug-free treatment for smoking cessation? A systematic review of the literature. Drug Alcohol Depend 2013;132(3):399–410.

58. Wayne PM, Kaptchuk TJ. Challenges inherent to t'ai chi research: part II—defining the intervention and optimal study design. J Altern Complement Med 2008;14(2):191–7.

59. Cramer H, Ward L, Saper R, et al. The safety of yoga: a systematic review and meta-analysis of randomized controlled trials. Am J Epidemiol 2015;182(4): 281–93.

60. Knoops KT, de Groot LC, Kromhout D, et al. Mediterranean diet, lifestyle factors, and 10-year mortality in elderly European men and women: the HALE project. JAMA 2004;292(12):1433–9.

61. Chainani-Wu N, Weidner G, Purnell DM, et al. Changes in emerging cardiac biomarkers after an intensive lifestyle intervention. Am J Cardiol 2011;108(4): 498–507.

62. Knowler WC, Barrett-Connor E, Fowler SE, et al. Reduction in the incidence of type 2 diabetes with lifestyle intervention or metformin. N Engl J Med 2002; 346(6):393–403.
63. Loef M, Walach H. Fruit, vegetables and prevention of cognitive decline or dementia: a systematic review of cohort studies. J Nutr Health Aging 2012;16(7): 626–30.
64. Morris MC, Tangney CC, Wang Y, et al. MIND diet slows cognitive decline with aging. Alzheimers Dement 2015;11(9):1015–22.
65. Katz D, Meller S. Can we say what diet is best for health? Annu Rev Public Health 2014;35:83–103.
66. Willett WC, Stampfer MJ. Current evidence on healthy eating. Annu Rev Public Health 2013;34:77–95.
67. Tapsell LC, Neale EP, Satija A, et al. Foods, nutrients, and dietary patterns: interconnections and implications for dietary guidelines. Adv Nutr 2016;7(3):445–54.
68. Campbell TC, Campbell TM. The China study. Dallas (TX): Benbella Books; 2005.
69. Wolever RQ, Reardon B, Hannan T. The mindful diet. New York: Scribner; 2015.
70. Wansink B, Hanks AS, Kaipainen K. Slim by design: kitchen counter correlates of obesity. Health Educ Behav 2016;43(5):552–8.
71. Pollan M. In defense of food: an eater's manifesto. New York: Penguin; 2008.
72. Hays NP, Roberts SB. Aspects of eating behaviors "disinhibition" and "restraint" are related to weight gain and BMI in women. Obesity 2008;16(1):52–8.
73. Fiore M, Jaen C, Baker T. Treating tobacco use and dependence: 2008 update. Clinical practice guideline. Rockville (MD): U.S. Department of Health and Human Services, Public Health Service; 2008.
74. Patnode CD, Henderson JT, Thompson JH, et al. Behavioral counseling and pharmacotherapy interventions for tobacco cessation in adults, including pregnant women: a review for the U.S. preventive services task force. Rockville (MD): Agency for Healthcare Research and Quality; 2015.
75. Graham AL, Carpenter KM, Cha S, et al. Systematic review and meta-analysis of internet interventions for smoking cessation among adults. Subst Abuse Rehabil 2016;7:55–69.
76. Donker T, Petrie K, Proudfoot J, et al. Smartphones for smarter delivery of mental health programs: a systematic review. J Med Internet Res 2013;15(11):e247.
77. Jacobson NS, Martell CR, Dimidjian S. Behavioral activation treatment for depression: returning to contextual roots. Clin Psychol Sci Pract 2001;8(3):255–70.
78. Kanter JW, Manos RC, Bowe WM, et al. What is behavioral activation? A review of the empirical literature. Clin Psychol Rev 2010;30(6):608–20.
79. Lejuez CW, Hopko DR, Hopko SD. A brief behavioral activation treatment for depression. Treatment manual. Behav Modif 2001;25(2):255–86.
80. Bovend'Eerdt TJ, Botell RE, Wade DT. Writing SMART rehabilitation goals and achieving goal attainment scaling: a practical guide. Clin Rehabil 2009;23(4): 352–61.
81. Hayes SC, Luoma JB, Bond FW, et al. Acceptance and commitment therapy: model, processes and outcomes. Behav Res Ther 2006;44(1):1–25.
82. Leeuw M, Goossens ME, Linton SJ, et al. The fear-avoidance model of musculoskeletal pain: current state of scientific evidence. J Behav Med 2007;30(1):77–94.
83. Venance SL, Cannon SC, Fialho D, et al. The primary periodic paralyses: diagnosis, pathogenesis and treatment. Brain 2006;129(Pt 1):8–17.
84. Levitt JO. Practical aspects in the management of hypokalemic periodic paralysis. J Transl Med 2008;6(1):1.

Integrative Medicine for the Treatment of Persistent Pain

Marni G. Hillinger, MD[a],*, Ruth Q. Wolever, PhD[b,c],
Lindsey C. McKernan, PhD[a,b], Roy Elam, MD[a]

KEYWORDS

- Chronic pain • Persistent pain • Integrative health • Acupuncture • Yoga • Massage
- Mindfulness meditation

KEY POINTS

- Integrative health modalities can provide useful tools in the management of persistent pain in the primary care setting.
- A relationship-centered approach is recommended, whereby the practitioner and patient devise a plan together. It is of utmost importance to acknowledge and treat both the physiologic and psychosocial components of chronic pain.
- Managing expectations and collaborative goal setting around improvements in function and quality of life at each visit are important in promoting self-efficacy.
- The authors recommend focusing on no more than 2 to 3 modalities at a given time because each modality can take time and sometimes a financial commitment on the part of the patient.
- Integrative health modalities can be safely used and may provide patients with hope and empowerment. It is highly recommended that the patient work alongside trained professionals for a given modality and/or an interprofessional team.

Disclosures: None (M.G. Hillinger, L.C. McKernan and R. Elam); R.Q. Wolever serves as the Chief Science Officer to eMindful, Inc, serves on the Executive Committee for the nonprofit National Consortium for Credentialing Health and Wellness Coaches, holds a contract with Nokia, and has grants from the US Air Force and the National Heart, Lung, and Blood Institute for research that entails health coaching and mindfulness, respectively. She is also the coauthor of *The Mindful Diet*. Additional funding relevant to health coaching and mindfulness in the 3 years before the submission of this article includes grants from the National Institute of Deafness and Communication Disorders, the Bravewell Philanthropic Collaborative, and the Duke Center for Personalized and Precision Medicine.

[a] Department of Physical Medicine and Rehabilitation, Osher Center for Integrative Medicine at Vanderbilt, Vanderbilt University Medical Center, 3401 West End Avenue, Suite 380, Nashville, TN 37203, USA; [b] Department of Psychiatry & Behavioral Sciences, Vanderbilt University Medical Center, 3401 West End Avenue, Suite 380, Nashville, TN 37203, USA; [c] Department of Physical Medicine and Rehabilitation, Osher Center for Integrative Medicine at Vanderbilt, Vanderbilt University Medical Center, Vanderbilt University School of Nursing, 3401 West End Avenue, Suite 380, Nashville, TN 37203, USA
* Corresponding author:
E-mail address: marni.hillinger@vanderbilt.edu

INTRODUCTION

Persistent pain is among the most common reasons for seeking medical care and the symptomatology is often complex, involving physical, social, psychological, and spiritual manifestations. Integrative strategies can provide a holistic approach to symptom management while also empowering patients. This method often involves synergizing conventional and integrative modalities. An individualized, relationship-centered approach, which meets the patient where they are, can be helpful in determining which modalities may be used synergistically. Concomitant with decreasing pain intensity, treatment goals should include a patient's personal functional goals to optimize quality of life. Setting expectations for treatment early on and using health coaching strategies may additionally benefit formulation of an optimal treatment plan.

Typically, an integrative health intake for chronic pain involves a comprehensive discussion of all relevant topics in the patient's life, using a holistic model such as the Wheel of Health (**Fig. 1**). This discussion, along with collaborative goal setting and treatment planning, encourages patients to be active participants in their care. Engaging patients in active self-care is linked to improvements in outcomes, including increased self-efficacy, decreased health care costs, and higher patient satisfaction.[1,2] Multimodal treatment plans are typically devised collaboratively at the end of the visit and follow-up arranged to assess progress.

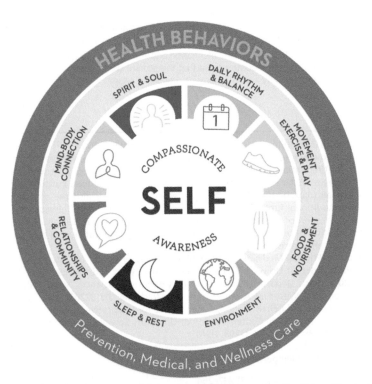

Fig. 1. Wheel of Health. (*Courtesy of* Osher Center for Integrative Medicine, Vanderbilt University Medical Center, Nashville, TN, 2015; with permission.)

MOVEMENT AND EXERCISE

In devising an integrative approach to pain management, practitioners may use a variety of movement practices, including physical therapy, yoga, and tai chi.

Physical Therapy

Physical therapy interventions are commonly used in patients suffering from common chronic pain conditions such as neck pain and pelvic floor pain. Active exercise physiotherapy interventions for neck pain, including strengthening, stretching, and aerobic exercises, improve outcomes as well as strength, function, quality of life, and pain control.[3] A supervised program of this nature may be of more benefit than an unsupervised home exercise program.[4] For chronic pelvic pain, pelvic floor physical therapy with trigger-point release is quite beneficial. In a study of 374 subjects enrolled in a 6-day clinic followed by a 6-month program for pelvic floor therapy program, pelvic floor therapy with trigger point release demonstrated a 36.9% reduction in medication use ($P<.001$) and reduction in overall symptoms.[5]

In addition to traditional 1-on-1 physical therapy, chronic pain patients benefit from functional restoration programs. A randomized controlled trial (RCT) of 132 adults with chronic low back pain compared outcomes following 5-week programs of active individual physical therapy to those from a functional restoration program.[6] Although the investigators did not find significant differences in pain scores, there were significant improvements in specific physical measures and endurance in the functional restoration group.

Yoga

Yoga (referring to asana practice) is an integrative modality that can help improve flexibility, balance, and strength, while simultaneously promoting self-awareness and the relaxation response.[7,8] Although many styles of yoga asana exist in the United States, therapeutically oriented yoga, such as viniyoga, in the authors' experience may be most appropriate in the chronic pain population.

There is growing interest in examining the effectiveness of yoga for low back pain because low back pain remains one of the most common reasons in the United States for seeking medical care.[9] Recent systematic reviews on yoga interventions for low back pain demonstrated that they can be safely implemented and may reduce both pain and disability.[7,8] In fact, there is strong evidence for short-term and moderate evidence for long-term effectiveness of yoga for chronic low back pain.[8] Moreover, yoga may be a cost-effective intervention for chronic or recurrent low back pain.[10] Although ongoing trials continue to investigate differences between yoga, physical therapy, and education for those with chronic low back pain, the optimal dosage and type of yoga necessary to produce meaningful clinical outcomes is still unclear.[11]

Although the evidence is still limited, a recent systematic review pooling 3 RCTs on yoga for chronic neck pain found that yoga may be beneficial.[12] Compared with controls, the review noted greater improvement in pain intensity and functional disability in the yoga groups.[12] Although greater rigor is needed in these trials, previous reviews have also noted improvements in pain intensity, disability, and health-related quality of life related to yoga for neck pain.[13]

In addition to helping those with low back pain and neck pain, yoga may result in clinically relevant improvements for other types of patients. A diverse range of musculoskeletal disorders, including osteoarthritis, rheumatoid arthritis, and fibromyalgia, show benefits in pain and functional outcomes with the use of yoga.[14,15] Importantly, yoga may also be effective across diverse and lower socioeconomic populations.[16]

Overall, a trial of gentle yoga, such as viniyoga, with a practitioner trained in yoga therapy is considered safe and may be beneficial for those with chronic back pain and those with several other musculoskeletal and spine disorders.

Patients experiencing chronic pain understandably demonstrate fear avoidance in regard to movement and this is observed with yoga as well.[17] Fear avoidance can often be modulated by managing expectations of pain up front. Qualitative research shows that, over the course of treatment, providers can positively shift patients toward greater acceptance of chronic pain and the need to move for greater self-care to prevent or mitigate flare-ups.[18]

Tai Chi

Tai chi, a gentle, ancient martial and healing art, involves "flowing circular movement of the upper limbs, constant weight shifting of lower limbs, meditation, breathing, moving of qi (the internal energy in Chinese belief), and various techniques to train mind-body control."[19] A review of tai chi for chronic pain in the treatment of osteoarthritis, fibromyalgia, rheumatoid arthritis, low back pain, and headache demonstrated improvements in measures of psychological well-being, including anxiety and depression scores, with no concern for patient safety.[19] In patients with knee osteoarthritis, there is particularly strong evidence for tai chi in not only improving psychological well-being but also in modulating pain scores and function.[19] Similarly, a rigorous RCT of tai chi in those with chronic low back pain demonstrated improvements in function and pain.[20] Notably, tai chi may be particularly useful for those with fibromyalgia, improving pain scores, functional outcomes, sleep, and self-efficacy.[21,22] The authors recommend a trial of tai chi with a trained practitioner, especially for the fibromyalgia population.

Massage Therapy

Heterogeneity in massage therapy styles and dosage has limited the ability to draw sound conclusions from research on the impact of massage therapy in patients with multiple chronic pain conditions. For example, a Cochrane review published in 2015 examined 25 different studies of the efficacy of massage therapy for low back pain patients.[23] Although the evidence was rated low to very low because of the elevated risk of bias, patients with acute, subacute, and chronic lower back pain receiving massage therapy demonstrated improvements in the short term. Small, nonrandomized trials have corroborated this when comparing physical therapy and massage therapy for nonspecific low back pain; both modalities improved function and pain scores.[24] Similarly, short-term improvements have been demonstrated in fibromyalgia.[25]

In an effort to gain insight into an optimal dose of massage therapy, RCTs have begun to systematically evaluate dose. For example, an RCT of individuals with chronic neck pain randomized subjects into a waitlist control or 1 of 5 dose levels for a 4-week course of massage (30 minutes 2 or 3 times per week, or 60 minutes once, 2 or 3 times per week). In comparison to controls, 60-minute massage treatments 2 to 3 times per week increased function and decreased pain.[26] Similarly, a 2-phase randomized trial on the same population assigned subjects to 4 weeks of massage at the same 5-dose levels, then secondarily randomized participants for a booster phase. During the booster phase, subjects received either 60 minutes of massage once per week or no further massage.[27] Subgroup analyses examining outcomes by initial and booster treatments revealed that the booster dose was only effective in subjects with neck pain who were initially randomized to a 60-minute massage group.[27] The take-home message for clinicians is that 60 minutes of massage per week seems to be the best recommendation, and that 10 weeks is more helpful than 4 weeks of such.

Although the optimal dose of massage therapy remains unclear, patients do seem to benefit, at least in the short term. Furthermore, they tend to seek it out. Because chronic pain patients seeking integrative medicine use massage therapy second only to acupuncture,[28] it is useful that no major adverse reactions are associated with massage therapy.[23] The authors often recommend this approach if there is a high suspicion of myofascial-type pain syndromes.

ACUPUNCTURE

A part of traditional Chinese Medicine, acupuncture is thought to be more than 2000 years old.[29] It involves placing thin needles at specific locations along energy pathways, known as meridians (**Fig. 2**), to influence qi, which is considered to be life-force energy. Disease has been attributed to improper energy flow. Thus, achieving proper energy flow is thought to positively affect health.[29] Over the past 50 years, there has been much interest in understanding the potential physiologic mechanisms of acupuncture among the western medical research community. For example, acupuncture has been shown to likely involve activation of the sensory system with subsequent regulation of neurotransmitters, neurohormones, and various other neuromodulators.[30] Changes on neuroimaging have been demonstrated with both electroacupuncture and manual acupuncture in comparison with sham

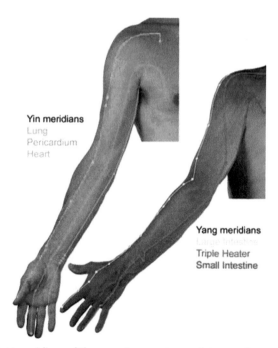

Yin meridians
Lung
Pericardium
Heart

Yang meridians
Large Intestine
Triple Heater
Small Intestine

Fig. 2. Acupuncture meridians of the arm. Acupuncture points were located by palpation in a living subject, according to anatomic guidelines provided in a major reference acupuncture textbook (Cheng, 1987).[31] Connective tissue planes associated with Yin meridians are more inward and deep, compared with the generally outward and superficial planes associated with Yang meridians. (*From* Langevin HM, Yandow JA. Relationship of acupuncture points and meridians to connective tissue planes. Anat Rec 2002;269(6):257–65; with permission.)

acunpuncture.[32] In addition, acupuncture may be a cost-effective treatment with the cost per quality-adjusted life year indicating possible benefit.[33]

A systematic review of 29 RCTs of acupuncture for chronic pain found that acupuncture was superior to both sham and no-acupuncture control groups for those with neck and low back pain, osteoarthritis, headache, and shoulder pain.[34] The effect remained after excluding outlying sets of RCTs with potential bias. Additionally, results withstood various sensitivity analyses. Hence, acupuncture is recommended for the treatment of chronic pain. Compared with sham acupuncture, true acupuncture demonstrates modest but significant results.

For chronic low back pain, acupuncture has particular promise.[35–37] Compared with sham acupuncture, several RCTs have shown that manual acupuncture improves pain scores, measures of disability, and depression.[35–37] Acupuncture in general is well-accepted, well-tolerated, and without significant adverse events.[36] In addition, it seems that acupuncture can be combined with traditional rehabilitation in low back pain patients to enhance improvements in function.[36]

For osteoarthritis, there is more equivocal evidence regarding the efficacy of acupuncture. Although a recent RCT of subjects older than 50 years old with chronic knee osteoarthritis failed to show significant benefit in primary outcomes,[38] the study was criticized for its methodology. A meta-analysis and review on acupuncture in osteoarthritis published in the same year concluded that "the use of acupuncture is associated with significant reductions in pain intensity, improvement in functional mobility and quality of life."[39]

In general, acupuncture is the most used approach for patients with chronic pain seeking care at integrative medicine clinics.[28] Based on the current available evidence, acupuncture is typically well-tolerated, safe, and can be a useful tool in the practitioner's armamentarium.

MIND-BODY STRATEGIES

Mind-body strategies have been shown to promote both structural and functional brain changes.[40] Thus, a growing body of evidence suggests they may help improve outcomes for the chronic-pain patient population, especially those with signs and symptoms of central sensitization.[40] These therapies include mindfulness meditation, hypnosis, biofeedback, and cognitive behavioral therapy (CBT) strategies. Central sensitization may play a role in many different pain syndromes, such as fibromyalgia, osteoarthritis, headache, and other neuropathic pain syndromes.[41]

Mindfulness Meditation

Mindfulness meditation has been commonly studied in the treatment of chronic pain. Mindfulness, historically a Buddhist practice, helps to cultivate moment-to-moment awareness with the hopes of decreasing suffering and promoting well-being. Although mindfulness practices differ, most include 3 tenets: (1) observing the present moment by attending to the objective qualities, (2) maintaining one's attention to a single focus (breath, sound, feeling) without judgment, and (3) remaining open to what arises in that moment.[42] As thoughts and emotions enter one's mind, they are observed, without judgment. Mindfulness-Based Stress Reduction (MBSR), developed by Dr. Jon Kabat-Zinn[43] is an 8-week intensive course using mindfulness strategies to help decrease stress; it has been taught since 1979. Chronic pain was one of the early research targets for this modality. Dr. Kabat-Zinn[43] conducted a study of 51 chronic pain subjects in 1982 to determine the efficacy of MBSR. He found that the intervention group had significant decreases in the perception of pain, with at least half of them reporting pain reductions of at least 50%. This finding was corroborated in subsequent studies.[42,44]

Meta-analytic and systematic reviews demonstrate that mindfulness-based treatments consistently decrease anxiety and depression, and improve well-being.[44–46] A 2013 review found that 10 of 16 studies (8 controlled, 8 uncontrolled) on mindfulness-based interventions (MBIs) generally showed effectiveness for reduced pain intensity.[42] In addition, findings were strongest in the controlled trials and more consistently positive in the clinical pain samples.[42] Several mechanisms have been proposed to explain why mindfulness strategies may mitigate pain intensity (**Fig. 3**).

Recently, a landmark RCT compared the efficacy of MBSR, CBT, and usual care for 342 subjects with chronic low back pain.[47] At 26 weeks, there were clinically meaningful improvements in both function and pain scores in both the CBT and MBSR groups in comparison with those who received usual care. At 52 weeks, both primary outcome measures were sustained in the MBSR group. This trial provides compelling evidence that programs like MBSR may be cost-effective, viable, long-term options to care for those suffering with chronic low back pain. The authors highly recommend mindfulness-based therapies for patients with persistent pain.

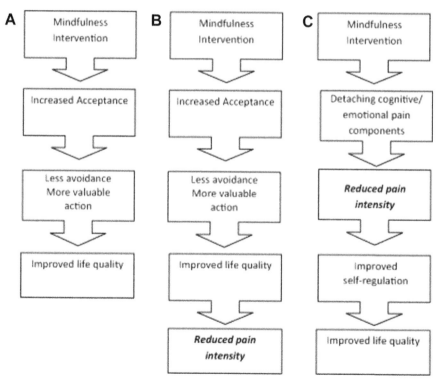

Fig. 3. Suggested mechanisms of change involved in MBIs. (*A*) Traditional view: MBIs improve life quality by increasing acceptance without necessarily change pain perception. (*B*) Suggested mechanism: MBIs increase acceptance, which in turn led to behavioral change that results in improved quality of life and reduced pain. (*C*) MBIs influence pain perception directly, which then mediate change in self-regulation and improved quality of life. (*From* Reiner K, Tibi L, Lipsitz JD. Do mindfulness-based interventions reduce pain intensity? A critical review of the literature. Pain Med 2013;14(2):239; with permission.)

Hypnosis

Hypnosis shows promise as a modality useful in the treatment of chronic pain and further study in this area is needed. This technique uses increased concentration and a heightened sense of awareness directed to suggestions related to feelings, behavior, and the physiologic state.[48] Despite heterogeneity among hypnotherapy protocols and a need for improved patient follow-up, a review of 13 studies examining the effectiveness of hypnosis to treat chronic pain demonstrated consistent improvements in pain scores.[49] Similarly, a recent RCT of veterans with low back pain that compared biofeedback to 3 hypnosis groups also demonstrated significantly improved pain scores among the hypnosis groups.[50] The study further concluded that a short course of self-hypnosis might be as effective as a longer treatment course. Moreover, active techniques, such as self-hypnosis, may have further benefit because allow for a greater sense of control and self-reliance.[49]

Biofeedback

Biofeedback makes use of real-time physiologic, typically auditory or visual, cues to help a patient self-monitor the response to pain.[51] Some of the most common physiologic measures are heart rate variability or skin temperature. Although a prior review reported low-quality evidence for biofeedback for low back pain subjects in the short term,[52] a recent pilot study of 20 adults with low back pain demonstrated decreased fear avoidance behavior and decreased pain intensity after using a specific titrated biofeedback protocol.[51] Improved outcomes were demonstrated at follow-up and at 3 months. Neurofeedback, which is a type of biofeedback that uses electroencephalography, also shows promise for the chronic pain population. One study performed neurofeedback while simultaneously collecting functional MRI (fMRI) data and demonstrated downregulation of blood oxygen level–dependent fMRI signals in most subjects.[53] This suggests that neurofeedback may serve as an important modality in self-regulation of pain. Frank and colleagues[54] provided an overview of the proposed efficacy of biofeedback for various conditions and concluded level 4 evidence (efficacious) for both chronic pain and headache.

Cognitive Behavioral Therapy

Several recent review studies concluded that CBT is a useful adjunct in the treatment of chronic pain.[55,56] Although CBT has demonstrated only small effects in terms of pain improvement and disability, it is effective for improving mood and decreasing catastrophising.[55] CBT may also be beneficial in regard to minimizing kinesiophobia in comparison with other modalities.[57] Knoerl and colleagues[56] concluded several key findings from their review of this modality, including the concept that the proper dose of CBT is not known, that online CBT may be comparable to traditional approaches, and that future studies should include an evaluation of the impact of CBT on anxiety, quality of life, sleep, treatment satisfaction, global impression of change, and fatigue. Internet-delivered CBT programs have also demonstrated efficacy and may help to improve access to these services.[58–60] In the authors' experience, CBT is often a key component in the integrative care plan for the chronic pain population.

BIOFIELD THERAPIES OR ENERGY HEALING

Biofield therapies are a broad term encompassing modalities grounded in the concept that subtle energy may influence the mind and body. Some of the most commonly used therapies include Reiki, therapeutic touch, and healing touch.

Varying conclusions have been drawn regarding the efficacy of these healing modalities in the treatment of pain. One systematic review examined the evidence for biofield therapies in various patient populations,[61] including 13 studies related to different pain syndromes. The investigators summarized that biofield studies examining impact for pain populations demonstrated level 1 evidence (strong) for these therapies to decrease measures of pain intensity. In contrast, they found only level 4 evidence (equivocal) for these therapies affecting more comprehensive assessments of pain (affective measures). Although there have been variations in length of treatment across studies, there is evidence for decreased use of pain medications when using these strategies.[62] Interestingly, a Cochrane review performed in 2008 demonstrated that more advanced practitioners yielded greater improvements in pain that could not be attributed to placebo effect alone.[63]

There is ongoing interest in further research investigating the use of these modalities for musculoskeletal concerns. A pilot study examining the impact of healing touch on pain and mobility in those with osteoarthritis demonstrated significant improvements in both pain intensity and life interference,[64] whereas another study showed improvements in shoulder range of motion.[65] Biofield modalities may hold promise as adjunctive treatments for pain. Further research is needed to elucidate the mechanisms and outcomes of these modalities in management of chronic pain.

THE ROLE OF SLEEP

Although more mechanistic research is needed, a reciprocal relationship does exist between chronic pain and sleep; worsening or improving one seems to have a similar impact on the other.[66,67] Integrative medicine treatment of sleep disorders in chronic pain patients include CBT for insomnia (CBT-I), mindfulness meditation, and various pharmacologic and supplemental therapies.

CBT-I is a safe and effective treatment of chronic insomnia that does not involve use of medication. For providers trying to minimize the use of narcotics or anxiolytics, CBT-I is particularly helpful. When compared with medications, CBT-I is as effective, and its effects may be more durable than medications.[68] It improves sleep habits and schedules, and focuses on correcting inaccurate perceptions and beliefs regarding sleep and insomnia that tend to worsen sleep difficulties.[69] Compared with control interventions, strong RCTs demonstrate that CBT-I improves insomnia secondary to chronic pain in pain disorders other than fibromyalgia.[66,67] Similarly, CBT for pain improves sleep disorders.[67] Although more severe cases may require weekly or biweekly visits with a psychologist trained in CBT-I, there is a highly-researched online version (www.myshuti.com/) with apps that can be easily recommended to patients.[70]

Integrative medicine practitioners also emphasize the role of sleep health versus symptom suppression and, as such, focus on the impact of lifestyle factors on sleep. Primary care providers should underline the importance of a daily relaxation routine and can train patients in simple relaxation techniques such as the 4-7-8 breath.[71] Sleep hygiene routines may be reviewed, with emphasis on the need for daily physical activity, and limitations in alcohol and caffeine consumption.

Mind-body approaches can also be helpful for improving sleep. A systematic review and meta-analysis of RCTs for MBIs targeting chronic pain found an effect size of 1.32 (95% CI -1.19–3.82) for sleep quality.[72] A recent systematic review found that mind-body therapies, including mindfulness meditation and hypnosis or imagery, improve both sleep and pain in fibromyalgia, although the number of studies measuring sleep was limited.[73] Although more rigorous trials are needed, a recent, fairly large (n = 269), longitudinal cohort study found preliminary evidence that both a traditional multidisciplinary pain management program and an education and mindfulness-based cognitive therapy approach improved pain intensity and health-related quality of life among women with chronic pain.[74] At 4 weeks, the traditional program showed greater improvement in pain intensity, whereas the mindfulness condition showed greater improvement in sleep quality.[74] Given improvement in both sleep and pain, with slight differences in which symptom set improved more depending on the treatment, primary care practitioners may do well to make recommendations based on the relative distress levels expressed by patients for each symptom set.

DIETARY MANAGEMENT STRATEGIES

The role of an anti-inflammatory diet, most commonly a Mediterranean diet, in modulating pain has been investigated, most frequently in the arthritis population.[75] Models of the Mediterranean diet have demonstrated anti-inflammatory activity via the arachidonic acid cascade, modulating proinflammatory genes and various immune cells.[75,76] A Mediterranean diet is high in vegetables, fruits, fish, olive oil and other monounsaturated oils. A Cochrane review performed in 2009 found that dietary effects on rheumatoid arthritis were uncertain given the limited number of studies available and risks of bias.[77] Although further studies are needed to determine the efficacy of anti-inflammatory diets in the treatment of chronic pain, the authors recommend a trial of a whole-foods, plant-based diet, such as a Mediterranean diet, given the implications for other chronic conditions such as cardiovascular disease and diabetes prevention. Please see Ruth Q. Wolever and colleagues article, "Integrative Medicine Strategies for Changing Health Behaviors: Support for Primary Care," in this issue.

HERBS AND SUPPLEMENTS

Although an in depth review of all vitamins, minerals, and botanic medicines is beyond the scope of this article, the authors focus on some of the most commonly used agents which are affordable and for which significant evidence exists to promote their use.

Several culinary herbs have been examined to determine their potential anti-inflammatory properties and, in turn, help manage pain. Two of the most common are *Curcuma longa* (turmeric) and *Zingiber officinale* (ginger). In recent years, there has been growing interest in turmeric in the treatment of pain associated with osteoarthritis, with a recent review demonstrating promising results.[78] This is likely related to laboratory evidence showing that curcumin functions as a selective cyclooxygenase-2 (COX-2) inhibitor.[79] A head-to-head clinical trial of curcumin supplementation in comparison with ibuprofen in the treatment of knee osteoarthritis demonstrated a similar treatment effect of each medication, with less gastrointestinal adverse events associated with curcumin.[80] Meriva, a lecithin delivery form of curcumin, has been studied in combination with glucosamine versus chondroitin and glucosamine for knee osteoarthritis. An observational study of 124 subjects demonstrated that those treated with Meriva plus glucosamine had significant improvements in physical function and walking endurance in comparison to those treated with glucosamine plus chondroitin.[81] Evidence for the use of ginger in the treatment of pain has demonstrated mixed results.[82] A review of 7 studies concluded that, although there is a need for future robust trials examining the potential pain-reducing effects of ginger, the available evidence does tentatively support its use as an anti-inflammatory.[83]

Glucosamine sulfate and chondroitin are 2 dietary supplements that gained recognition after early clinical trials demonstrated efficacy in controlling progression of knee osteoarthritis.[84,85] Since that time, studies have demonstrated mixed results. A large double-blind clinical RCT of subjects with osteoarthritis of the knee showed statistically significant reductions in joint space narrowing when taken in combination with glucosamine and chondroitin in comparison with placebo or single-treatment allocations.[86] However, none of the treatment groups showed statistically significant decreases in pain in comparison with placebo. A recent Cochrane review examined the efficacy of chondroitin alone or in combination with glucosamine; the investigators concluded that short-term studies demonstrated small to moderate improvements in pain related to osteoarthritis in comparison with placebo, with no significant safety concerns identified.[87]

An additional Cochrane review, performed in 2014, examined evidence for supplementation for osteoarthritis.[88] The investigators concluded that the proprietary product made of a combination of one-third avocado and two-thirds soybean unsaponifiables (ASU) demonstrated moderate to high improvements in pain in the short term. In addition, they noted that the herb *Boswellia serrata* showed trends toward benefit that warrants further investigation.[88]

There have been significant efforts examining the role of vitamin D in pain processing that involve complex pathophysiologic pathways. Earlier studies have demonstrated that high rates of hypovitaminosis D are prevalent in subjects with fibromyalgia and chronic pain.[89] Vitamin D is actually a hormone that can be endogenously produced by the human skin and is available in very few dietary sources.[90] Several review studies have concluded that, although there seems to be a trend toward vitamin D supplementation and decreased pain, there is a need for further randomized control trials.[90,91]

Polyunsaturated fatty acids, which include omega-3 and omega-6 fatty acids, are considered essential dietary nutrients. Omega-3 fatty acids include alpha-linolenic acid (ALA), eicosapentaenoic acid (EPA), and docosahexaenoic acid (DHA). EPA and DHA are often found in cold water fish whereas, ALA can be found in certain nut and seed oils (eg, flaxseed, pumpkin seed).[92] The impact of these fatty acids has been examined for several pain-related disorders and it is thought that omega-3 fatty acids may have an anti-inflammatory effect.[93] Ramsden and colleagues[94] performed an RCT examining the impact of omega-3 fatty acid supplementation for the treatment of chronic headaches. There was a significant reduction in measures of headache intensity pain, in addition to increased markers of antinociceptive lipid mediators.

There has also been recent interest investigating the role of omega-3 fatty acids in managing pain in arthritic conditions.[95,96] An RCT of 202 subjects with knee osteoarthritis demonstrated pain improvements with both high-dose and low-dose omega-3 fatty acids.[96] Although some initial human studies look promising, a recent review demonstrates the need for further long-term studies.[95]

CASE STUDY

This case serves as an example of how an integrative plan can be used in a real patient setting.

Background

JH is a 45-year-old married, white man with refractory complex regional pain syndrome in his right shoulder and arm. He was referred to integrative medicine after no longer responding to interventional therapies for pain. He had undergone a series of procedures and traditional interventions for pain relief without much benefit. At initial evaluation, JH reported uncontrolled pain averaging 8 to 10 throughout the day. He struggled to fall asleep and could not rest for more than 2 hours at a time. In addition, he acknowledged a "short fuse" and being quick to anger, which also worsened his pain. He expressed concern that he would have a "heart attack" because his blood pressure significantly spiked in times of anger or pain increase. Through examining his case from the Wheel of Health (see **Fig. 1**), JH's primary needs involved mind-body intervention, sleep and rest, and spirit.

Integrative Medicine Treatment Plan

- His integrative treatment plan, led by a nurse practitioner, involved regular medical massage, individual yoga therapy, participation in a telephone-based pain coaching program, and clinical hypnosis for pain control.
- JH followed all treatment recommendations and was highly engaged.
- After establishing regular massage, an at-home yoga practice, and weekly pain coaching, he underwent 10 sessions of clinical hypnosis.
  - Hypnosis was directed at JH being less bothered by pain, feeling more in control over his body during waves of pain (eg, suggestions of pleasant numbness and cooling sensations to address the burning or sharp pain in his neck and arms). JH's hypnosis sessions were recorded and also used during his massage therapy.

Subjective outcomes

- Increased ability to fall asleep at night through yoga practice and self-hypnosis
- Improved ability to relax and think when angered, as opposed to reacting
- Decreased feelings of isolation and increased connectedness with others who experienced similar health-related difficulties through his participation in the pain coaching program.

Objective outcomes

- Using the McGill Pain Questionnaire–Short Form (SF-MPQ-2),[97] his overall pain score went from 171 to 134 over 10 weeks, which is a 22% change (**Fig. 4**).
- This change was most reflected in his report of neuropathic pain, which was 37% lower at follow-up and consistent with what is considered clinically meaningful in similar measures (see **Fig. 4**).[98]

Follow-up

JH continues to meet with his integrative nurse practitioner, receive regular massage, and have occasional booster sessions in yoga and clinical hypnosis to maintain treatment gains.

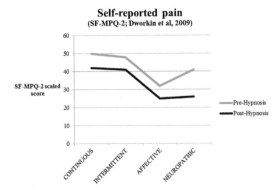

Fig. 4. Self- reported pain before and after hypnosis based on the SF-MPQ-2.

REFERENCES

1. Marks R, Allegrante JP, Lorig K. A review and synthesis of research evidence for self-efficacy-enhancing interventions for reducing chronic disability: implications for health education practice (part I). Health Promot Pract 2005;6(1):37–43.
2. Charmel PA, Frampton SB. Building the business case for patient-centered care. Healthc Financ Manage 2008;62(3):80–5. Available at: http://www.ncbi.nlm.nih.gov/pubmed/19097611. Accessed August 16, 2016.
3. O'Riordan C, Clifford A, Van De Ven P, et al. Chronic neck pain and exercise interventions: frequency, intensity, time, and type principle. Arch Phys Med Rehabil 2014;95(4):770–83.
4. Evans R, Bronfort G, Schulz C, et al. Supervised exercise with and without spinal manipulation performs similarly and better than home exercise for chronic neck pain: a randomized controlled trial. Spine (Phila Pa 1976) 2012;37(11):903–14.
5. Anderson RU, Harvey RH, Wise D, et al. Chronic pelvic pain syndrome: reduction of medication use after pelvic floor physical therapy with an internal myofascial trigger point wand. Appl Psychophysiol Biofeedback 2015;40(1):45–52.
6. Roche G, Ponthieux A, Parot-Shinkel E, et al. Comparison of a functional restoration program with active individual physical therapy for patients with chronic low back pain: a randomized controlled trial. Arch Phys Med Rehabil 2007;88(10):1229–35.
7. Chang DG, Holt JA, Sklar M, et al. Yoga as a treatment for chronic low back pain: A systematic review of the literature. J Orthop Rheumatol 2016;3(1):1–8. Available at: http://www.ncbi.nlm.nih.gov/pubmed/27231715.
8. Cramer H, Lauche R, Haller H, et al. A systematic review and meta-analysis of yoga for low back pain. Clin J Pain 2013;29(5):450–60.
9. Friedly J, Standaert C, Chan L. Epidemiology of spine care: the back pain dilemma. Phys Med Rehabil Clin N Am 2010;21(4):659–77.
10. Sherman KJ, Cherkin DC, Wellman RD, et al. A randomized trial comparing yoga, stretching, and a self-care book for chronic low back pain. Arch Intern Med 2011;171(22):2019–26.
11. Saper RB, Sherman KJ, Delitto A, et al. Yoga vs. physical therapy vs. education for chronic low back pain in predominantly minority populations: study protocol for a randomized controlled trial. Trials 2014;15:67.
12. Kim S-D. Effects of yoga on chronic neck pain: a systematic review of randomized controlled trials. J Phys Ther Sci 2016;28(7):2171–4.
13. Cramer H, Lauche R, Hohmann C, et al. Randomized-controlled trial comparing yoga and home-based exercise for chronic neck pain. Clin J Pain 2013;29(3):216–23.
14. Langhorst J, Klose P, Dobos GJ, et al. Efficacy and safety of meditative movement therapies in fibromyalgia syndrome: a systematic review and meta-analysis of randomized controlled trials. Rheumatol Int 2013;33(1):193–207.
15. Ward L, Stebbings S, Cherkin D, et al. Yoga for functional ability, pain and psychosocial outcomes in musculoskeletal conditions: a systematic review and meta-analysis. Musculoskeletal Care 2013;11(4):203–17.
16. Stein KM, Weinberg J, Sherman KJ, et al. Participant characteristics associated with symptomatic improvement from yoga for chronic low back pain. J Yoga Phys Ther 2014;4(1):151.
17. Combs MA, Thorn BE. Yoga attitudes in chronic low back pain: Roles of catastrophizing and fear of movement. Complement Ther Clin Pract 2015;21(3):160–5.

18. Eaves ER, Sherman KJ, Ritenbaugh C, et al. A qualitative study of changes in expectations over time among patients with chronic low back pain seeking four CAM therapies. BMC Complement Altern Med 2015;15:12.

19. Peng PWH. Tai Chi and chronic pain. Reg Anesth Pain Med 2012;37(4):372–82.

20. Hall AM, Maher CG, Lam P, et al. Tai chi exercise for treatment of pain and disability in people with persistent low back pain: a randomized controlled trial. Arthritis Care Res (Hoboken) 2011;63(11):1576–83.

21. Jones KD, Sherman CA, Mist SD, et al. A randomized controlled trial of 8-form Tai chi improves symptoms and functional mobility in fibromyalgia patients. Clin Rheumatol 2012;31(8):1205–14.

22. Wang C, Schmid CH, Rones R, et al. A randomized trial of tai chi for fibromyalgia. N Engl J Med 2010;363(8):743–54.

23. Furlan AD, Giraldo M, Baskwill A, et al. Massage for low-back pain. Cochrane Database Syst Rev 2015;(9):CD001929.

24. Kamali F, Panahi F, Ebrahimi S, et al. Comparison between massage and routine physical therapy in women with sub acute and chronic nonspecific low back pain. J Back Musculoskelet Rehabil 2014;27(4):475–80.

25. Terry R, Perry R, Ernst E. An overview of systematic reviews of complementary and alternative medicine for fibromyalgia. Clin Rheumatol 2012;31(1):55–66.

26. Sherman KJ, Cook AJ, Wellman RD, et al. Five-week outcomes from a dosing trial of therapeutic massage for chronic neck pain. Ann Fam Med 2014;12(2):112–20.

27. Cook AJ, Wellman RD, Cherkin DC, et al. Randomized clinical trial assessing whether additional massage treatments for chronic neck pain improve 12- and 26-week outcomes. Spine J 2015;15(10):2206–15.

28. Abrams DI, Dolor R, Roberts R, et al. The BraveNet prospective observational study on integrative medicine treatment approaches for pain. BMC Complement Altern Med 2013;13:146.

29. Beal MW. Acupuncture and Oriental body work: traditional and biomedical concepts in holistic care: history and basic concepts. Holist Nurs Pract 2000;14(3):69–78. Available at: http://www.ncbi.nlm.nih.gov/pubmed/12119630. Accessed July 31, 2016.

30. Soligo M, Nori SL, Protto V, et al. Acupuncture and neurotrophin modulation. Int Rev Neurobiol 2013;111:91–124.

31. Cheng X. Chinese acupuncture and moxibustion. Beijing (China): Foreign Language Press; 1987.

32. Scheffold BE, Hsieh C-L, Litscher G. Neuroimaging and neuromonitoring effects of electro and manual acupuncture on the central nervous system: a literature review and analysis. Evid Based Complement Alternat Med 2015;2015:641742.

33. Ambrósio EMM, Bloor K, MacPherson H. Costs and consequences of acupuncture as a treatment for chronic pain: a systematic review of economic evaluations conducted alongside randomised controlled trials. Complement Ther Med 2012;20(5):364–74.

34. Vickers AJ, Cronin AM, Maschino AC, et al. Acupuncture for chronic pain: individual patient data meta-analysis. Arch Intern Med 2012;172(19):1444–53.

35. Cho Y-J, Song Y-K, Cha Y-Y, et al. Acupuncture for chronic low back pain: a multi-center, randomized, patient-assessor blind, sham-controlled clinical trial. Spine (Phila Pa 1976) 2013;38(7):549–57.

36. Weiss J, Quante S, Xue F, et al. Effectiveness and acceptance of acupuncture in patients with chronic low back pain: results of a prospective, randomized, controlled trial. J Altern Complement Med 2013;19(12):935–41.

37. Molsberger AF, Mau J, Pawelec DB, et al. Does acupuncture improve the ortho-pedic management of chronic low back pain–a randomized, blinded, controlled trial with 3 months follow up. Pain 2002;99(3):579–87. Available at: http://www.ncbi.nlm.nih.gov/pubmed/12406534.
38. Hinman RS, McCrory P, Pirotta M, et al. Acupuncture for chronic knee pain: a ran-domized clinical trial. JAMA 2014;312(13):1313–22.
39. Manyanga T, Froese M, Zarychanski R, et al. Pain management with acupuncture in osteoarthritis: a systematic review and meta-analysis. BMC Complement Altern Med 2014;14:312.
40. Davidson RJ, McEwen BS. Social influences on neuroplasticity: stress and inter-ventions to promote well-being. Nat Neurosci 2012;15(5):689–95.
41. Woolf CJ. Central sensitization: implications for the diagnosis and treatment of pain. Pain 2011;152(3 Suppl):S2–15.
42. Reiner K, Tibi L, Lipsitz JD. Do mindfulness-based interventions reduce pain in-tensity? A critical review of the literature. Pain Med 2013;14(2):230–42.
43. Kabat-Zinn J. An outpatient program in behavioral medicine for chronic pain pa-tients based on the practice of mindfulness meditation: theoretical considerations and preliminary results. Gen Hosp Psychiatry 1982;4(1):33–47. Available at: http://www.ncbi.nlm.nih.gov/pubmed/7042457.
44. la Cour P, Petersen M. Effects of mindfulness meditation on chronic pain: a ran-domized controlled trial. Pain Med 2015;16(4):641–52.
45. Gotink RA, Chu P, Busschbach JJV, et al. Standardised mindfulness-based inter-ventions in healthcare: an overview of systematic reviews and meta-analyses of RCTs. PLoS One 2015;10(4):e0124344.
46. Goyal M, Singh S, Sibinga EMS, et al. Meditation programs for psychological stress and well-being: a systematic review and meta-analysis. JAMA Intern Med 2014;174(3):357–68.
47. Cherkin DC, Sherman KJ, Balderson BH, et al. Effect of Mindfulness-Based Stress Reduction vs cognitive behavioral therapy or usual care on back pain and functional limitations in adults with chronic low back pain: a randomized clin-ical trial. JAMA 2016;315(12):1240–9.
48. Elkins G, Johnson A, Fisher W. Cognitive hypnotherapy for pain management. Am J Clin Hypn 2012;54(4):294–310.
49. Elkins G, Jensen MP, Patterson DR. Hypnotherapy for the management of chronic pain. Int J Clin Exp Hypn 2007;55(3):275–87.
50. Tan G, Rintala DH, Jensen MP, et al. A randomized controlled trial of hypnosis compared with biofeedback for adults with chronic low back pain. Eur J Pain 2015;19(2):271–80.
51. Weeks DL, Whitney AA, Tindall AG, et al. Pilot randomized trial comparing inter-session scheduling of biofeedback results to individuals with chronic pain: influ-ence on psychologic function and pain intensity. Am J Phys Med Rehabil 2015;94(10 Suppl 1):869–78.
52. Henschke N, Ostelo RW, van Tulder MW, et al. Behavioural treatment for chronic low-back pain. In: Henschke N, editor. Cochrane Database of systematic reviews. Chichester (United Kingdom): John Wiley & Sons, Ltd; 2010.
53. Guan M, Ma L, Li L, et al. Self-regulation of brain activity in patients with posther-petic neuralgia: a double-blind randomized study using real-time fMRI neuro-feedback. PLoS One 2015;10(4):e0123675.
54. Frank DL, Khorshid L, Kiffer JF, et al. Biofeedback in medicine: who, when, why and how? Ment Health Fam Med 2010;7(2):85–91. Available at: http://www.ncbi.nlm.nih.gov/pubmed/22477926. Accessed July 30, 2016.

55. Williams AC, Eccleston C, Morley S. Psychological therapies for the management of chronic pain (excluding headache) in adults. Cochrane Database Syst Rev 2012;(11):CD007407.

56. Knoerl R, Lavoie Smith EM, Weisberg J. Chronic pain and cognitive behavioral therapy: an integrative review. West J Nurs Res 2016;38(5):596–628.

57. Monticone M, Cedraschi C, Ambrosini E, et al. Cognitive-behavioural treatment for subacute and chronic neck pain. Cochrane Database Syst Rev 2015;(5):CD010664.

58. Dear BF, Titov N, Perry KN, et al. The Pain Course: a randomised controlled trial of a clinician-guided Internet-delivered cognitive behaviour therapy program for managing chronic pain and emotional well-being. Pain 2013;154(6):942–50.

59. Eccleston C, Fisher E, Craig L, et al. Psychological therapies (Internet-delivered) for the management of chronic pain in adults. Cochrane Database Syst Rev 2014;(2):CD010152.

60. Carpenter KM, Stoner SA, Mundt JM, et al. An online self-help CBT intervention for chronic lower back pain. Clin J Pain 2012;28(1):14–22.

61. Jain S, Mills PJ. Biofield therapies: helpful or full of hype? A best evidence synthesis. Int J Behav Med 2010;17(1):1–16.

62. Fazzino DL, Griffin MTQ, McNulty RS, et al. Energy healing and pain: a review of the literature. Holist Nurs Pract 2010;24(2):79–88.

63. So PS, Jiang Y, Qin Y. Touch therapies for pain relief in adults. Cochrane Database Syst Rev 2008;(4):CD006535.

64. Lu D-F, Hart LK, Lutgendorf SK, et al. The effect of healing touch on the pain and mobility of persons with osteoarthritis: a feasibility study. Geriatr Nurs 2013;34(4):314–22.

65. Baldwin AL, Fullmer K, Schwartz GE. Comparison of physical therapy with energy healing for improving range of motion in subjects with restricted shoulder mobility. Evid Based Complement Alternat Med 2013;2013:329731.

66. Roehrs TA. Workshop Participants. Does effective management of sleep disorders improve pain symptoms? Drugs 2009;69(Suppl 2):5–11.

67. Smith MT, Haythornthwaite JA. How do sleep disturbance and chronic pain interrelate? Insights from the longitudinal and cognitive-behavioral clinical trials literature. Sleep Med Rev 2004;8(2):119–32.

68. Mitchell MD, Gehrman P, Perlis M, et al. Comparative effectiveness of cognitive behavioral therapy for insomnia: a systematic review. BMC Fam Pract 2012;13:40.

69. Foundation NS. Cognitive-behavioral therapy for insomnia. Available at: https://sleepfoundation.org/sleep-news/cognitive-behavioral-therapy-insomnia. Accessed January 1, 2016.

70. Virginia U of. BeHealth Solutions. Available at: http://www.myshuti.com/. Accessed January 1, 2016.

71. Naiman R. Integrative medicine. In: Rackel D, editor. Integrative medicine. 3rd edition. Philadelphia: Elsevier; 2012. p. 65–76.

72. Bawa FLM, Mercer SW, Atherton RJ, et al. Does mindfulness improve outcomes in patients with chronic pain? Systematic review and meta-analysis. Br J Gen Pract 2015;65(635):e387–400.

73. Lauche R, Cramer H, Häuser W, et al. A systematic overview of reviews for complementary and alternative therapies in the treatment of the fibromyalgia syndrome. Evid Based Complement Alternat Med 2015;2015:610615.

74. Björnsdóttir SV, Arnljótsdóttir M, Tómasson G, et al. Health-related quality of life improvements among women with chronic pain: comparison of two multidisciplinary interventions. Disabil Rehabil 2016;38(9):828–36.

75. Oliviero F, Spinella P, Fiocco U, et al. How the Mediterranean diet and some of its components modulate inflammatory pathways in arthritis. Swiss Med Wkly 2015; 145:w14190.

76. Totsch SK, Waite ME, Sorge RE. Chapter fifteen – dietary influence on pain via the immune system. Prog Mol Biol Transl Sci 2015;131:435–69.

77. Hagen KB, Byfuglien MG, Falzon L, et al. Dietary interventions for rheumatoid arthritis. Cochrane Database Syst Rev 2009;(1):CD006400.

78. Peddada KV, Peddada KV, Shukla SK, et al. Role of curcumin in common musculoskeletal disorders: a review of current laboratory, translational, and clinical data. Orthop Surg 2015;7(3):222–31.

79. Goel A, Boland CR, Chauhan DP. Specific inhibition of cyclooxygenase-2 (COX-2) expression by dietary curcumin in HT-29 human colon cancer cells. Cancer Lett 2001;172(2):111–8. Available at: http://www.ncbi.nlm.nih.gov/pubmed/11566484. Accessed July 19, 2016.

80. Kuptniratsaikul V, Dajpratham P, Taechaarpornkul W, et al. Efficacy and safety of Curcuma domestica extracts compared with ibuprofen in patients with knee osteoarthritis: a multicenter study. Clin Interv Aging 2014;9:451–8.

81. Belcaro G, Dugall M, Luzzi R, et al. Meriva®+Glucosamine versus Condroitin+‴ Glucosamine in patients with knee osteoarthritis: an observational study. Eur Rev Med Pharmacol Sci 2014;18(24):3959–63. Available at: http://www.ncbi.nlm.nih.gov/pubmed/25555891. Accessed July 19, 2016.

82. White B. Ginger: an overview. Am Fam Physician 2007;75(11):1689–91. Available at: http://www.ncbi.nlm.nih.gov/pubmed/17575660. Accessed July 19, 2016.

83. Terry R, Posadzki P, Watson LK, et al. The use of ginger (Zingiber officinale) for the treatment of pain: a systematic review of clinical trials. Pain Med 2011; 12(12):1808–18.

84. Pavelká K, Gatterová J, Olejarová M, et al. Glucosamine sulfate use and delay of progression of knee osteoarthritis: a 3-year, randomized, placebo-controlled, double-blind study. Arch Intern Med 2002;162(18):2113–23. Available at: http://www.ncbi.nlm.nih.gov/pubmed/12374520. Accessed July 19, 2016.

85. Reginster JY, Deroisy R, Rovati LC, et al. Long-term effects of glucosamine sulphate on osteoarthritis progression: a randomised, placebo-controlled clinical trial. Lancet 2001;357(9252):251–6.

86. Fransen M, Agaliotis M, Nairn L, et al. Glucosamine and chondroitin for knee osteoarthritis: a double-blind randomised placebo-controlled clinical trial evaluating single and combination regimens. Ann Rheum Dis 2015;74(5):851–8.

87. Singh JA, Noorbaloochi S, MacDonald R, et al. Chondroitin for osteoarthritis. Cochrane Database Syst Rev 2015;(1):CD005614.

88. Cameron M, Chrubasik S. Oral herbal therapies for treating osteoarthritis. Cochrane Database Syst Rev 2014;(5):CD002947.

89. Plotnikoff GA, Quigley JM. Prevalence of severe hypovitaminosis D in patients with persistent, nonspecific musculoskeletal pain. Mayo Clin Proc 2003;78(12): 1463–70.

90. Shipton EE, Shipton EA. Vitamin D deficiency and pain: clinical evidence of low levels of vitamin d and supplementation in chronic pain states. Pain Ther 2015; 4(1):67–87.

91. Straube S, Derry S, Moore RA, et al. Vitamin D for the treatment of chronic painful conditions in adults. Cochrane Database Syst Rev 2010;(1):CD007771.

92. Nadtochiy SM, Redman EK. Mediterranean diet and cardioprotection: the role of nitrite, polyunsaturated fatty acids, and polyphenols. Nutrition 2011;27(7–8): 733–44.
93. Zhang MJ, Spite M. Resolvins: anti-inflammatory and proresolving mediators derived from omega-3 polyunsaturated fatty acids. Annu Rev Nutr 2012;32: 203–27.
94. Ramsden CE, Faurot KR, Zamora D, et al. Targeted alteration of dietary n-3 and n-6 fatty acids for the treatment of chronic headaches: a randomized trial. Pain 2013;154(11):2441–51.
95. Boe C, Vangsness CT. Fish oil and osteoarthritis: current evidence. Am J Orthop (Belle Mead NJ) 2015;44(7):302–5. Available at: http://www.ncbi.nlm.nih.gov/pubmed/26161757. Accessed August 6, 2016.
96. Hill CL, March LM, Aitken D, et al. Fish oil in knee osteoarthritis: a randomised clinical trial of low dose versus high dose. Ann Rheum Dis 2016;75(1):23–9.
97. Dworkin RH, Turk DC, Revicki DA, et al. Development and initial validation of an expanded and revised version of the Short-form McGill Pain Questionnaire (SF-MPQ-2). Pain 2009;144(1–2):35–42.
98. Farrar JT, Young JP, LaMoreaux L, et al. Clinical importance of changes in chronic pain intensity measured on an 11-point numerical pain rating scale. Pain 2001; 94(2):149–58. Available at: http://www.ncbi.nlm.nih.gov/pubmed/11690728.

Integrative Medicine for Gastrointestinal Disease

Michelle L. Dossett, MD, PhD, MPH[a],*, Ezra M. Cohen, MD[b], Jonah Cohen, MD[c]

KEYWORDS

- Complementary therapies • Integrative medicine • Digestive system diseases
- Gastroesophageal reflux disease • Inflammatory bowel disease
- Irritable bowel syndrome • Liver disease • Nausea

KEY POINTS

- Patients with gastrointestinal conditions frequently use integrative medicine, and evidence of efficacy of specific therapies for certain conditions is growing.
- Promising results have been achieved with mind–body therapies, acupuncture, diet, and some dietary supplements, including probiotics and specific herbs in distinct gastrointestinal conditions.
- The most commonly studied conditions are gastroesophageal reflux disease, inflammatory bowel disease, irritable bowel syndrome, nonalcoholic fatty liver disease, and nausea and vomiting.

INTRODUCTION

Gastrointestinal (GI) conditions account for substantial morbidity, mortality, and health care costs in the United States.[1] Approximately 42% of the US adult population with GI conditions have used integrative therapies over the course of a given year.[2] Interest in, and research on, integrative approaches for addressing GI conditions is growing, in part owing to the recognition of the importance of the gut microbiome on human health, the effects of stress on the enteric nervous system, and their interrelationship.[3] Although an exhaustive review of integrative approaches for managing GI disease is

Disclosure: Dr M.L. Dossett was supported by K23AT009218 from the National Center for Complementary and Integrative Health (NCCIH). The content is solely the responsibility of the authors and does not necessarily represent the official views of Harvard University and its affiliated academic health care centers or the National Institutes of Health.
a Division of General Internal Medicine, Benson-Henry Institute for Mind Body Medicine, Massachusetts General Hospital, 151 Merrimac Street, 4th Floor, Boston, MA 02114, USA; b Division of Immunology, Department of Rheumatology, Boston Children's Hospital, 300 Longwood Avenue, Boston, MA 02115, USA; c Division of Gastroenterology and Hepatology, Beth Israel Deaconess Medical Center, 330 Brookline Avenue, Dana 501, Boston, MA 02215, USA
* Corresponding author.
E-mail address: mdossett@mgh.harvard.edu

outside of the scope this work, herein we focus on the more common and studied approaches for addressing common GI disorders.

GASTROESOPHAGEAL REFLUX DISEASE

Gastroesophageal reflux disease (GERD) is one of the most prevalent health-related conditions in the Western world, with prevalence estimates ranging from 20% to 40%.[4,5] GERD is primarily a clinical diagnosis, characterized by symptoms of heartburn and acid reflux. It is associated with decreased health-related quality of life and significant health care costs and lost productivity.[6,7] Several integrative therapies may help to reduce symptoms.

Acupuncture

Two studies from China suggest that acupuncture (4 points stimulated daily for 6 weeks with a 2- to 3-day break between each week of stimulation) can significantly reduce esophageal acid and bile reflux and improve GERD-related symptoms.[8,9] Another study found that for individuals with ongoing GERD symptoms despite once daily proton pump inhibitor therapy, addition of acupuncture (10 sessions over 4 weeks) was more effective than doubling the proton pump inhibitor dose.[8,10] Many patients with GERD also have functional dyspepsia, and acupuncture treatment seems to be effective for those symptoms as well, perhaps through a centrally mediated mechanism.[11]

Mind–Body Therapies

Anxiety and depression are known to increase reports of GERD symptoms, and patients who respond less well to proton pump inhibitor therapy are more likely to suffer from psychological distress.[8] In small studies, hypnotherapy, biofeedback, and muscle relaxation techniques have been shown to improve GERD symptoms.[8] In a recent randomized, controlled trial (RCT) of diaphragmatic breathing exercises for patients with nonerosive GERD, subjects were instructed to practice for 30 minutes daily and were given a recording with instructions and relaxing music.[12] After 4 weeks, those practicing the breathing exercises had a significant decrease in esophageal acid exposure by esophageal manometry and improvements in quality of life, whereas there were no changes in the control group. In those still practicing at 9 months, proton pump inhibitor use was decreased.

Herbs and Dietary Supplements

Melatonin is synthesized in the GI tract and is an important gut motility signal. Two studies suggest that melatonin may be as or more effective than omeprazole 20 mg in reducing GERD-related symptoms.[10] One study examined 3 mg of melatonin daily, the other examined 6 mg of melatonin in combination with several vitamins and amino acids. The only side effect noted in the latter study was somnolence.

STW 5 (Iberogast) is a commercial formula that includes 9 botanicals: *Iberis amara, Matricaria chamomilla, Carum carvi, Mentha piperita, Glycyrrhiza glabra, Melissa officinalis, Chelidonium majus, Silybum marianum,* and *Angelica archangelica.*[10] In 3 studies of functional dyspepsia that included patients with GERD symptoms, those receiving STW 5 were more likely to have improvement in symptoms than those receiving placebo. STW 5 was most effective for epigastric pain, retrosternal pain, and acid regurgitation. Adverse events were similar to placebo and included dermatitis, angioedema, digestive intolerance, and 1 case of allergic asthma. The product has been sold in Germany for 40 years and has a good safety profile.

Raft-forming agents include alginate, pectin, and carbenoxolone (a synthetic derivative of glycyrrhizin). When these compounds come in contact with gastric acid, they form polymers and float to the surface of the stomach contents, providing a barrier that protects the esophagus from acid reflux.[10] These agents lack major side effects and are useful in treating mild to moderate GERD.

Some patients take deglycyrhiziniated licorice, chamomile, slippery elm, marshmallow root, D-limonene, and/or betaine. These products are part of the herbal and naturopathic medicine traditions for GERD treatment; however, there are no rigorous studies evaluating their efficacy. Herbs from the mint family (eg, peppermint, spearmint) can reduce lower esophageal sphincter pressure and may exacerbate reflux.[10,13]

Nutrition and Lifestyle Interventions

Studies of the effects of diet on heartburn and reflux symptoms have often yielded contradictory results, perhaps because different foods or nutrients exacerbate symptoms in different individuals.[10,13] Foods that have been associated with increased GERD-related symptoms include fatty foods, fried foods, spicy foods, citrus, tomato-based products, and alliums (eg, onion, garlic). Chocolate, peppermint, coffee, carbonated beverages, and alcohol can all decrease lower esophageal sphincter tone and may play a role. In addition, consumption of fewer meals with a large meal in the evening is associated with increased GERD symptoms.[13] Weight loss (obesity increases the risk of GERD) and elevating the head of the bed can help to decrease symptoms.[10]

Summary

There is good evidence for acupuncture, raft-forming agents, Iberogast, weight loss, and elevating the head of the bed for reducing GERD-related symptoms. There is reasonable evidence to consider mind–body approaches (especially if stress may be playing a role), melatonin, and dietary modification.

INFLAMMATORY BOWEL DISEASE

Inflammatory bowel disease (IBD) includes both ulcerative colitis (UC) and Crohn's disease (CD). The use of integrative medicine among patients with IBD is common, with current or past use ranging from 21% to 60% of patients.[14] The most commonly used modalities are homeopathy, herbal products, and probiotics, followed by specific diets and traditional Chinese medicine and acupuncture.[15] However, there are few studies for most of these modalities and, of those that are available, most are pilot studies with small numbers of subjects. We review the most studied therapies.

Herbal Medicines

Two recent reviews examined herbal products for IBD.[14,16] The best evidence is for *Plantago ovata* and curcumin in UC maintenance therapy and *Artemisia absinthium* (wormwood) in CD. *Aloe vera*, *Boswellia serrata*, wheat grass, *Andrographis paniculata*, silymarin, cannabis, evening primrose oil, mastic gum, and a few herbal combinations have all been studied, but there are insufficient data to make conclusions about effectiveness.

In an open-label trial of 105 patients with UC in remission, *P ovata* seeds (10 g twice daily) were as effective as mesalamine in maintaining remission at 12 months. Subjects receiving *P ovata* had higher levels of butyrate in their stool. Side effects were few, mainly constipation and bloating.[14,16]

Curcumin is a phytochemical present in turmeric and has potent antiinflammatory activity. In a double-blind, RCT of 89 patients with quiescent UC, subjects were randomized to curcumin 1 g twice daily or placebo with sulfasalazine or mesalamine. After 6 months, the curcumin group had a significantly lower rate of relapse as well as lower clinical activity index and endoscopic index compared with the placebo group.[14,16]

Two studies of *A absinthium* in patients with active CD have suggested benefit.[14,16] In 1 trial, 40 patients were randomized to receive *A absinthium* 500 mg 3 times daily or placebo in addition to prednisone. After 8 weeks, there was near complete clinical remission in 65% of the intervention subjects and none within the placebo group. *A absinthium* was also steroid sparing. In another study, *A absinthium* treatment was associated with reductions in tumor necrosis factor-α and improvements in quality of life. In both studies, adverse events were similar in the intervention and comparison groups.

Three studies of *Tripterygium wilfordii* (Thunder God Vine) suggest that it is as or more effective than sulfasalazine or mesalamine for the prevention of postoperative relapse (clinically and endoscopically) in CD.[16] Although well-tolerated in these studies, there is concern about potential side effects and toxicity of the plant.[17]

Probiotics

Providing recommendations on the use of probiotics in IBD is challenging given the small numbers of subjects in most studies and the wide variety of organisms used. A recent review concluded that evidence suggests that the probiotic combination VSL#3 is effective in inducing remission in mild to moderate UC (alone or combined with conventional therapies) and that *Escherichia coli* Nissle 1917 strain is effective in maintaining remission in UC.[18] There are insufficient data on the use of probiotics in CD to provide recommendations.

Fish Oil

Fish oil contains omega-3 fatty acids known to have antiinflammatory properties. A Cochrane review examining the effects of fish oil on induction of remission in patients with UC concluded that there were insufficient data to determine whether fish oil is effective for inducing remission in UC.[19] A more recent Cochrane review examined the evidence for omega-3 fatty acids in maintenance of remission in CD and concluded that based on 2 large, high-quality RCTs, omega-3 fatty acids are likely ineffective.[20]

Mind–Body Therapies

Studies of several different mind–body interventions, including mindfulness-based stress reduction, relaxation therapy, hypnotherapy, and comprehensive lifestyle programs, have been studied in patients with UC and CD, mostly in those with inactive disease.[16,21] Stress is a risk factor for disease flare. In general, these studies suggest improvements in quality of life, and sometimes anxiety and pain, but did not change laboratory parameters or reduce disease activity, although these studies may have been underpowered to detect the latter.

Traditional Chinese Medicine and Acupuncture

Two studies have suggested benefit with acupuncture and moxibustion in patients with active UC or CD with regard to disease activity, but did not show improvement in quality of life or symptoms. Additional studies of acupuncture and moxibustion have been conducted but were of such poor methodologic quality that no definitive conclusion can be made.[14]

Nutrition

The Internet contains conflicting information on dietary approaches to ameliorate IBD, and data suggest that patients and clinicians have differing attitudes toward the role of diet and dietary modifications.[22,23] Importantly, patients with IBD commonly have both protein–energy and micronutrient deficiencies that can adversely affect patient outcomes.[24] Epidemiologic studies have suggested that diets high in sucrose, animal fats, and fast foods are risk factors for the development of IBD, whereas diets rich in unsaturated fats, fruits, vegetables, and whole grains are protective. Food additives such as maltodextrin, carageenans, titanium dioxide, and aluminum silicates have been shown to injure enterocytes or alter enteric immune responses in animal models. Exclusive enteral nutrition has clear benefits for inducing remission in patients with active CD. There are emerging data that the specific carbohydrate diet (eliminates all dietary disaccharides, oligosaccharides, and polysaccharides) and a low FODMAP diet (fermentable oligosaccharides, disaccharides, monosaccharides, and polyols; **Table 1**) may help to reduce symptoms in patients with IBD.[25,26] Single studies have demonstrated some improvement with a semivegetarian diet, gluten-free diet, or allergen elimination diet. Given the potential for elimination/exclusion diets to exacerbate nutritional deficiencies, we recommend that patients work with a nutritionist or registered dietician who has expertise in helping patients with IBD.

Table 1 Low and high FODMAP foods	
Low FODMAP Foods	**High FODMAP Foods**
Broccoli	Garlic
Cabbage	Onions
Carrots	Artichoke
Collard greens	Asparagus
Kale	Black beans
Olives	Cauliflower
Radish	Mushrooms
Red peppers	Soy beans
Spinach	Apples
Bananas	Avocado
Blueberries	Mango
Beef	Wheat
Chicken	Cashews
Tuna	Rye
Gluten-free breads	Granola
Alcohol	Honey
Coffee	Beer
Tofu	Dairy

For additional information see: http://www.ibsdiets.org/fodmap-diet/fodmap-food-list/.
Abbreviation: FODMAP, fermentable oligosaccharides, disaccharides, monosaccharides, and polyols.

Summary

In UC, there is good evidence for *P ovata* (10 g twice daily), curcumin (1 g twice daily), and *E coli* Nissle 1917 for maintenance therapy and VSL#3 for inducing remission. In active CD, there is good evidence for exclusive enteral nutrition and *A absinthium* (500 mg 3 times daily) for inducing remission. In IBD in general, there is reasonable evidence to consider mind–body approaches, acupuncture, the specific carbohydrate diet, and/or the low FODMAP diet for symptom reduction. Although there are good data for *T wilfordii* in CD, there is concern about potential toxicity and more data are needed.

IRRITABLE BOWEL SYNDROME

Irritable bowel syndrome (IBS) is a functional bowel disorder characterized by chronic abdominal pain and altered bowel habits in the absence of any organic etiology.[27] In North America and Europe, its prevalence is around 12%.[28,29] IBS likely has multifactorial roots related to alterations in GI motility, alterations in fecal flora, visceral hypersensitivity, previous infections, inflammation, bacterial overgrowth, and food sensitivity.[30] IBS accounts for a significant number of primary care visits and up to 50% of all referrals to general gastroenterologists.[31] IBS subtypes include IBS with predominant constipation, IBS with predominant diarrhea, and IBS with mixed bowel habits. Certain treatments may work better than others for specific IBS subtypes; however, the integrative medicine literature largely does not distinguish between IBS subtypes.

Testing

IBS is a diagnosis of exclusion, and alarm features (eg, nocturnal or progressive abdominal pain or diarrhea, rectal bleeding in the absence of documented bleeding hemorrhoids or anal fissures, unintentional weight loss, or laboratory abnormalities such as anemia, elevated inflammatory markers, or electrolyte disturbances) should always be evaluated.[32] Clinicians must also exclude concomitant IBD, infection, malignancy, microscopic colitis, small intestinal bacterial overgrowth, lactose or fructose intolerance, and celiac disease among other entities, however, overlap between IBS and these entities does exist.[33] Appropriate testing depends on the patients' symptoms and context. Some patients may specifically ask about complete stool analyses, food allergy or food sensitivity tests, and intestinal permeability tests. Food allergy testing is particularly challenging given the potential for false-positive and false-negative results, and requires careful interpretation.[34] Providers can consider training in functional medicine to learn more or refer to an integrative medicine center that incorporates functional medicine testing.

Mind–Body Therapies

A metaanalysis of yoga for IBS found significant reductions in bowel symptoms and anxiety, although the heterogeneity of controls, multiple sources of potential bias, and inadequate reporting of randomization methods tempered this conclusion.[35] A metaanalysis evaluating 7 RCTs of hypnosis found a significant improvement in abdominal pain at 3 months, although performance bias (salutary effects of the provider–patient interaction) and difficulties with blinding likely contribute to positive effects.[36] A larger metaanalysis of psychological therapies (mindfulness, relaxation, cognitive behavioral therapy, hypnosis, and stress reduction techniques) for IBS calculated a pooled risk ratio for improvement of 1.47, favoring psychological therapies.[37] These studies were quite heterogeneous, with different control arms and criteria for improvement. Meditation and mindfulness-based approaches also show promise in IBS with sustained symptom improvements in abdominal pain, quality of life, and other associated symptoms.[21,38,39] Given the favorable safety profile of mind–body therapies and the likelihood that some individuals will derive significant benefit, it is reasonable to recommend such practices for patients with IBS.

Special Diets and Dietary Supplements

The role of nutrition in the pathogenesis and management of IBS has evolved in recent years with increasing evidence supporting the recommendation of various dietary interventions. Notably, patients should be asked about their diet with special attention paid to the ingestion of caffeine, wheat, fruits, vegetables, dairy products, sweetened soft drinks, and chewing gum because these can mimic or exacerbate IBS symptoms.[40] Interesting, dietary restriction of gluten globally improves symptoms in IBS patients in whom celiac disease was excluded carefully.[41] Mechanistically, it has been shown that gluten alters bowel barrier functions in patients with IBS with predominant diarrhea.[42]

Low Fermentable Oligosaccharides, Disaccharides, Monosaccharides, and Polyols Diet

FODMAPs are short-chain carbohydrates that are absorbed incompletely in the small intestine, fermented in the colon, and associated with bloating, diarrhea, and abdominal pain. FODMAP reduction decreases the osmotic load and gas production in the distal small bowel and the proximal colon, providing symptomatic relief in patients with IBS. **Table 1** lists low and high FODMAP foods. A recent metaanalysis of 6 RCTs and 16 nonrandomized studies showed that a low FODMAP diet was associated with reduced abdominal pain, bloating, and improvement in overall symptom score.[43] Overall, up to 86% of patients with IBS may find improvement in their GI symptoms following the diet, including those of constipation and flatulence as well as abdominal pain, diarrhea, and bloating.[44] Although a low FODMAP diet seems to be safe for short-term use, long-term data are lacking and adherence can be challenging. Nutritional intervention by specialized dietitians may improve the success of the low FODMAP diet.

Dietary Fiber

Dietary fiber supplementation has long served as a standard component of IBS management; however, its optimal use can be nuanced given that certain forms of fiber, such as bran, in specific patients may exacerbate abdominal distention and flatulence.[45] Additionally, high amounts of dietary fiber can impair absorption of certain medications; thus, medications should be taken 1 hour before or 2 hours after fiber supplementation.[46] Additional information regarding soluble and insoluble fiber is presented in **Table 2** and a recent review.[47] Fiber should be most often considered in patients with IBS whose predominant symptom is constipation. It is believed that dietary fiber softens stool by drawing in water for easier passage. A recent systematic review and metaanalysis on the effect of fiber supplementation on IBS evaluated 14 RCTs involving 906 subjects and concluded that there was a significant benefit of soluble fiber in IBS with a number needed to treat of 7 subjects; however, no benefit was seen with wheat bran.[45] However, a Cochrane review evaluating 12 studies found no beneficial effect for bulking agents over placebo in improving abdominal pain, global assessment or symptom scores.[48] Interestingly, in constipation, prunes seem to be superior to psyllium for improving stool frequency and consistency.[49]

Table 2 Soluble and insoluble fiber	
Soluble Fiber	**Insoluble Fiber**
Absorbs water and reduces glycemic response and plasma cholesterol	Increases fecal bulk and decreases intestinal transit
Types include pectins and gums	Types include cellulose and lignin
Foods high in soluble fiber • Beans • Avocado • Peas • Oat • Psyllium • Passion fruit • Dried figs	Foods high in insoluble fiber • Wheat bran • Barley • Millet • Flaxseeds • Field beans • Parsnips • Apple

Probiotics

A systematic review of 19 RCTs in 1650 patients with IBS concluded that probiotics were significantly better than placebo with a number needed to treat of 4 subjects.[50] However, the most effective species and strains are uncertain based on heterogeneity in the studies. A more recent metaanalysis of 1793 patients demonstrated that probiotics reduce pain and global symptom severity in patients with IBS compared with placebo.[51] Although probiotics are felt to be safe with a generally favorable side effect profile aside from mild gas and bloating, there is a theoretic risk of causing infection in individuals with compromised immune systems.[52]

Peppermint Oil

Peppermint oil is derived from the peppermint plant and causes relaxation of GI smooth muscle through blockade of calcium channels.[53] Although peppermint oil is generally well-tolerated, smooth muscle relaxation can occur at both the intestinal level as well as the lower esophageal sphincter and thus lead to gastroesophageal reflux. Aside from heartburn, common adverse effects may include allergic reactions, blurred vision, perianal burning, nausea, and vomiting.[53] At very high doses, it has been associated with acute renal failure via interstitial nephritis. It may inhibit the cytochrome P450 1A2 system and thus medication interactions should be evaluated such as those of cyclosporine and statin drugs.[53] A metaanalysis of 4 RCTs with 392 subjects with IBS found peppermint oil to be superior to placebo for global symptom reduction (especially abdominal pain and diarrhea) compared with placebo with a number needed to treat to prevent persistent symptoms of 2.5.[54] More recently, a metaanalysis of 9 RCTs with 726 patients showed that peppermint oil was superior to placebo for global improvement of IBS symptoms.[55] In this analysis, the reported adverse events in the placebo-controlled studies were mild and transient, and included heartburn, dry mouth, belching, peppermint taste, rash, dizziness, headache, increased appetite, and a cold perianal sensation. Peppermint oil is best taken in the form of enteric-coated capsules (containing 0.2 mL of oil), which reduces the risk of heartburn and the recommended dosage for adults is 1 to 2 capsules 3 times per day before meals.[53]

Acupuncture

A clear consensus on the effects of acupuncture in IBS has been challenging owing to small, heterogeneous, and methodologically unsound trials. A Cochrane review of 17

RCTs with 1806 subjects found no benefit of acupuncture relative to a credible sham acupuncture control on IBS symptom severity or IBS-related quality of life.[56] However, even "sham" acupuncture may have clinical effects because needles are often placed into the skin. Moreover, subgroup analyses revealed that acupuncture was more effective than either pharmacotherapy (relative risk, 1.28; 5 studies, 449 patients) or no specific therapy (relative risk, 2.11; 2 studies, 181 patients). In this analysis, there was 1 adverse event (ie, syncope) associated with acupuncture. Other side effects that have been reported are often mild and transient, including aching at the sites of needle insertion and dizziness; however, more serious rare events have been reported including bruising, infection, and bleeding.[57]

Summary

There is good evidence for mind–body therapies, a low FODMAP diet, probiotics, and enteric-coated peppermint oil (0.2–0.4 mL 3 times per day for abdominal pain) for reducing IBS-related symptoms. There is reasonable evidence to consider soluble fiber supplementation (especially for constipation), a trial of gluten elimination, and acupuncture.

LIVER DISEASE

Nonalcoholic fatty liver disease (NAFLD) is perhaps the most common liver disorder with prevalence estimates of more than 20% in North America and Europe and increasing rates in other countries.[58] NAFLD is associated with obesity and the metabolic syndrome. Lifestyle modification is critical; however, a growing number of studies suggest potential benefits with herbs and dietary supplements. Fewer data are available for hepatitis C and other liver diseases.

Herbal Medicines and Vitamin E

A systematic review of 419 studies of traditional Chinese medicine herbal combinations (246 different herbs overall) in patients with NAFLD concluded that overall there were improvements in laboratory values and steatosis on imaging and that traditional Chinese medicine provides modest benefit in NAFLD.[59] A Cochrane review examined 77 RCTs of 6753 participants that included 75 different herbal medicine products.[58] Some products had positive effects on liver enzymes (aspartate aminotransferase, alanine aminotransferase), ultrasound imaging, and computed tomography results. There was no differences between the herbal medicine and control groups in terms of adverse effects. No definitive conclusions could be made owing to a high risk of bias and the limited number of studies testing individual herbs.

Another review specifically examined silymarin, a lipophilic extract from the milk thistle plant.[60] Seven studies of varying doses of silymarin with or without vitamin E and other antioxidants were examined in patients with NAFLD. In 1 study, 138 patients received treatment or placebo for 12 months. Side effects were mild and included diarrhea, dysgeusia, and pruritus. The authors concluded that there was good clinical evidence for silymarin at 140 mg/d combined with vitamin E in the treatment of NAFLD. A major challenge is that extraction and standardization methods for the compounds used in these studies has not been described adequately. Another metaanalysis concluded that oral silymarin had no benefit on aminotransferase levels or viral load in patients with chronic hepatitis C infection.[61] Finally, vitamin E may improve liver enzymes in NAFLD, nonalcoholic steatohepatitis, and chronic hepatitis C; however, dosing varied greatly in the studies examined.[62]

Probiotics

A review of probiotic use in patients with a variety of different liver conditions (hepatic encephalopathy, NAFLD, alcoholic liver disease, hepatocellular carcinoma, and patients undergoing liver surgery) concluded that probiotics show promise in reducing the incidence of hepatic encephalopathy, improving serum liver enzymes and inflammatory markers, and reducing postoperative infections.[63] In a review of probiotics for NAFLD, the authors found that probiotic administration reduced serum aminotransferase levels, total cholesterol, tumor necrosis factor-α, and improved insulin resistance.[64] Another review of 10 studies of probiotics for NAFLD found similar benefits including improvements in ultrasound imaging-based fatty liver scores.[65] However, given the variety of products used, it is unclear which organisms or dose is most effective.

Summary

There is good evidence for weight loss, silymarin (140 mg/d) combined with vitamin E, and probiotics for patients with NAFLD. There are insufficient data to recommend any specific therapy for chronic hepatitis C virus infection.

NAUSEA AND VOMITING

Integrative therapies have been used for the treatment of nausea and vomiting in a variety of settings. Here we present the most studied therapies.

Ginger (Zingiber officinale)

Ginger is one of the most well-known and studied herbal treatments for nausea. Gingerols and shogaols are thought be among its pharmacoactive constituents, and may have anticholinergic and antiserotonergic effects.[66] Evidence suggests that ginger may be effective in reducing morning sickness, postoperative nausea and vomiting, and antiretroviral-induced nausea and vomiting.[67] Doses range from 1 to 2 g/d. A metaanalysis of 12 studies concluded that ginger is likely safe and may be effective in reducing nausea associated with pregnancy.[68] Another metaanalysis of ginger in pregnancy included 6 studies and 508 subjects, and concluded a 5-fold pooled likelihood of improvement with 4 consecutive days of 1 g/d.[69] A study of 102 patients with human immunodeficiency virus infection randomized to ginger or placebo at the initiation of antiretroviral therapy resulted in 90% of the placebo group experiencing some degree of nausea versus 56% of the ginger group ($P = .001$).[70] A metaanalysis in chemotherapy-induced nausea and vomiting found no difference in the incidence and severity of nausea and vomiting in the ginger groups versus placebo or metoclopramide.[71] These results are difficult to interpret because there were only 5 trials and comparison groups included both placebo and active controls. Overall, ginger is likely effective for a variety of conditions producing nausea.

Vitamin B₆ (Pyridoxine)

A study comparing vitamin B₆ with ginger found ginger more effective for reducing nausea, but equally effective for reducing vomiting associated with pregnancy.[72] Another study found that ginger and vitamin B₆ both significantly reduced nausea in pregnancy equivalently.[73] A Cochrane review concluded that vitamin B₆ is possibly effective in reducing pregnancy-associated nausea, but that data are insufficient.[74] Dosing in studies ranged from 10 to 25 mg every 8 hours to 50 mg/d. Vitamin B₆ has not been studied extensively in other conditions producing nausea. Vitamin B₆ has a long record of safety; however, there are reports of B_6 toxicity leading to peripheral neuropathy.[75]

Aromatherapy

Aromatherapy, typically in the form of ginger or peppermint oil, has also been used to reduce nausea. A recent qualitative review found that these 2 oils were most commonly used and may be effective, although all studies suffered from significant design flaws.[76] A Cochrane review of 9 trials (6 RCTs and 3 controlled clinical trials) concluded that isopropyl alcohol was more effective than saline for postoperative nausea but less effective than standard antiemetics.[77] There was insufficient evidence to evaluate studies of peppermint oil. A more recent study randomized 301 patients to normal saline, 70% isopropyl alcohol, ginger oil or a blend of oils including peppermint and they found a significant reduction in nausea and antiemetic use in the ginger and blend group but not isopropyl alcohol.[78]

Acupuncture and Acupressure

A reductionist approach to studying acupuncture is difficult because of the nuances of individual treatment and the different points that may be stimulated. Nevertheless, 1 point in particular, the PC6 point (located 2 ½ to 3 fingerbreadths from the wrist crease up the arm, **Fig. 1**), has emerged with the most supportive evidence for use in reducing nausea. A metaanalysis concluded that acupuncture at PC6 is likely effective for reducing postoperative nausea, but that there are insufficient data to support efficacy for other points with or without PC6.[79] A Cochrane review of 59 trials involving 7667 subjects examined acupuncture stimulation at PC6 for the prevention of postoperative nausea and vomiting.[80] The authors found low-quality evidence for efficacy of PC6 over sham, and moderate quality evidence that there was no difference between acupressure and antiemetics. Finally, a recent systematic review evaluating 29 trials of acustimulation (acupressure, acupuncture, auricular stimulation, or moxibustion) in nausea associated with pregnancy found some evidence of benefit; however, the authors urged caution given the heterogeneity of the studies and poor blinding.[81]

Summary

There is good evidence for ginger (1–2 g/d) in reducing nausea and vomiting and vitamin B_6 (10–25 mg 3 times a day or 50 mg/d) in reducing nausea and vomiting

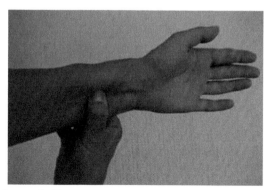

Fig. 1. PC6 point. (*From* Blackburn J, Spencer R. Postoperative nausea and vomiting. Anaesthesia & Intensive Care Medicine 2015;16:452–56; with permission.)

associated with pregnancy. There is reasonable evidence to consider use of ginger or peppermint oil as aromatherapy or acupuncture.

SUMMARY

An increasing number of studies support the use of integrative medicine approaches for reducing nausea and vomiting, symptoms associated with GERD, IBD, and IBS, as well as steatosis associated with NALFD. The majority of these approaches have excellent safety profiles and are unlikely to interfere with pharmaceuticals, making them particularly attractive options. In some cases, data suggest that therapies may be broadly beneficial (eg, probiotics in IBS), but there is as yet insufficient information to recommend specific dosing or agents. Categories of integrative medicine approaches that seem to show the most promise in GI conditions include mind–body therapies, acupuncture, diet, probiotics, and specific dietary supplements and herbs.

REFERENCES

1. Peery AF, Crockett SD, Barritt AS, et al. Burden of gastrointestinal, liver, and pancreatic diseases in the United States. Gastroenterology 2015;149(7): 1731–41.e3.
2. Dossett ML, Davis RB, Lembo AJ, et al. Complementary and alternative medicine use by US adults with gastrointestinal conditions: results from the 2012 National Health Interview Survey. Am J Gastroenterol 2014;109(11):1705–11.
3. Konturek PC, Brzozowski T, Konturek SJ. Stress and the gut: pathophysiology, clinical consequences, diagnostic approach and treatment options. J Physiol Pharmacol 2011;62(6):591–9.
4. Cohen E, Bolus R, Khanna D, et al. GERD symptoms in the general population: prevalence and severity versus care-seeking patients. Dig Dis Sci 2014;59(10): 2488–96.
5. Agréus L, Svärdsudd K, Talley NJ, et al. Natural history of gastroesophageal reflux disease and functional abdominal disorders: a population-based study. Am J Gastroenterol 2001;96(10):2905–14.
6. Tack J, Becher A, Mulligan C, et al. Systematic review: the burden of disruptive gastro-oesophageal reflux disease on health-related quality of life. Aliment Pharmacol Ther 2012;35(11):1257–66.
7. Rubenstein JH, Chen JW. Epidemiology of gastroesophageal reflux disease. Gastroenterol Clin North Am 2014;43(1):1–14.
8. Maradey-Romero C, Kale H, Fass R. Nonmedical therapeutic strategies for non-erosive reflux disease. J Clin Gastroenterol 2014;48(7):584–9.
9. Zhang C, Qin Y, Guo B. Clinical study on the treatment of gastroesophageal reflux by acupuncture. Chin J Integr Med 2010;16(4):298–303.
10. Patrick L. Gastroesophageal reflux disease (GERD): a review of conventional and alternative treatments. Altern Med Rev 2011;16(2):116–33.
11. Ford AC, Moayyedi P. Dyspepsia. Curr Opin Gastroenterol 2013;29(6):662–8.
12. Eherer AJ, Netolitzky F, Högenauer C, et al. Positive effect of abdominal breathing exercise on gastroesophageal reflux disease: a randomized, controlled study. Am J Gastroenterol 2012;107(3):372–8.
13. Jarosz M, Taraszewska A. Risk factors for gastroesophageal reflux disease: the role of diet. Przeglad Gastroenterol 2014;9(5):297–301.
14. Langhorst J, Wulfert H, Lauche R, et al. Systematic review of complementary and alternative medicine treatments in inflammatory bowel diseases. J Crohns Colitis 2015;9(1):86–106.

15. Joos S. Review on efficacy and health services research studies of complementary and alternative medicine in inflammatory bowel disease. Chin J Integr Med 2011;17(6):403–9.

16. Triantafyllidi A, Xanthos T, Papalois A, et al. Herbal and plant therapy in patients with inflammatory bowel disease. Ann Gastroenterol 2015;28(2):210–20.

17. Thunder God Vine. NCCIH. Available at: https://nccih.nih.gov/health/tgvine. Accessed August 16, 2016.

18. Cammarota G, Ianiro G, Cianci R, et al. The involvement of gut microbiota in inflammatory bowel disease pathogenesis: potential for therapy. Pharmacol Ther 2015;149:191–212.

19. De Ley M, de Vos R, Hommes DW, et al. Fish oil for induction of remission in ulcerative colitis. Cochrane Database Syst Rev 2007;(4):CD005986.

20. Lev-Tzion R, Griffiths AM, Leder O, et al. Omega 3 fatty acids (fish oil) for maintenance of remission in Crohn's disease. Cochrane Database Syst Rev 2014;(2):CD006320.

21. Kuo B, Bhasin M, Jacquart J, et al. Genomic and clinical effects associated with a relaxation response mind-body intervention in patients with irritable bowel syndrome and inflammatory bowel disease. PLoS One 2015;10(4):e0123861.

22. Hou JK, Lee D, Lewis J. Diet and inflammatory bowel disease: review of patient-targeted recommendations. Clin Gastroenterol Hepatol 2014;12(10):1592–600.

23. Holt DQ, Strauss BJ, Moore GT. Patients with inflammatory bowel disease and their treating clinicians have different views regarding diet. J Hum Nutr Diet 2017;30(1):66–72.

24. Wędrychowicz A, Zając A, Tomasik P. Advances in nutritional therapy in inflammatory bowel diseases: review. World J Gastroenterol 2016;22(3):1045–66.

25. Shah ND, Parian AM, Mullin GE, et al. Oral diets and nutrition support for inflammatory bowel disease: what is the evidence? Nutr Clin Pract 2015;30(4):462–73.

26. Lee D, Albenberg L, Compher C, et al. Diet in the pathogenesis and treatment of inflammatory bowel diseases. Gastroenterology 2015;148(6):1087–106.

27. Mearin F, Lacy BE, Chang L, et al. Bowel Disorders. Gastroenterology 2016; 150(6):1393–407.e5.

28. Wilson S, Roberts L, Roalfe A, et al. Prevalence of irritable bowel syndrome: a community survey. Br J Gen Pract 2004;54(504):495–502.

29. Lovell RM, Ford AC. Global prevalence of and risk factors for irritable bowel syndrome: a meta-analysis. Clin Gastroenterol Hepatol 2012;10(7):712–21.e4.

30. Deiteren A, de Wit A, van der Linden L, et al. Irritable bowel syndrome and visceral hypersensitivity : risk factors and pathophysiological mechanisms. Acta Gastroenterol Belg 2016;79(1):29–38.

31. Everhart JE, Renault PF. Irritable bowel syndrome in office-based practice in the United States. Gastroenterology 1991;100(4):998–1005.

32. Ford AC, Bercik P, Morgan DG, et al. Validation of the Rome III criteria for the diagnosis of irritable bowel syndrome in secondary care. Gastroenterology 2013;145(6):1262–70.e1.

33. Schmulson MW, Chang L. Diagnostic approach to the patient with irritable bowel syndrome. Am J Med 1999;107(5A):20S–6S.

34. Stukus DR, Mikhail I. Pearls and pitfalls in diagnosing IgE-mediated food allergy. Curr Allergy Asthma Rep 2016;16(5):34.

35. Schumann D, Anheyer D, Lauche R, et al. Effect of yoga in the therapy of irritable bowel syndrome: a systematic review. Clin Gastroenterol 2016;14(12):1720–31.

36. Lee HH, Choi YY, Choi M-G. The efficacy of hypnotherapy in the treatment of irritable bowel syndrome: a systematic review and meta-analysis. J Neurogastroenterol Motil 2014;20(2):152–62.

37. Ford AC, Quigley EMM, Lacy BE, et al. Effect of antidepressants and psychological therapies, including hypnotherapy, in irritable bowel syndrome: systematic review and meta-analysis. Am J Gastroenterol 2014;109(9):1350–65 [quiz: 1366].

38. Aucoin M, Lalonde-Parsi M-J, Cooley K. Mindfulness-based therapies in the treatment of functional gastrointestinal disorders: a meta-analysis. Evid Based Complement Altern Med 2014;2014:140724.

39. Lakhan SE, Schofield KL. Mindfulness-based therapies in the treatment of somatization disorders: a systematic review and meta-analysis. PLoS One 2013;8(8): e71834.

40. Longstreth GF, Thompson WG, Chey WD, et al. Functional bowel disorders. Gastroenterology 2006;130(5):1480–91.

41. Biesiekierski JR, Newnham ED, Irving PM, et al. Gluten causes gastrointestinal symptoms in subjects without celiac disease: a double-blind randomized placebo-controlled trial. Am J Gastroenterol 2011;106(3):508–14 [quiz: 515].

42. Vazquez-Roque MI, Camilleri M, Smyrk T, et al. A controlled trial of gluten-free diet in patients with irritable bowel syndrome-diarrhea: effects on bowel frequency and intestinal function. Gastroenterology 2013;144(5):903–11.e3.

43. Marsh A, Eslick EM, Eslick GD. Does a diet low in FODMAPs reduce symptoms associated with functional gastrointestinal disorders? A comprehensive systematic review and meta-analysis. Eur J Nutr 2016;55(3):897–906.

44. Nanayakkara WS, Skidmore PM, O'Brien L, et al. Efficacy of the low FODMAP diet for treating irritable bowel syndrome: the evidence to date. Clin Exp Gastroenterol 2016;9:131–42.

45. Moayyedi P, Quigley EMM, Lacy BE, et al. The effect of fiber supplementation on irritable bowel syndrome: a systematic review and meta-analysis. Am J Gastroenterol 2014;109(9):1367–74.

46. Michelfelder AJ, Lee KC, Bading EM. Integrative medicine and gastrointestinal disease. Prim Care 2010;37(2):255–67.

47. Mudgil D, Barak S. Composition, properties and health benefits of indigestible carbohydrate polymers as dietary fiber: a review. Int J Biol Macromol 2013;61: 1–6.

48. Ruepert L, Quartero AO, de Wit NJ, et al. Bulking agents, antispasmodics and antidepressants for the treatment of irritable bowel syndrome. Cochrane Database Syst Rev 2011;(8):CD003460.

49. Lever E, Cole J, Scott SM, et al. Systematic review: the effect of prunes on gastrointestinal function. Aliment Pharmacol Ther 2014;40(7):750–8.

50. Moayyedi P, Ford AC, Talley NJ, et al. The efficacy of probiotics in the treatment of irritable bowel syndrome: a systematic review. Gut 2010;59(3):325–32.

51. Didari T, Mozaffari S, Nikfar S, et al. Effectiveness of probiotics in irritable bowel syndrome: updated systematic review with meta-analysis. World J Gastroenterol 2015;21(10):3072–84.

52. Boyle RJ, Robins-Browne RM, Tang MLK. Probiotic use in clinical practice: what are the risks? Am J Clin Nutr 2006;83(6):1256–64 [quiz: 1446–7].

53. Kligler B, Chaudhary S. Peppermint oil. Am Fam Physician 2007;75(7):1027–30.

54. Ford AC, Talley NJ, Spiegel BMR, et al. Effect of fibre, antispasmodics, and peppermint oil in the treatment of irritable bowel syndrome: systematic review and meta-analysis. BMJ 2008;337:a2313.

55. Khanna R, MacDonald JK, Levesque BG. Peppermint oil for the treatment of irritable bowel syndrome: a systematic review and meta-analysis. J Clin Gastroenterol 2014;48(6):505–12.
56. Manheimer E, Cheng K, Wieland LS, et al. Acupuncture for treatment of irritable bowel syndrome. Cochrane Database Syst Rev 2012;(5):CD005111.
57. Wu J, Hu Y, Zhu Y, et al. Systematic review of adverse effects: a further step towards modernization of acupuncture in China. Evid Based Complement Altern Med 2015;2015:432467.
58. Liu ZL, Xie LZ, Zhu J, et al. Herbal medicines for fatty liver diseases. Cochrane Database Syst Rev 2013;(8):CD009059.
59. Shi K-Q, Fan Y-C, Liu W-Y, et al. Traditional Chinese medicines benefit to nonalcoholic fatty liver disease: a systematic review and meta-analysis. Mol Biol Rep 2012;39(10):9715–22.
60. Milosević N, Milanović M, Abenavoli L, et al. Phytotherapy and NAFLD–from goals and challenges to clinical practice. Rev Recent Clin Trials 2014;9(3):195–203.
61. Yang Z, Zhuang L, Lu Y, et al. Effects and tolerance of silymarin (milk thistle) in chronic hepatitis C virus infection patients: a meta-analysis of randomized controlled trials. Biomed Res Int 2014;2014:941085.
62. Ji H-F, Sun Y, Shen L. Effect of vitamin E supplementation on aminotransferase levels in patients with NAFLD, NASH, and CHC: results from a meta-analysis. Nutrition 2014;30(9):986–91.
63. Minemura M, Shimizu Y. Gut microbiota and liver diseases. World J Gastroenterol 2015;21(6):1691–702.
64. Ma Y-Y, Li L, Yu C-H, et al. Effects of probiotics on nonalcoholic fatty liver disease: a meta-analysis. World J Gastroenterol 2013;19(40):6911–8.
65. Paolella G, Mandato C, Pierri L, et al. Gut-liver axis and probiotics: their role in non-alcoholic fatty liver disease. World J Gastroenterol 2014;20(42):15518–31.
66. Abdel-Aziz H, Windeck T, Ploch M, et al. Mode of action of gingerols and shogaols on 5-HT3 receptors: binding studies, cation uptake by the receptor channel and contraction of isolated guinea-pig ileum. Eur J Pharmacol 2006;530(1–2):136–43.
67. Marx W, Kiss N, Isenring L. Is ginger beneficial for nausea and vomiting? An update of the literature. Curr Opin Support Palliat Care 2015;9(2):189–95.
68. Viljoen E, Visser J, Koen N, et al. A systematic review and meta-analysis of the effect and safety of ginger in the treatment of pregnancy-associated nausea and vomiting. Nutr J 2014;13:20.
69. Thomson M, Corbin R, Leung L. Effects of ginger for nausea and vomiting in early pregnancy: a meta-analysis. J Am Board Fam Med 2014;27(1):115–22.
70. Dabaghzadeh F, Khalili H, Dashti-Khavidaki S, et al. Ginger for prevention of antiretroviral-induced nausea and vomiting: a randomized clinical trial. Expert Opin Drug Saf 2014;13(7):859–66.
71. Lee J, Oh H. Ginger as an antiemetic modality for chemotherapy-induced nausea and vomiting: a systematic review and meta-analysis. Oncol Nurs Forum 2013;40(2):163–70.
72. Ensiyeh J, Sakineh M. Comparing ginger and vitamin B6 for the treatment of nausea and vomiting in pregnancy: a randomised controlled trial. Midwifery 2009;25(6):649–53.
73. Sripramote M, Lekhyananda N. A randomized comparison of ginger and vitamin B6 in the treatment of nausea and vomiting of pregnancy. J Med Assoc Thai 2003;86(9):846–53.

74. Matthews A, Haas DM, O'Mathúna DP, et al. Interventions for nausea and vomiting in early pregnancy. Cochrane Database Syst Rev 2015;(9):CD007575.
75. Kulkantrakorn K. Pyridoxine-induced sensory ataxic neuronopathy and neuropathy: revisited. Neurol Sci 2014;35(11):1827–30.
76. Lua P, Zakaria N. A brief review of current scientific evidence involving aromatherapy use for nausea and vomiting. J Altern Complement Med 2012;18(6):534–40.
77. Hines S, Steels E, Chang A, et al. Aromatherapy for treatment of postoperative nausea and vomiting. Cochrane Database Syst Rev 2012;(4):CD007598.
78. Hunt R, Dienemann J, Norton HJ, et al. Aromatherapy as treatment for postoperative nausea: a randomized trial. Anesth Analg 2013;117(3):597–604.
79. Cheong KB, Zhang J, Huang Y, et al. The effectiveness of acupuncture in prevention and treatment of postoperative nausea and vomiting–a systematic review and meta-analysis. PLoS One 2013;8(12):e82474.
80. Lee A, Chan SKC, Fan LTY. Stimulation of the wrist acupuncture point PC6 for preventing postoperative nausea and vomiting. Cochrane Database Syst Rev 2015;(11):CD003281.
81. Van den Heuvel E, Goossens M, Vanderhaegen H, et al. Effect of acustimulation on nausea and vomiting and on hyperemesis in pregnancy: a systematic review of Western and Chinese literature. BMC Complement Altern Med 2016;16:13.

Integrative Medicine and Mood, Emotions and Mental Health

Anuj K. Shah, MD, MPH[a],*, Roman Becicka, MD[b],
Mary R. Talen, PhD[a], Deborah Edberg, MD[a],
Sreela Namboodiri, MD[a]

KEYWORDS

- Integrative medicine • Mood management • Herbal therapies
- Diet and supplements • Meaning and purpose • Spirituality • Mind-body therapies
- Physical therapies • Emotional regulation

KEY POINTS

- An integrative approach to patients with mental health concerns or mood complaints involves the presentation and consideration of several different therapeutic modalities.
- Modalities include traditional allopathic pharmacotherapy and psychotherapy but also include spiritual assessments, herbal therapies, nutritional support, movement and physical manipulative therapies, mind-body therapies, and others.

INTRODUCTION

Is allopathic medicine the answer to human suffering? Medical practice is often a tool to address disruptions in the biological system but only sometimes does it focus directly on the suffering itself. It is only one tool among many that can be used to help people manage their suffering. Integrative approaches to health and well-being can help health professionals with multiple ways to help patients in need according to where they are on their journey and why they are seeking consultation. This article presents an overview of diverse approaches to the most common mental health complaints of the authors' patients: anxiety and depression. The aim is to provide some ready-to-use tools for these conditions that can supplement the allopathic approach, including guidance on the use of herbs, nutritional support, mind-body therapies, physical therapies, and behavioral therapies. These interventions are not just for those patients who have failed or are fearful of allopathic medicine. These integrative approaches can be first-line approaches when aligned with a patient's beliefs and culture and, based on evidence, as alternative methods for managing mental health and promoting well-being.

[a] Northwestern Family Medicine Residency, Erie Family Health Center, 2750 W North Avenue, Chicago, IL 60647, USA; [b] Feinberg School of Medicine, Northwestern University, 303 E Chicago Avenue, Chicago, IL 60610, USA
* Corresponding author.
E-mail address: ashah@eriefamilyhealth.org

Prim Care Clin Office Pract 44 (2017) 281–304
http://dx.doi.org/10.1016/j.pop.2017.02.003
0095-4543/17/Published by Elsevier Inc.

OVERVIEW

In modern Western medicine, physical health care has been divorced from mental health care. Integrative approaches are an important avenue for reconnecting the mind-body-spirit to human functioning. This article proposes a holistic definition of mental health from an integrative medicine perspective and depicts the salient factors and dynamics in this model. A patient-centered example provides the backdrop for how to attend to mood and mental health issues to weave together the different integrative health aspects of care from assessment through intervention. A variety of modalities that have the strongest evidence for effective treatment are discussed.

THE CONTEXT: PREVALENCE OF MENTAL DISORDERS IN PRIMARY CARE

There is strong evidence that primary care is the de facto behavioral health services and care system.[1,2] It has been estimated that 43% to 60% of patients with mental health problems are solely treated in primary care setting. Studies have also shown that the most effective response to these patients with both medical and mental health symptoms is in developing collaborative, integrated care models in primary care practices.[2–4]

Depression, anxiety, panic, somatization, and substance abuse are the most frequently cited mental health disorders in primary care[4]; 80% of people who come to primary care because of emotional and social distress come to their physician about physical signs of mood instability and stress-related symptoms. A majority of patients have no clear organic cause for their physical complaints of depression or anxiety and almost a third of patients present with multiple unexplainable symptoms.[3] Pharmacology is the most common treatment intervention recommended for emotionally distressed patients, although less than half of patients follow through with treatment. Consequently, integrative medicine holds promise in expanding options for treating mental health symptoms.

Integrative and Integrated Behavioral Health Distinctions

Integrated health care and integrative health care are 2 terms that often create confusion and need to be differentiated. Integrative health care expands and incorporates treatment modalities that are wider than allopathic interventions for the health of whole persons (mind, body, and spirit). Integrated health care refers to the collaboration between mental-behavioral health and other auxiliary providers (eg, nutritionists and dentists) with medical providers at the level of health care teams and services within an organizational system. There are areas of overlap between integrative and integrated care, especially in treatments that focus on lifestyle and behavioral interventions. This article focuses on integrative care provided within the context of a strong therapeutic relationship.

Mental Health and Integrative Care: A Case Example

Ms Zayas is a 36-year-old Latina. She has 3 children, ages 15, 12, and 9. She lives with her husband, who works long hours and is rarely home, and her mother, who helps care for the children but suffers from diabetes, hypertension, and heart disease. Ms Zayas has had a fairly stable health history except for hypertension and obesity. She comes to a clinic with complaints of fatigue, restless sleep, and vague aches and pains. On further inquiry she acknowledges feeling depressed about her current situation—financial worries and feeling trapped at home and sedentary.

Setting the Tone for Integrative Clinical Care and Mental Health

One of the goals with an integrative approach to patient care is addressing a patient not as an organism with various pathologies but as an individual. An examination of an individual's well-being should explore an individual's life purpose, meaning, and goals. Conversely, an approach to a person's *dis*-ease must address how this disruption has affected his or her journey toward those life purpose. This disruption, whether true, perceived, or subconscious, is a source of stress and can manifest itself as altered mood, such as dysthymic or anxious disorders. To address these aspects of a person's care, direct questions about meaning and purpose are valuable and enlightening. Simple questions (**Table 1**) can open the door to a rich conversation and guide treatment plans in practical ways.

Clinical Protocol

An integrative assessment can be constructed through 4 steps: framing the conversation, symptom identification and normalization, engaging the spirit, and therapeutic approach.

Step 1: framing the conversation

Ms Zayas goes on to describe her various physical complaints. She has had several months of intermittent headaches associated with upper back pain and neck pain. These episodes of pain can last up to several hours, and are alleviated by taking a nap or going for a walk. She also has been having crampy abdominal pain and bloating, worse if she has been too busy to eat a proper meal. She does not feel like her "old self." Finally, Ms Zayas complains of difficulty falling asleep. After a long day of working with her family, she finds herself tossing and turning most of the night, re-examining all of the actions of the day before and what she needs to accomplish the next day.

One of the challenges in addressing mental health issues is explaining the intricate interactions between physical, emotional, and social functioning for a patient. Using an integrative perspective, a provider can provide a basic understanding of the tridirectional interplay between body, mind, and spirit (**Fig. 1**). Examples and drawings can relate how sensations in the body have an impact on thoughts and moods as well as having an impact on purpose in life—spiritual being. Presented in a concrete way, the inter-relationships are more understandable and natural for patients. This is often

Table 1
Sample questions for patients

Inquiry into Meaning	Relating Meaning with Current Circumstances	Building a Therapeutic Plan
• What brings you joy? • What gives your life meaning? • What is most important to you in your life? • What is your life purpose? • What are your goals in life? • What makes you happiest?	• How have your current symptoms affected your practice? • How has your perspective changed since the start of your symptoms? • How do your symptoms relate to these aspects of your life?	• What can we do to help you practice your joy more often/more easily? • What are your barriers to meeting your goals, and how can we overcome them?

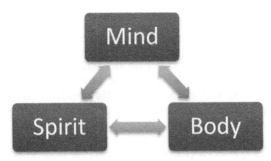

Fig. 1. Mind-body-spirit diagram.

instructive for patients who suffer from and focus on somatic sensations related to mood disorders. Explaining this dynamic interdependent, tridirectional model helps circumvent any implications that the "physical symptoms are all in your head." In framing this approach, it is helpful to use visual illustrations, to actively engage the patient in the conversation, and check for understanding.

Step 2: symptom identification and normalization

After a thorough history and a complete physical examination, the provider has ruled out many red flags for most worrisome organic causes of sleep disturbance, headache, and abdominal pain. She would like to do some basic laboratory tests to be sure but highly suspects that the symptoms are related to her depressed mood and stress.

Once the framework has been set, body sensations and mood symptoms can be listed and organized to help validate a patient's current experiences. This is especially helpful in circumstances where patients feel overwhelmed by their current state or have had a hard time expressing all of their many symptoms to providers in the past. The provider can use checklists (**Table 2**) or the diagram already drawn from the framework conversation. Listing these common manifestations of mood disturbances (somatization) can help to validate a patient's own physical symptoms and normalize the condition.

Any concerning physical symptom deserves an appropriate diagnostic work-up to rule out organic causes, but caution is also warranted to avoid further anxiety or catastrophizing by ordering too many tests. It may be important to allow a patient to

Table 2
Symptom checklists for patient validation

Mind-Mood Symptoms	Body Symptoms	Spirit/Meaning/Purpose
• Depression • Sadness • Worry • Panic • Anxiety • Stress • Fear	• Headaches, sleep disturbance (insomnia or hypersomnia), changes in energy level • Joint pains, muscle aches • Appetite changes (too much or too little), bowel changes (diarrhea or constipation), digestive issues (dyspepsia, abdominal pain, bloating) • Pelvic pain, dysuria, polyuria • Pruritis, hives • Palpitations, shortness of breath	• Hopeless • Isolation • Lack of safety • Loss of purpose

prioritize which symptoms are most pressing. This serves as a provider's guide to the order in which diagnostic work-up is handled and where to focus therapeutic approaches.

Step 3: engaging the spirit

Once symptoms re identified, it is important to explore how the myriad symptoms (both mental and physical) have had an impact on the patient's life. Simple reflective statements can go a long way: "It must be so difficult for you to have all of these symptoms. How has this affected your life?"

Ms. Zayas has felt that she has recently been more short with her children, quick to lose her temper, and easy to frustrate. Her mood and lack of energy have affected her relationship with her partner, with whom she has not had sexual desire in several months. She worries that this strain may disrupt her family even further.

Step 4: therapeutic approach

The provider should emphasize a commitment to treating not only individual symptoms in isolation but also the whole patient: mind, body, and spirit. Furthermore, the provider can also reflect that symptomatic relief is not as valuable as investigating a true cause and dealing with the root of the symptoms.

> I could prescribe you 4 different medications: 1 for your headaches, 1 for your belly pain, 1 for your insomnia, and 1 for your mood. Each medication has its own side effects and can interact with other medications. Doing so, we are only treating symptoms and not caring for the whole you.

An alternative model presented is an integrative one, which may include a diverse array of both allopathic and integrative therapies, using choices based on evidence (discussed later) (**Fig. 2**).

Patients should be informed that using more than 1 modality of therapeutics may be more powerful than any one alone. Drawing a figure may help frame an integrative approach to therapeutics. A patient is asked to choose which of the petals of the flower resonate best, knowing that the modalities may work synergistically. There is significant overlap in many of the petals. For example, yoga can be viewed as a mind-body therapy while also having value as a physical exercise and, for some, as a spiritual practice. The more petals that a patient feels comfortable engaging, the more well-rounded the therapeutic plan becomes.

> "Some patients may choose to take medications, change their diet, and do exercise. Others feel like they would like to see a counselor and try acupuncture. Which of these modalities feels right to you?" Ms Zayas agrees that she does not want to be "on a bunch of medications" for different symptoms and instead is interested in pursuing physical activity, herbal therapies, and nutritional support.

SCIENTIFIC OVERVIEW OF TREATMENT APPROACHES

This section summarizes the clinical evidence for 5 major integrative treatment approaches for managing moods: spirituality, herbs and supplements, nutrition, mind-body therapies, and leisure activities.

Spirituality

The term, *spirituality*, generally refers to those aspects of a person's life that give meaning and purpose and a sense of the transcendence in life.[5,6] Research strongly supports that having spiritual and religious beliefs is associated with greater

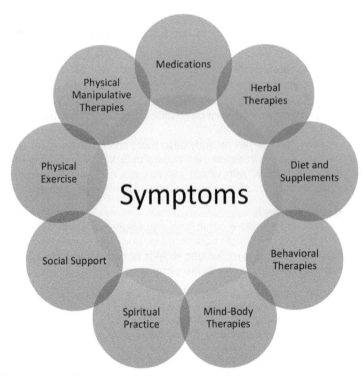

Fig. 2. Integrative model.

well-being, improved ability to cope with stress, better health outcomes, better mental health, and a sense of self and well-being[7,8] Consequently, attending to the spiritual beliefs and practices of patients can be a catalyst to address the emotional health and well-being of individuals.

Herbs

There are a host of herbs used throughout different cultures to help alleviate anguish, depression, and fear along with heightening emotional experiences. This section reviews the most common and well researched herbs for depression and anxiety. **Table 3** summarizes the indications, dosing, strength of evidence, and side effects for each of these herbs.

St. John's wort

St. John's wort (SJW) refers to the flowering plant *Hypericum perforatum*. The mechanism of action of SJW is unclear. In a recent review, researchers found antidepressant activity for multiple compounds within SJW, including hyperforin, hypericin, pseudohypericin, and several flavonoids, leading to the conclusion that the total extract containing multiple bioactive compounds contributes to the antidepressant activity.[9] Numerous trials have studied the effects of SJW on depression. In a Cochrane review, SJW was found superior to placebo and equivalent to antidepressants.[10,11] Despite these positive results, the American Psychiatric Association does not strongly endorse SJW, citing the significant heterogeneity in trial outcomes and the 2 prominent American studies that failed to show SJW superior to placebo for major depression.[12] Instead, it has been recommended that SJW be an option for patients who prefer complementary and alternative therapies, with the caveat that its evidence of efficacy is modest at best. The pooled evidence suggests SJW is efficacious for depression and its use should be encouraged in patients who refuse psychotherapy or antidepressants.

The data supporting SJW for other mood disorders, such as anxiety or bipolar disorders, are less compelling. A randomized controlled trial (RCT) found no difference between SJW and placebo.[13] According to a recent review, no RCTs have been done evaluating its use in generalized anxiety disorder, bipolar disorder, or posttraumatic stress disorder (PTSD), and a high-quality RCT showed no efficacy for social phobia.[14] Thus depression is the only disorder in which multiple high-quality studies have established the efficacy of SJW.

SJW is well tolerated: an analysis of 5570 patients found no difference between SJW and placebo in adverse events and found significantly more adverse events occurring in patients treated with paroxetine (relative risk 2.4).[15] Drug-drug interactions of SJW, however, may be more complicated and warrant caution. As an inducer of cytochrome P450 3A4, coingestion of SJW can have an impact on the plasma level of several statins, omeprazole, warfarin, verapamil, and oral contraceptives.[16] Although important to consider these interactions, not all of them serve as absolute contraindications to SJW.

Kava

Kava, typically used for patients with anxiety disorders, is an extract from the rhizome of *Piper methysticum*.[17] The precise mechanism of kava is unknown; however, the leading theory is that kavalactones interact with γ-aminobutyric acid (GABA) type A receptors.[18] A Cochrane review and another meta-analysis found that patients who were given kava had significantly reduced scores on the Hamilton Anxiety Rating Scale (HAM-A) compared with placebo.[17,19] Kava is relatively safe despite fears of hepatotoxicity. Furthermore, there are few substantiated cases of hepatotoxicity in Cochrane reviews.[17] Although this issue is one to monitor, the current evidence suggests there is low risk for hepatotoxicity when kava is taken in a safe and regulated manner.

Withania somnifera

Withania somnifera, commonly known as ashwagandha, is used in Ayurvedic medicine for a wide range of ailments and is considered an anti-inflammatory, antioxidant, adaptogen, and anxiolytic.[20] Its use as an anxiolytic is promising, but dosing in research studies have varied, from 150 mg of root extract capsules daily to 4 g of powdered root granules 3 times daily.[21]

Ginseng

The *Panax* genus includes *P ginseng* (Asian or Korean ginseng) and *Panax quinquefolius* (American ginseng). *P ginseng* is commonly used to improve cognition, alertness, and well-being and seems to effect the hypothalamic pituitary axis as well as modulate dopamine and serotonin.[14,22,23] *P quinquefolius* seems to have more of an anxiolytic effect.[24] There is overall a lack of consistent evidence for the use of either species in mood disorders, and individual response may be variable (eg, stimulant for some and anxiolytic for others). A variety of adverse side effects have been attributed to both species of herb, although side effects are rare.[22]

Rhodiola rosea

Rhodiola rosea has been used in traditional Scandanavian and Russian medicine as a psychostimulant for depression and fatigue.[25] Its active ingredient acts as a

Table 3
Herbs: dose, use, strength of evidence, and cautions

Herb	Dose/Administration	Uses	Strength of Evidence	Cautions
SJW	Usual dosing (for depression): 300 mg PO TID for up to 6 wk Studied: 500–1200 mg PO daily, 0.3%–0.5% standardized hyperforin extract	Depression	Good	Inducer of cytochrome P450 3A4: several herb-drug interactions Risk of serotonin syndrome if used in combination with other seritenergic medications
Kava	140–800 mg daily of 70% Standardized extract, usual dose 50–100 mg PO TID Root tea: 2–4 g root/150 mL water, served 1 cup PO daily TID	Anxiety	Good	Reports of hepatotoxicity
Valeriana officinalis (valerian root)	2–3 g dry root (decoction in water) 300–900 mg PO extract prior to bedtime[27]	Insomnia, restlessness	Good	Valerian decoctions have a pungent aroma, unpleasant to most Can cause headache or grogginess Should not be used in pregnancy, lactation, or in children <3 y
Lavendula angustifolia (lavender)	1–2 tsp dry herb/1 cup water (tea) Extract of 100 g dried flowers. 10-g dried leaves, or 1–4 drops essential oil in 1 L hot water[31]	Anxiety, insomnia, depression (adjuvant)	Limited, but promising.[23,31]	Essential oils NOT generally recommended for ingestion- only topical or aromatherapy[27] Topical use may cause contact dermatitis or allergic reaction
Humulus lupulus (Hops)	0.5 g dried herb as needed.[31]	Anxiety, insomnia	Poor in vivo	Sedation, contact dermatitis
Melissa officinalis (lemon balm)	Tea of 1.5–4.5 g dried leaf in 150 mL water[31] Aromatherapy oil	Anxiety, insomnia	Promising, limited	Very safe, possible gastrointestinal upset in high oral doses. Contact dermatitis and irritation possible with topical use[29]

P ginseng (Asian ginseng, Korean ginseng) P quinquefolius (American ginseng)	0.5–2 g dry root daily (limit to 1 g daily for long-term use) 200–600 mg extract daily[22]	Anxiety, depression (adaptogen)	Poor	Several reported adverse effects, including changes in vaginal bleeding, insomnia, euphoria, mania, headache, vertigo, and Stevens-Johnson syndrome[22]
R rosea (rose root, arctic root, golden root)	Depression: 340–680 mg extract daily[28] Anxiety: 170 mg BID Adaptogen: 100–300 mg rosavins and salidroside 3 times daily[27,100]	Depression, possible anxiolysis (adaptogen)	Promising, few data	Limited evidence, but so far good safety and well tolerated
Matricaria recutita (chamomile)	50 g crude flower per 1 L water[31] Anxiety: 220–1100 mg daily for 8 wk[100]	Anxiety, stress, insomnia	Promising, few data	Very good safety profile
Withania somnifera (ashwagandha, winter cherry, Indian ginseng)	Root extract capsules 150 mg–300 mg PO daily to twice daily[21] Granules of root extract 1–6 g daily to TID, up to 12 g total/d[27]	Anxiety, stress, adaptogen	Promising, few data	Good safety profile[20]

monoamine oxidase A inhibitor as well as inhibiting cortisol and normalizing effects of serotonin.[26] It is primary use as an antidepressant and stimulant, although it may also reduce anxiety.[14,27] The research on *R rosea* is limited and most studies are poorly designed or have limited power. There is some evidence, however, that its antidepressant properties are promising and it is well tolerated.[28]

Lemon balm
Melissa officinalis (lemon balm) is used topically, as aromatherapy, and ingested, primarily as a tea. It has a long history of traditional uses, primarily in Europe and the Middle Eastern cultures.[29] Lemon balm has cholinergic receptor-binding properties and patients using it have reported improved memory and increased calmness compared with placebo.[30]

Hops
The sedating and anxiolytic properties of hops was first noticed by reports that farm workers who pick the flowers for beer production suffered from fatigue while working.[31] Aromatic compounds released during the harvesting have been subsequently noted to act as an agonist to the melatonin receptor.[23,26] The compounds that are present at fresh-picking are highly volatile, however, and are not present in high concentrations in the dried form of the plant limiting its therapeutic potential.[31]

Lavender
Lavender is well known for its calming effects as an aromatherapy and is popular in candles, soaps, and other home products. True lavender is the species of flower *Lavendula angustifolia*. Animal studies demonstrate similar effects on GABA receptors as benzodiazepines and barbiturates, increasing sedation. Lavender aromatherapy has also been shown to effect electroencephalographic potentials in humans, corresponding to sedation and relaxation.[31] Few studies have been done on oral doses of lavender, although a small double-blind RCT demonstrated that 1:5 lavender tincture (50% alcohol) was associated with improvement in Hamilton Anxiety Rating Scale (HAM-D) depression scores when administered as an adjunctive therapy to standard pharmacotherapy.[32] Aromatherapy studies are also promising but are difficult to evaluate given the inability to blind patients to the study design.[31] Given its overall safety, it is a safe adjunct for insomnia and anxiety. Allergic reactions to even small exposures are possible, and all patients should generally be advised against ingesting essential oils.[27]

Matricaria recutita
Matricaria recutita (chamomile) is often used in teas for insomnia, and there is some limited evidence that chamomile may have anxiolytic effects.[33] Active compounds from the flowers have been found to have benzodiazepine-like properties, binding GABA receptors, whereas other components also serve a neuroendocrine function and affect monoamine neurotransmission.[23] As a safe herb in tea, it is reasonable to suggest it as a part of a broader plan or adjunctive therapy for sleep and muscle tension. As with many of the anxiolytic and sedative herbs, it is commonly found in combination with others in commercially available teas; however, higher doses are needed for therapeutic effects.[30]

Genus Valeriana
Genus *Valeriana* is found worldwide, with more than 250 species. The root of *Valeriana officinalis* is most studied for its sedative and hypnotic properties; it acts as a GABA agonist, partial serotonin agonist, and adenosine-1 receptor modulator.[23] Use of valerian extract has been shown to result in significant electroencephalographic waveform

changes corresponding to sedation, improved sleep quality, and reduced sleep latency.[31] Because it is highly sedating, it is a reasonable adjunct for patients with anxiety and coexisting insomnia.

Supplements/Vitamins/Minerals

Omega-3

Omega-3 fatty acids are polyunsaturated fatty acids that are present at significant levels in some nuts, seeds, and fish. Fish oil has 2 specific omega-3 fatty acids as its bioactive components: docosahexaenoic acid (DHA) and eicosapentaenoic acid (EPA).[34] The mechanism of omega-3 fatty acids is not certain, but proposed theories have suggested it alters neurotransmitter receptor concentrations, has therapeutic anti-inflammatory effects, or it has a positive impact on neuronal plasticity.[35]

Data suggest omega-3 fatty acids have a statistically significant effect on depression. A Cochrane review looking at RCTs involving omega-3 fatty acids found a significant decrease in depressive symptoms.[36] Several studies have indicated higher EPA dosage (more than 60%) is associated with improved outcome.[37] Several small RCTs have found decreased anxiety scores in various patient populations taking combinations of EPA and DHA, but larger RCTs for specific disorders are needed before recommendations can be made.[35] Current evidence suggests a similar rate of adverse events when taking omega-3 fatty acids as placebo.[36]

S-adenosylmethionine

S-adenosylmethionine (SAM-e) is a cosubstrate used in cellular pathways that involve methylation, transulfuration, and aminopropylation.[38] The mechanism of SAM-e is unclear, but postulated theories include that its antidepressant effects are secondary to phospholipid methylation, DNA methylation, or neurotransmitter synthesis.[38] Regarding efficacy, numerous RCTs have found SAM-e superior to placebo and equivalent to antidepressants for treating depression.[38–40] SAM-e also has potential as an augmenter for treatment-resistant depression, with 1 RCT finding adjunctive SAM-e to significantly improve HAM-D response and remission rates.[41] Overall SAM-e has been tolerated significantly better than tricyclic antidepressants but does result in occasional complaints of gastrointestinal symptoms, headaches, fatigue, and anxiety (**Table 4**).[38]

Relaxation Response and Mood

Mind-body medicine practices are a diverse group of clinical practices that focus on the interactions between the brain, mind, body, and behavior, with the goal of harnessing the power of the mind to affect physical functioning and promote health. The most common practices for the stress reduction and enhancing the relaxation response are meditation, mindfulness, yoga, progressive muscle relaxation (PMR), biofeedback, and hypnosis. The goals of these practices are to alleviate stress and enhance the relaxation response through intentional and focused cognitive processes.

Mindfulness-based stress reduction

Over the past 2 decades, a structured intervention called mindfulness-based stress reduction (MBSR) has become an empirically supported, gold standard mind-body medicine approach for helping people reduce stress and manage disease and treatment related sequelae across multiple medical conditions.[42–45] Based primarily on the instruction of mindfulness meditation and yoga, MBSR is a group-based, 8-week program that was developed at the University of Massachusetts Stress Reduction Clinic under the direction of Jon Kabat-Zinn.[46] As a nonreligious practice, MBSR

Table 4
Herbs and supplements

Name	Dose	Use	Strength of Evidence	Cautions
Folate	Folic acid 200–500 μg/d, folinic acid 15–30 mg/d, or 5-methyltetrahydrofolate 15–90 mg/d[101]	Depression	Good[101,102]	Large doses can mask vitamin B_{12} deficiency
Magnesium	200–450 mg/d of elemental magnesium used in studies; recommended upper limit of 350 mg/d[103–106]	Depression	Good[104–106]	Most common side effect is diarrhea with possible abdominal cramping and nausea if taken above 360 mg/d[103] Caution in individuals with renal impairment[103]
Melatonin	0.5–6 mg/d for depression[107] 3–15 mg dose 60–90 min prior to surgery for preoperative anxiety[108]	Preoperative anxiety Depression	Good[107,108]	Headaches, dizziness, drowsiness and nausearates similar to placebo[109]
Zinc	7–25 mg/d of elemental zinc taken orally[110]	Depression[110] Attention-deficit/hyperactivity disorder[111] Obsessive-compulsive disorder[112]	Good[110–112]	Gastrointestinal symptoms and headaches have been reported.[113]
Serotonin or L-tryptophan	1 g/d L-tryptophan orally or 3 g/d serotonin orally[114–116]	Depression	Good[26,114,117]	Epigastric pain, dizziness, and diarrhea may occur.[114]

Vitamin D	No consensus. Trials range from 400 IU/ to 1-time doses of 500,000 IU.[118,119]	Depression	Poor[118,120,121]	None
Dehydroepiandrosterone	Most studies use 90 mg/d but has been used up to 450 mg/d[122–124]	Depression	Good[122–125]	Occasional dermatologic issues, such as acne[122–124,126]
Omega-3 fatty acids or fish oil	Oral supplement of 1–4 g/d with at least 60% EPA with 400 mg to 2000 mg EPA in excess of DPA[36,127]	Depression Anxiety	Excellent for depression[36,37] Good for anxiety[35]	Prescribe cautiously in patients with prostate cancer, given there is a potential association.[128]
SAM-e	150–400 mg/d parenterally or 1600–3200 mg/d orally[38,40]	Depression	Good[38–41]	Tolerated better than tricyclic antidepressants, but occasional complaints of gastrointestinal symptoms, headaches, fatigue, and anxiety have been reported.[38]
N-acetylcysteine	1–1.5 g twice/d orally[129]	Depression Anxiety Bipolar	Excellent for depression[129] Limited for anxiety[130] Good for bipolar[130]	Slight risk of nausea, heartburn, and joint pain[129]

facilitates the cultivation of nonjudgmental, moment-to-moment awareness through a process of attentional single-focus called mindfulness. Numerous RCTs have been conducted on MBSR across different disease groups and clinical conditions, including mental health dysfunction.[21] These studies have demonstrated that MBSR can lead to significant reductions in emotional distress (depression and anxiety) and pain and improvements in sleep and overall health-related quality of life.[47–50]

Progressive muscle relaxation

PMR is another strategy used to develop the relaxation response and promote healthier emotional functioning. This technique is designed for individuals to practice tightening and loosening muscle groups with the goal of easing muscle tension throughout the body. Individuals who practice this technique gain the capacity to reduce their anxiety symptoms and stress for cancer patients and caregivers.[51,52] In a meta-analysis, PMR and relaxation techniques were less effective than cognitive behavior therapy in managing depression but better than no treatment.[53,54]

Hypnosis

Hypnosis is a form of relaxation that has been an effective treatment of state anxiety (eg, prior to tests, surgery, procedures, irritable bowel syndrome, and headaches). It is a form of relaxation training that incorporates suggestions and guidance from a trained provider to improve an individual's functioning. The evidence for using hypnosis, however, to treat generalized anxiety, PTSD, or phobias is not well established [55,56] A small number of limited studies suggest that hypnosis may be effective for the treatment of depression.[57]

Biofeedback

Biofeedback and neurofeedback are techniques that use monitoring systems via noninvasive electrical devices to record physiologic measures, such as heart rate, respiration, skin temperature, and blood flow. These feedback monitoring systems can be used to train individuals to modify their brain and body patterns by focusing on ways to alter their physical and cognitive activity and create a less stressful, aroused physiologic state.[58] Biofeedback is usually an adjunct treatment of patients with mental health disorders and has been shown that in combination with other treatments it can decrease stress and reduce anxiety.[59] Autogenic training and heart rate variability are 2 specific forms of biofeedback that have a small number of studies that demonstrate their effectiveness in treating anxiety or depression.[60]

Manipulative Physical Therapies and Energy Medicine

Massage

Massage therapy (MT) typically refers to manipulating the body's soft tissues.[61] Massage sessions range from 15 minutes to 90 minutes and most studies that have assessed their use in mood disorder have involved between 5 and 32 total sessions given once or twice per week. The mechanism of MT is unclear, although 1 review suggests its presumed psychological benefits are due to pressure leading to a vagal nerve–mediated relaxation response.[42] A recent open-label study found MT more effective than placebo and light touch at reducing HAM-D scores.[43] Another RCT analyzing MT for generalized anxiety disorder found no difference in outcome between MT, thermotherapy, and being placed in a relaxing room.[44] More research is needed to determine the effectiveness of MT in adult or pediatric populations for anxiety or depressive disorders. The only significant adverse event with MT is that 10% of patients report muscle soreness after treatment, suggesting MT has a benign side-effect profile.[45]

Osteopathic manipulative treatment and chiropractic manipulation

Osteopathic manipulative treatment (OMT) refers to a range of techniques that can include soft tissue stretching, spinal manipulation, and resisted isometric stretches.[46] Sessions reported in the literature typically ranged from 15 minutes to 30 minutes and were given from daily to weekly for a total of 3 sessions to 7 sessions.[62–64] Few data on the efficacy of OMT are available. One blinded RCT found OMT used as an adjunct to paroxetine and psychotherapy significantly improved depressive symptoms; however, small sample sizes and potential demographic differences limit the conclusions that can be drawn from this study.[63] A study on OMT for medical students found it significantly reduced fatigue but did not alter stress or depression whereas a study of patients with cystic fibrosis found no relation between OMT and anxiety.[62,64] High-quality studies with power analyses are necessary before the relationship between OMT and anxiety or depressive disorders can be determined.

Chiropractic therapy involves passive manual maneuvers in which 3-joint complexes are carried outside of their normal physiologic range without compromising anatomic integrity.[65] Data on the effectiveness of chiropractic therapy for the management of chronic anxiety or depressive conditions are limited to 2 case studies.[48,66] Chiropractic therapy is relatively safe, with 1 RCT showing no significant difference in rate of adverse events between chiropractic therapy and sham treatment.[49]

Reiki

Reiki is an energy medicine technique originating in Japan in which trained healers pass healing energy to a patient through direct physical contact or intention from a distance.[50] Most research studies consist of one to two 30-minute to 45-minute sessions per week for a total of 6 to 16 sessions.[67] A Cochrane review evaluating the impact of reiki on depression and anxiety identified 3 RCTs, none of which has shown a statistically significant impact.[67] A more recent crossover study suggests reiki may reduce burnout in mental health clinicians; however, further high-quality studies are necessary to establish if reiki has a significant effect on stress, depression, or anxiety disorders.[68]

Procedural therapies

Acupuncture

Acupuncture is one part of traditional Chinese medicine dating back to the first century BCE. The classical Eastern teaching of acupuncture relies on the unhindered flow of vital energy translated as *qi* (pronounced "chee") through specific channels, or meridians, in the body. Acupuncture relies on the use of small, thin needles to stimulate the flow of qi. The risks of acupuncture are minimal and include infection generally caused by using unsterilized needles or the extremely rare possibility of puncturing an organ if inserted too deeply. Western medicine has slowly come to accept and incorporate acupuncture as an appropriate mode of therapy for various conditions. A World Health Organization consensus article in 2003 endorsed the use of acupuncture for various types of medical conditions, including depression, as well as supporting likely benefit for anxiety disorders, schizophrenia, and addiction.[69–73] Since that time an increase in literature has arisen, confirming the benefit of acupuncture for depression, in particular, as an adjunct to traditional treatment with selective serotonin reuptake inhibitors. Some smaller promising studies have shown benefits for generalized anxiety as well as PTSD.[74,75]

Bright light therapies

Bright light therapies have been another treatment of depression that has strong evidence for seasonal affective disorder, moderate support for nonseasonal depression, and as an adjunctive treatment to other forms of drug resistant depression.[76–79] Bright light therapies generally suggest that patients use a broad spectrum light (10,000 lux) placed 40.64 cm to 60.96 cm away from the face for 20 minutes to 30 minutes every day for 2 weeks to 5 weeks to alleviate symptoms of depression.[80,81] The standards for administering bright light therapies are not well defined, however, and studies have not used uniform dosing for the intensity, frequency, and duration of this treatment.[79,82] Consequently, the guidelines for the dosing of this treatment still need to be evaluated and standardized.[77]

Leisure activities

The positive effects of physical activity on depression has been the focus of numerous studies. Physical activity in nonclinical groups of adolescents and adults improves symptoms of depressive symptoms.[83,84] Physical activity alone and in combination with medication for treatment of depression has been shown effective with adolescents, adults, older adults, and schizophrenics.[85–88] Physical activity for anxiety disorders yields a more mixed picture. Exercise can exacerbate anxiety in some studies while alleviating anxiety symptoms in others.[86,89] Leisure activities and supportive or art therapies have been shown to have mostly a positive effect on emotional and mental health. Laughter therapies, for example, have had positive effects on depression and insomnia, especially with seniors.[90–92] Dance and music therapy have also been used to treat depression and enhance healthy expression of emotions.[93,94] The studies on the overall effectiveness of dance-movement therapies has limited evidence, however, to demonstrate its effectiveness.[95] Bibliotherapy, where patients read personal narratives or self-help books, have some promising approaches to enhance treatments of depression.[96–98] Pet therapy has achieved more recognition in the treatment of depression and loneliness. Encouraging elderly or isolated individuals to have a pet has been show to decrease loneliness and depression and enhance quality of life.[99] In general, these alternative psychosocial-oriented approaches to treatment are promising approaches that could be included in patient care to not only treat depression and anxiety but also enhance well-being and emotional health.

SUMMARY

Integrative medicine holds a treasure chest of opportunities and interventions to support, manage, and treat an individual's mental and emotional health. This model of care is centered on exploring a patient's purpose and meaning in life and using person-centered and collaborative communication between patients and providers to investigate a range of therapeutic options. Although the options are considerable, the evidence to support these types of interventions is limited. Spirituality and MBSR have the strongest foundation for empiric support for mood and mental health. A vast majority of studies in the area of herbs, supplements, relaxation, and expressive therapies have significant limitations in the recruitment of and limited number of subjects, poor sampling strategies, poor quality of research design, and poor power within studies to determine statistical significance. Consequently, there needs to be concerted effort to support the research to develop an evidence base for these treatments so that clinicians are armed with the data needed to guide patients to their optimal emotional health.

REFERENCES

1. Baird M, Blount A, Brungardt S, et al. Joint principles: integrating behavioral health care into the patient-centered medical home. Ann Fam Med 2014; 12(2):183–5.

2. Blount A. Getting mental health care where it is needed. Fam Syst Health 2013; 31(2):117–8.
3. Kessler R. Identifying and screening for psychological and comorbid medical and psychological disorders in medical settings. J Clin Psychol 2009;65(3): 253–67.
4. Kessler R, Miller BF, Kelly M, et al. Mental health, substance abuse, and health behavior services in patient-centered medical homes. J Am Board Fam Med 2014;27(5):637–44.
5. Bonelli RM, Koenig HG. Mental disorders, religion and spirituality 1990 to 2010: a systematic evidence-based review. J Relig Health 2013;52(2):657–73.
6. Koenig HG. Research on religion, spirituality, and mental health: a review. Can J Psychiatry 2009;54(5):283.
7. Koenig HG, Berk LS, Daher NS, et al. Religious involvement is associated with greater purpose, optimism, generosity and gratitude in persons with major depression and chronic medical illness. J Psychosom Res 2014;77(2):135–43.
8. Moreira-Almeida A, Koenig HG, Lucchetti G. Clinical implications of spirituality to mental health: review of evidence and practical guidelines. Rev Bras Psiquiatr 2014;36(2):176–82.
9. Butterweck V, Schmidt M. St. John's wort: role of active compounds for its mechanism of action and efficacy. Wien Med Wochenschr 2007;157(13–14):356–61.
10. Linde K, Berner MM, Kriston L. St John's wort for major depression. Cochrane Database Syst Rev 2008;(4):CD000448.
11. Gartlehner G, Gaynes BN, Amick HR, et al. Comparative benefits and harms of antidepressant, psychological, complementary, and exercise treatments for major depression: an evidence report for a clinical practice guideline from the American College of Physicians. Ann Intern Med 2016;164(5):331–41.
12. Freeman MP, Fava M, Lake J, et al. Complementary and alternative medicine in major depressive disorder: the American Psychiatric Association Task Force report. J Clin Psychiatry 2010;71(6):669–81.
13. Kobak KA, Taylor LV, Bystritsky A, et al. St John's wort versus placebo in obsessive-compulsive disorder: results from a double-blind study. Int Clin Psychopharmacol 2005;20(6):299–304.
14. Sarris J. St. John's wort for the treatment of psychiatric disorders. Psychiatr Clin North Am 2013;36(1):65–72.
15. Kasper S, Gastpar M, Moller HJ, et al. Better tolerability of St. John's wort extract WS 5570 compared to treatment with SSRIs: a reanalysis of data from controlled clinical trials in acute major depression. Int Clin Psychopharmacol 2010;25(4): 204–13.
16. Izzo AA. Drug interactions with St. John's Wort (Hypericum perforatum): a review of the clinical evidence. Int J Clin Pharmacol Ther 2004;42(3):139–48.
17. Pittler MH, Ernst E. Kava extract for treating anxiety. Cochrane Database Syst Rev 2003;(1):CD003383.
18. Chua HC, Christensen ET, Hoestgaard-Jensen K, et al. Kavain, the Major constituent of the anxiolytic kava extract, potentiates GABAA receptors: functional characteristics and molecular mechanism. PLoS One 2016;11(6):e0157700.
19. Witte S, Loew D, Gaus W. Meta-analysis of the efficacy of the acetonic kava-kava extract WS1490 in patients with non-psychotic anxiety disorders. Phytother Res 2005;19(3):183–8.
20. Kulkarni SK, Dhir A. Withania somnifera: an Indian ginseng. Prog Neuropsychopharmacol Biol Psychiatry 2008;32(5):1093–105.

21. Pratte MA, Nanavati KB, Young V, et al. An alternative treatment for anxiety: a systematic review of human trial results reported for the Ayurvedic herb ashwagandha (Withania somnifera). J Altern Complement Med 2014;20(12):901–8.
22. Ernst E. The risk-benefit profile of commonly used herbal therapies: Ginkgo, St. John's Wort, Ginseng, Echinacea, Saw Palmetto, and Kava. Ann Intern Med 2002;136(1):42–53.
23. Sarris J, Panossian A, Schweitzer I, et al. Herbal medicine for depression, anxiety and insomnia: a review of psychopharmacology and clinical evidence. Eur Neuropsychopharmacol 2011;21(12):841–60.
24. Scholey A, Ossoukhova A, Owen L, et al. Effects of American ginseng (Panax quinquefolius) on neurocognitive function: an acute, randomised, double-blind, placebo-controlled, crossover study. Psychopharmacology 2010;212(3):345–56.
25. Romm AJ. In: Hardy ML, Mills S, editors. Botanical medicine for women's health. Saint Louis (MO): Churchill Livingstone; 2010. p. iv.
26. Sarris J, Murphy J, Mischoulon D, et al. Adjunctive nutraceuticals for depression: a systematic review and meta-analyses. Am J Psychiatry 2016;173(6):575–87.
27. Low Dog T. Botanical foundations. In: Medicine ACfI, editor. Fellowship in integrative medicine 2017 fall. Univeristy of Arizona; 2016.
28. Amsterdam JD, Panossian AG. Rhodiola rosea L. as a putative botanical antidepressant. Phytomedicine 2016;23(7):770–83.
29. Shakeri A, Sahebkar A, Javadi B. Melissa officinalis L. - A review of its traditional uses, phytochemistry and pharmacology. J Ethnopharmacol 2016;188:204–28.
30. Kennedy DO, Wake G, Savelev S, et al. Modulation of mood and cognitive performance following acute administration of single doses of Melissa officinalis (Lemon balm) with human CNS nicotinic and muscarinic receptor-binding properties. Neuropsychopharmacology 2003;28(10):1871–81.
31. Schulz V, Telger TC, Hansel R, et al. Rational phytotherapy: a reference guide for physicians and pharmacists. Berlin: Springer; 2004.
32. Akhondzadeh S, Kashani L, Fotouhi A, et al. Comparison of Lavandula angustifolia Mill. tincture and imipramine in the treatment of mild to moderate depression: a double-blind, randomized trial. Prog Neuropsychopharmacol Biol Psychiatry 2003;27(1):123–7.
33. Amsterdam JD, Li Y, Soeller I, et al. A randomized, double-blind, placebo-controlled trial of oral Matricaria recutita (chamomile) extract therapy for generalized anxiety disorder. J Clin Psychopharmacol 2009;29(4):378–82.
34. Yang JR, Han D, Qiao ZX, et al. Combined application of eicosapentaenoic acid and docosahexaenoic acid on depression in women: a meta-analysis of double-blind randomized controlled trials. Neuropsychiatr Dis Treat 2015;11:2055–61.
35. Su KP, Matsuoka Y, Pae CU. Omega-3 polyunsaturated fatty acids in prevention of mood and anxiety disorders. Clin Psychopharmacol Neurosci 2015;13(2):129–37.
36. Appleton KM, Sallis HM, Perry R, et al. Omega-3 fatty acids for depression in adults. Cochrane Database Syst Rev 2015;(11):CD004692.
37. Martins JG, Bentsen H, Puri BK. Eicosapentaenoic acid appears to be the key omega-3 fatty acid component associated with efficacy in major depressive disorder: a critique of Bloch and Hannestad and updated meta-analysis. Mol Psychiatry 2012;17(12):1144–9 [discussion: 1163–7].
38. Papakostas GI. Evidence for S-adenosyl-L-methionine (SAM-e) for the treatment of major depressive disorder. J Clin Psychiatry 2009;70(Suppl 5):18–22.

39. De Berardis D, Orsolini L, Serroni N, et al. A comprehensive review on the efficacy of S-adenosyl-L-methionine in major depressive disorder. CNS Neurol Disord Drug Targets 2016;15(1):35–44.
40. Mischoulon D, Price LH, Carpenter LL, et al. A double-blind, randomized, placebo-controlled clinical trial of S-adenosyl-L-methionine (SAMe) versus escitalopram in major depressive disorder. J Clin Psychiatry 2014;75(4):370–6.
41. Papakostas GI, Mischoulon D, Shyu I, et al. S-adenosyl methionine (SAMe) augmentation of serotonin reuptake inhibitors for antidepressant nonresponders with major depressive disorder: a double-blind, randomized clinical trial. Am J Psychiatry 2010;167(8):942–8.
42. Field T. Massage therapy research review. Complement Ther Clin Pract 2014; 20(4):224–9.
43. Poland RE, Gertsik L, Favreau JT, et al. Open-label, randomized, parallel-group controlled clinical trial of massage for treatment of depression in HIV-infected subjects. J Altern Complement Med 2013;19(4):334–40.
44. Sherman KJ, Ludman EJ, Cook AJ, et al. Effectiveness of therapeutic massage for generalized anxiety disorder: a randomized controlled trial. Depress Anxiety 2010;27(5):441–50.
45. Cambron JA, Dexheimer J, Coe P, et al. Side-effects of massage therapy: a cross-sectional study of 100 clients. J Altern Complement Med 2007;13(8): 793–6.
46. Franke H, Franke JD, Fryer G. Osteopathic manipulative treatment for nonspecific low back pain: a systematic review and meta-analysis. BMC Musculoskelet Disord 2014;15:286.
47. CADTH Rapid Response Reports. Mindfulness interventions for the treatment of post-traumatic stress disorder, generalized anxiety disorder, depression, and substance use disorders: a review of the clinical effectiveness and guidelines. Ottawa (Ontario): Canadian Agency for Drugs and Technologies in Health; 2015.
48. Elster EL. Treatment of bipolar, seizure, and sleep disorders and migraine headaches utilizing a chiropractic technique. J Manipulative Physiol Ther 2004;27(3): E5.
49. Walker BF, Hebert JJ, Stomski NJ, et al. Outcomes of usual chiropractic. The OUCH randomized controlled trial of adverse events. Spine 2013;38(20): 1723–9.
50. Rakel D. Integrative medicine. Philadelphia: Elsevier Saunders; 2012.
51. Charalambous A, Giannakopoulou M, Bozas E, et al. A randomized controlled trial for the effectiveness of progressive muscle relaxation and guided imagery as anxiety reducing interventions in breast and prostate cancer patients undergoing chemotherapy. Evid Based Complement Alternat Med 2015;2015: 270876.
52. Choi YK. The effect of music and progressive muscle relaxation on anxiety, fatigue, and quality of life in family caregivers of hospice patients. J music Ther 2010;47(1):53–69.
53. Hashim HA, Hanafi Ahmad Yusof H. The effects of progressive muscle relaxation and autogenic relaxation on young soccer players' mood states. Asian J Sports Med 2011;2(2):99–105.
54. Jorm AF, Morgan AJ, Hetrick SE. Relaxation for depression. Cochrane database Syst Rev 2008;(4):CD007142.
55. Pelissolo A. Hypnosis for anxiety and phobic disorders: a review of clinical studies. Presse Med 2016;45(3):284–90.

56. Hammond DC. Hypnosis in the treatment of anxiety- and stress-related disorders. Expert Rev Neurother 2010;10(2):263–73.

57. Shih M, Yang YH, Koo M. A meta-analysis of hypnosis in the treatment of depressive symptoms: a brief communication. Int J Clin Exp Hypn 2009;57(4):431–42.

58. CADTH Rapid Response Reports. Neurofeedback and biofeedback for mood and anxiety disorders: a review of the clinical evidence and guidelines - an update. Ottawa (ON): Canadian Agency for Drugs and Technologies in Health; 2014.

59. Schoenberg PL, David AS. Biofeedback for psychiatric disorders: a systematic review. Appl psychophysiology biofeedback. 2014;39(2):109–35.

60. Lee J, Kim JK, Wachholtz A. The benefit of heart rate variability biofeedback and relaxation training in reducing trait anxiety. Hanguk Simni Hakhoe Chi Kongang 2015;20(2):391–408.

61. Hollis M. Massage for therapists: a guide to soft tissue therapy. 3rd edition. Ames (IA): Wiley-Blackwell; 2009.

62. Swender DA, Thompson G, Schneider K, et al. Osteopathic manipulative treatment for inpatients with pulmonary exacerbations of cystic fibrosis: effects on spirometry findings and patient assessments of breathing, anxiety, and pain. J Am Osteopath Assoc 2014;114(6):450–8.

63. Plotkin BJ, Rodos JJ, Kappler R, et al. Adjunctive osteopathic manipulative treatment in women with depression: a pilot study. J Am Osteopath Assoc 2001;101(9):517–23.

64. Wiegand S, Bianchi W, Quinn TA, et al. Osteopathic manipulative treatment for self-reported fatigue, stress, and depression in first-year osteopathic medical students. J Am Osteopath Assoc 2015;115(2):84–93.

65. Ernst E. Manual therapies for pain control: chiropractic and massage. Clin J Pain 2004;20(1):8–12.

66. Tsai JF. A case of chiropractic manipulation immediately relieving depression with chronic pain. J Altern Complement Med 2009;15(6):611–2.

67. Joyce J, Herbison GP. Reiki for depression and anxiety. Cochrane Database Syst Rev 2015;(4):CD006833.

68. Rosada RM, Rubik B, Mainguy B, et al. Reiki reduces burnout among community mental health clinicians. J Altern Complement Med 2015;21(8):489–95.

69. Acupuncture: Review and Analysis of Reports on Controlled Clinical Trials. World Health Organization; 2002.

70. Andreescu C, Mulsant BH, Emanuel JE. Complementary and alternative medicine in the treatment of bipolar disorder–a review of the evidence. J Affect Disord 2008;110(1–2):16–26.

71. Au DW, Tsang HW, Ling PP, et al. Effects of acupressure on anxiety: a systematic review and meta-analysis. Acupunct Med 2015;33(5):353–9.

72. Bae H, Bae H, Min BI, et al. Efficacy of acupuncture in reducing preoperative anxiety: a meta-analysis. Evid Based Complement Alternat Med 2014;2014:850367.

73. Goyata SL, Avelino CC, Santos SV, et al. Effects from acupuncture in treating anxiety: integrative review. Rev Bras Enferm 2016;69(3):602–9.

74. Chan YY, Lo WY, Yang SN, et al. The benefit of combined acupuncture and antidepressant medication for depression: A systematic review and meta-analysis. J Affect Disord 2015;176:106–17.

75. Bazzan AJ, Zabrecky G, Monti DA, et al. Current evidence regarding the management of mood and anxiety disorders using complementary and alternative medicine. Expert Rev Neurother 2014;14(4):411–23.

76. Al-Karawi D, Jubair L. Bright light therapy for nonseasonal depression: meta-analysis of clinical trials. J Affect Disord 2016;198:64–71.

77. Nussbaumer B, Kaminski-Hartenthaler A, Forneris CA, et al. Light therapy for preventing seasonal affective disorder. Cochrane Database Syst Rev 2015;(11):CD011269.

78. Camardese G, Leone B, Serrani R, et al. Augmentation of light therapy in difficult-to-treat depressed patients: an open-label trial in both unipolar and bipolar patients. Neuropsychiatr Dis Treat 2015;11:2331–8.

79. Golden RN, Gaynes BN, Ekstrom RD, et al. The efficacy of light therapy in the treatment of mood disorders: a review and meta-analysis of the evidence. Am J Psychiatry 2005;162(4):656–62.

80. Virk G, Reeves G, Rosenthal NE, et al. Short exposure to light treatment improves depression scores in patients with seasonal affective disorder: a brief report. Int J Disabil Hum Dev 2009;8(3):283.

81. Melrose S. Seasonal affective disorder: an overview of assessment and treatment approaches (Disease/Disorder overview). Depress Res Treat 2015;2015:178564.

82. Jonas DE, Cusack K, Forneris CA, et al. AHRQ comparative effectiveness reviews. Psychological and pharmacological treatments for adults with posttraumatic stress disorder (PTSD). Rockville (MD): Agency for Healthcare Research and Quality (US); 2013.

83. Melo MC, Daher Ede F, Albuquerque SG, et al. Exercise in bipolar patients: a systematic review. J Affect Disord 2016;198:32–8.

84. Carter T, Morres ID, Meade O, et al. The effect of exercise on depressive symptoms in adolescents: a systematic review and meta-analysis. J Am Acad Child Adolesc Psychiatry 2016;55(7):580–90.

85. Danielsson L, Noras AM, Waern M, et al. Exercise in the treatment of major depression: a systematic review grading the quality of evidence. Physiother Theory Pract 2013;29(8):573–85.

86. Dauwan M, Begemann MJ, Heringa SM, et al. Exercise improves clinical symptoms, quality of life, global functioning, and depression in schizophrenia: a systematic review and meta-analysis. Schizophr Bull 2016;42(3):588–99.

87. Park SH, Han KS, Kang CB. Effects of exercise programs on depressive symptoms, quality of life, and self-esteem in older people: a systematic review of randomized controlled trials. Appl Nurs Res 2014;27(4):219–26.

88. Schuch FB, Vancampfort D, Rosenbaum S, et al. Exercise improves physical and psychological quality of life in people with depression: A meta-analysis including the evaluation of control group response. Psychiatry Res 2016;241:47–54.

89. Ensari I, Greenlee TA, Motl RW, et al. Meta-analysis of acute exercise effects on state anxiety: an update of randomized controlled trials over the past 25 years. Depress Anxiety 2015;32(8):624–34.

90. Foley E, Matheis R, Schaefer C. Effect of forced laughter on mood. Psychol Rep 2002;90(1):184.

91. Ko HJ, Youn CH. Effects of laughter therapy on depression, cognition and sleep among the community-dwelling elderly. Geriatr Gerontol Int 2011;11(3):267–74.

92. Konradt B, Hirsch RD, Jonitz MF, et al. Evaluation of a standardized humor group in a clinical setting: a feasibility study for older patients with depression. Int J Geriatr Psychiatry 2013;28(8):850–7.

93. Akandere M, Demir B. The effect of dance over depression. Coll Antropol 2011; 35(3):651–6.

94. Murrock CJ, Graor CH. Effects of dance on depression, physical function, and disability in underserved adults. J Aging Phys Act 2014;22(3):380–5.

95. Meekums B, Karkou V, Nelson EA. Dance movement therapy for depression. Cochrane Database Syst Rev 2015;(2):CD009895.

96. Moldovan R, Cobeanu O, David D. Cognitive bibliotherapy for mild depressive symptomatology: randomized clinical trial of efficacy and mechanisms of change. Clin Psychol psychotherapy 2013;20(6):482–93.

97. Naylor EV, Antonuccio DO, Litt M, et al. Bibliotherapy as a treatment for depression in primary care. J Clin Psychol Med Settings 2010;17(3):258–71.

98. Fanner D, Urquhart C. Bibliotherapy for mental health service users Part 1: a systematic review. Health Info Libr J 2008;25(4):237–52.

99. Creagan ET, Bauer BA, Thomley BS, et al. Animal-assisted therapy at Mayo Clinic: the time is now. Complement Ther Clin Pract 2015;21(2):101–4.

100. Natural Medicines. 2016. Available at: http://naturaldatabase.therapeuticresearch. com/home.aspx?cs=&s=ND&AspxAutoDetectCookieSupport=1. Accessed September 29, 2016.

101. Fava M, Mischoulon D. Folate in depression: efficacy, safety, differences in formulations, and clinical issues. J Clin Psychiatry 2009;70(Suppl 5):12–7.

102. Almeida OP, Ford AH, Flicker L. Systematic review and meta-analysis of randomized placebo-controlled trials of folate and vitamin B12 for depression. Int Psychogeriatr 2015;27(5):727–37.

103. Institute of Medicine Standing Committee on the Scientific Evaluation of Dietary Reference I. The National Academies Collection: reports funded by National Institutes of Health. Dietary reference Intakes for Calcium, Phosphorus, Magnesium, Vitamin D, and Fluoride. Washington, DC: National Academies Press (US) National Academy of Sciences; 1997.

104. Derom ML, Sayon-Orea C, Martinez-Ortega JM, et al. Magnesium and depression: a systematic review. Nutr Neurosci 2013;16(5):191–206.

105. Barragan-Rodriguez L, Rodriguez-Moran M, Guerrero-Romero F. Efficacy and safety of oral magnesium supplementation in the treatment of depression in the elderly with type 2 diabetes: a randomized, equivalent trial. Magnes Res 2008;21(4):218–23.

106. Walker AF, De Souza MC, Vickers MF, et al. Magnesium supplementation alleviates premenstrual symptoms of fluid retention. J Womens Health 1998;7(9): 1157–65.

107. Hansen MV, Danielsen AK, Hageman I, et al. The therapeutic or prophylactic effect of exogenous melatonin against depression and depressive symptoms: a systematic review and meta-analysis. Eur Neuropsychopharmacol 2014; 24(11):1719–28.

108. Hansen MV, Halladin NL, Rosenberg J, et al. Melatonin for pre- and postoperative anxiety in adults. Cochrane Database Syst Rev 2015;(4):CD009861.

109. Buscemi N, Vandermeer B, Hooton N, et al. The efficacy and safety of exogenous melatonin for primary sleep disorders. A meta-analysis. J Gen Intern Med 2005;20(12):1151–8.

110. Lai J, Moxey A, Nowak G, et al. The efficacy of zinc supplementation in depression: systematic review of randomised controlled trials. J Affect Disord 2012; 136(1–2):e31–9.
111. DiGirolamo AM, Ramirez-Zea M. Role of zinc in maternal and child mental health. Am J Clin Nutr 2009;89(3):940s–5s.
112. Sayyah M, Olapour A, Saeedabad Y, et al. Evaluation of oral zinc sulfate effect on obsessive-compulsive disorder: a randomized placebo-controlled clinical trial. Nutrition 2012;28(9):892–5.
113. Institute of Medicine Panel on M. Dietary reference intakes for vitamin A, vitamin K, arsenic, boron, chromium, copper, iodine, iron, manganese, molybdenum, nickel, silicon, vanadium, and zinc. Washington, DC: National Academies Press (US); 2001.
114. Shaw K, Turner J, Del Mar C. Tryptophan and 5-hydroxytryptophan for depression. Cochrane Database Syst Rev 2002;(1):CD003198.
115. van Praag HM, Korf J, Dols LC, et al. A pilot study of the predictive value of the probenecid test in application of 5-hydroxytryptophan as antidepressant. Psychopharmacologia 1972;25(1):14–21.
116. Thomson J, Rankin H, Ashcroft GW, et al. The treatment of depression in general practice: a comparison of L-tryptophan, amitriptyline, and a combination of L-tryptophan and amitriptyline with placebo. Psychol Med 1982;12(4):741–51.
117. Shaw K, Turner J, Del Mar C. Are tryptophan and 5-hydroxytryptophan effective treatments for depression? A meta-analysis. Aust N Z J Psychiatry 2002;36(4): 488–91.
118. Gowda U, Mutowo MP, Smith BJ, et al. Vitamin D supplementation to reduce depression in adults: meta-analysis of randomized controlled trials. Nutrition 2015;31(3):421–9.
119. Sanders KM, Stuart AL, Williamson EJ, et al. Annual high-dose vitamin D3 and mental well-being: randomised controlled trial. Br J Psychiatry 2011;198(5): 357–64.
120. Li G, Mbuagbaw L, Samaan Z, et al. Efficacy of vitamin D supplementation in depression in adults: a systematic review. J Clin Endocrinol Metab 2014; 99(3):757–67.
121. Shaffer JA, Edmondson D, Wasson LT, et al. Vitamin D supplementation for depressive symptoms: a systematic review and meta-analysis of randomized controlled trials. Psychosom Med 2014;76(3):190–6.
122. Schmidt PJ, Daly RC, Bloch M, et al. Dehydroepiandrosterone monotherapy in midlife-onset major and minor depression. Arch Gen Psychiatry 2005;62(2): 154–62.
123. Wolkowitz OM, Reus VI, Keebler A, et al. Double-blind treatment of major depression with dehydroepiandrosterone. Am J Psychiatry 1999;156(4):646–9.
124. Bloch M, Schmidt PJ, Danaceau MA, et al. Dehydroepiandrosterone treatment of midlife dysthymia. Biol Psychiatry 1999;45(12):1533–41.
125. Peixoto C, Devicari Cheda JN, Nardi AE, et al. The effects of dehydroepiandrosterone (DHEA) in the treatment of depression and depressive symptoms in other psychiatric and medical illnesses: a systematic review. Curr Drug Targets 2014; 15(9):901–14.
126. Crosbie D, Black C, McIntyre L, et al. Dehydroepiandrosterone for systemic lupus erythematosus. Cochrane Database Syst Rev 2007;(4):CD005114.
127. Sublette ME, Ellis SP, Geant AL, et al. Meta-analysis of the effects of eicosapentaenoic acid (EPA) in clinical trials in depression. J Clin Psychiatry 2011;72(12): 1577–84.

128. Fu YQ, Zheng JS, Yang B, et al. Effect of individual omega-3 fatty acids on the risk of prostate cancer: a systematic review and dose-response meta-analysis of prospective cohort studies. J Epidemiol 2015;25(4):261–74.
129. Fernandes BS, Dean OM, Dodd S, et al. N-Acetylcysteine in depressive symptoms and functionality: a systematic review and meta-analysis. J Clin Psychiatry 2016;77(4):e457–66.
130. Deepmala SJ, Slattery J, Kumar N, et al. Clinical trials of N-acetylcysteine in psychiatry and neurology: a systematic review. Neurosci Biobehav Rev 2015;55: 294–321.

Complementary and Integrative Interventions for Chronic Neurologic Conditions Encountered in the Primary Care Office

Danny Bega, MD, MSCI

KEYWORDS

- Complementary and alternative • Integrative • Dementia • Neuropathy • Migraine

KEY POINTS

- Chronic neurologic conditions are frequently managed in the primary care setting, and patients with these conditions are increasingly seeking nonconventional treatment options.
- There is evidence for the use of topical capsaicin and percutaneous electrical nerve stimulation in the treatment of diabetic neuropathy. There is some evidence for α-lipoic acid (ALA) and acupuncture, but further studies are needed.
- Healthy lifestyle, trigger avoidance, and acupuncture may reduce migraine frequency. Some patients may benefit from taking magnesium, coenzyme Q10 (CoQ10), riboflavin, butterbur, or feverfew, although these should be discussed with a health care provider first.
- Diet, exercise, cognitive training, and vascular risk monitoring may preserve cognitive function. Several low-risk, low-cost strategies may prevent delirium, including early mobilization, reorientation, education of nurses, avoidance of deliriogenic drugs, and avoidance of medical or physical restraints.

INTRODUCTION

Chronic neurologic diseases are commonly managed in the primary care setting. In 2013, the *Journal of the American Board of Family Medicine* published a report of the prevalence of chronic conditions managed in primary care practices.[1] Based on data from more than 600,000 patients, several neurologic conditions were identified among the 25 most prevalent encounters: migraine (5.6%), cerebrovascular disease (2.88%), dementia (1.1%), epilepsy (1.0%), and Parkinson disease (PD) (0.3%). The

Department of Neurology, Northwestern University Feinberg School of Medicine, 710 North Lake Shore Drive, Abbott Hall, 1124, Chicago, IL 60611, USA
E-mail address: danny.bega@northwestern.edu

Prim Care Clin Office Pract 44 (2017) 305–322
http://dx.doi.org/10.1016/j.pop.2017.02.004

prevalence of chronic neurologic symptoms is likely even higher when complications of common diseases like diabetes (11.9%) are taken into account. Chronic neurologic disease states highlight the current limitations of conventional medicine. With regard to neurodegenerative diseases like Alzheimer disease or Parkinson disease, the lack of neurorestorative therapies and the subsequent focus on symptom management and supportive care may lead to frustration among patients and their caregivers, dissatisfaction with health care, and a sense of loss of control over the future. For neurologic pain syndromes like migraine and neuropathy, chronic pharmacotherapy can be ineffective or have adverse effects. Furthermore, the impact and interplay of psychological stress on neurologic symptoms may be underestimated or overlooked when management is based on typology of disease rather than individual needs. Consequently, the conventional management of chronic neurologic conditions may fall short in making an adequate impact on quality of life.

There is a public demand for alternative solutions to the management of chronic neurologic diseases; 1 study found that approximately 30% of patients with conditions like migraine and memory loss use mind-body interventions, such as deep breathing exercises, meditation, and yoga.[2] For common chronic diseases in neurology, primary care providers (PCPs) are at the front lines of management and have a responsibility to guide their patients in making safe and effective choices, even if those choices strain the philosophic limits of conventional medical education. To this end, what follows is a review and summary of the scientific evidence for some of the most common complementary and integrative medicine (CIM) interventions used for 3 common neurologic conditions encountered in primary care offices – diabetic neuropathy, migraine, and dementia. Although numerous alternative therapies are touted as beneficial, this article's attention is restricted to randomized controlled trials (RCTs) and systematic reviews of the best studied or most popularly used modalities.

DIABETIC PERIPHERAL NEUROPATHY

The prevalence of diabetic peripheral neuropathy (DPN) in newly diagnosed patients with diabetes is estimated to be 8% and may be up to 59% in patients with long-standing disease.[3,4] DPN is characterized by a loss of nerve fibers and slowed nerve conduction that predispose a person to painful, tingling, or insensitive extremities and results in a large disease burden in terms of incapacity for work, poor quality of life, poor sleep, and consumption of health care resources.[5] The pathophysiology of DPN is complex and includes increased oxidative stress and advanced glycosylation, decreased nitric oxide and impaired endothelial function, impaired Na^+/K^+-ATPase activity, and homocysteinemia.[6] Reduced levels of nerve growth factors have also been noted in experimental models.[6]

Beyond blood glucose management, DPN treatment is typically focused on pain management. Despite many pharmaceutical options, a 2004 study reported that 43% of patients with neuropathy used CIM treatments, usually due to inadequate pain control[7]; 27% of CIM users thought their neuropathy symptoms improved with approaches, which included megavitamins (35%), acupuncture (30%), and herbal remedies (22%).

Nutraceuticals (Antioxidants and Supplements) for Diabetic Peripheral Neuropathy

Chronic elevations in plasma and nerve glucose levels contribute to nerve damage by several proposed mechanisms related to oxygen-free radical production and the formation of advanced glycosylation end products.[8] Reduced nerve perfusion and decreased production of prostaglandin vasodilators have been proposed as contributing factors with endoneurial hypoxia, ultimately leading to nerve dysfunction.[9] These mechanisms are the basis for the use of antioxidant supplements in the treatment of DPN, with the most commonly studied products ALA, vitamin E, vitamin D, and acetyl-L-carnitine (ALC).

α-Lipoic acid

ALA is an endogenous free radical scavenger found in mitochondria, which may reduce oxidation throughout the body, recycle other antioxidants, and improve nitric oxide–mediated endothelial vasodilation, thereby improving nerve blood flow.[9] ALA may also improve endothelial dysfunction through anti-inflammatory and antithrombotic mechanisms.[10] In a review of 15 RCTs,[11] 300 mg to 600 mg of daily intravenous ALA was associated with significant improvement in nerve conduction velocities and pain symptom ratings, although the reviewers concluded that these studies were largely of poor methodological quality. The largest RCT of ALA had more than 500 subjects treated for 6 months and found no significant difference in pain ratings with oral ALA compared with placebo,[12] although 2 subsequent placebo-controlled trials of shorter durations did show significant benefits in pain rating scales.[13,14] *ALA is approved for the treatment of DPN in some European countries, and, because studies have shown a limited side-effect profile, it can be considered a supplement for diabetic patients with neuropathy,[9] although higher-quality studies need to be conducted to confirm efficacy. Furthermore, patients and physicians need to be aware that ALA is a chelating agent with the potential to cause mineral shortages and caution should be used in patients taking other medications that chelate with ALA (ie, antacids) because these may need to be spaced apart.*

Vitamin E, vitamin D, and acetyl-L-carnitine

The data supporting other antioxidants are less robust than for ALA. At least 1 RCT was available on each of vitamin E, vitamin D, and ALC. In a 12-week RCT of 92 patients with DPN, vitamin E was shown to improve pain intensity as an adjunct to usual care,[15] although the treatment group also had a significant reduction in their blood sugar levels, which may confound the results. ALC tends to be deficient in diabetics[16]; clinical trials of ALC compared with placebo have shown inconsistent results with regards to pain outcomes and nerve conduction analyses.[17] Deficiencies of vitamin D have been associated with the presence and the severity of neuropathy.[18] In an 8-week RCT of 112 patients with DPN, statistically significant improvement in neuropathy symptoms was seen with vitamin D over placebo.[19] Another study reported similar benefits in pain scores but used an open-label design.[20] *Given the limited research on the effectiveness of ACL, vitamin D, and vitamin E, these supplements cannot be recommended for DPN at this time. Given the prevalence of vitamin D deficiency in this population, however, there may be benefit to screening and supplementing for those who are deficient.*

Acupuncture

The mechanism by which acupuncture may serve to relieve the symptoms of peripheral neuropathy remains unclear; however, acupuncture has been linked to substances that are associated with nervous system activity, such as release of β-endorphins, γ-aminobutyric acid, glutamate, adenosine, and nerve growth factors.[21,22] A review by Chen and colleagues[23] of 25 studies for acupuncture and DPM in Chinese literature included more than 1600 participants in total, but, due to the poor methodological quality of these studies, no conclusion could be made. In the English-language literature, 2 trials had conflicting results. In a 10-week study of 45 subjects, Garrow and colleagues[24] failed to demonstrate a significant benefit in pain with acupuncture over placebo. In a shorter study, which included 63 subjects, Tong and colleagues[25] did show improvement in subjective sensory complaints as well as nerve conduction measures in an acupuncture group compared with placebo. Similar benefits for nerve conduction measures were seen in a trial of acupuncture compared with best medical management.[26] *Although acupuncture seems safe, and many patients anecdotally describe benefit, there is not sufficient evidence to recommend it for patients with DPN at this time, given inconsistencies in the data.*

Capsaicin

Topical capsaicin formulations are widely used to manage pain.[27] Capsaicin is a natural alkaloid that is extracted from red chili peppers. It selectively binds to a receptor expressed on unmyelinated C-type nerve fibers and causes the release of the pain signaling chemical substance P. After repeated exposure to topical capsaicin, substance P is depleted from sensory nerve endings and cutaneous nociceptors may be desensitized.[28] Three placebo-controlled trials of capsaicin gel for DPN each evaluated the effects on pain reduction over an 8-week period. In the largest trial, which included 252 patients, pain intensity improved significantly with 0.075% capsaicin gel compared with placebo (38% vs 27%).[29] On the other hand, a study of 0.025% gel reported no significant difference in pain.[30] In a study comparing capsaicin to amitriptyline, a similar reduction in pain was found between groups but with fewer side effects in the group receiving capsaicin.[31] According to the American Academy of Neurology (AAN) guidelines, capsaicin has level B evidence for the treatment of DPN.[27] Low-concentration creams, lotions, and patches intended for daily skin application have been available in most countries since the early 1980s, and application site burning is the most common reason for discontinuation. Unlike many other botanical-based products, capsaicin is regulated as an over-the-counter product by the Food and Drug Administration and therefore meets manufacturing, safety, and clinical efficacy standards for over-the-counter products. *Although the clinical usefulness of capsaicin is not conclusive, it can be considered an option for monotherapy or as an adjunctive agent in combination with prescription drug therapy if side effects are tolerated. In some cases, lack of efficacy may be related to dosages that are too low, and in the studies that showed efficacy, a dosage of at least 0.075% was found beneficial.*

Conclusion

Although vitamins and supplements traditionally have been considered safe, there is little evidence to support or refute their usefulness in the treatment of neuropathy in the absence of specific vitamin deficiencies.[9] Whether antioxidant supplements are beneficial is also unclear, although the most evidence is available for ALA. Among herbal substances, topical capsaicin is the only substance to which the AAN guidelines attribute level B evidence for efficacy.[27] Chinese herbs were not covered by this review given the quality and complexity of the literature. The only nonpharmacologic treatment that achieves level B evidence by the AAN is percutaneous electrical nerve stimulation (based largely on a single class I study).[27] Although there is interest in acupuncture, strong evidence with which to guide recommendations is lacking.

MIGRAINE

Headache is a common medical complaint, accounting for 1 in 10 general practitioner consultations.[32] The prevalence of migraine in the general population is approximately

6% in men and 15% in women, and it is common for patients to present to their PCPs before consulting a specialist. Traditionally, pharmacologic treatments are first-line in migraine therapy.[33] Shortcomings of existing treatment options substantiate the great need for CIM treatment strategies, and various studies report the prevalence of CIM use in patients with migraine, anywhere from 28% to 82%.[34,35] The most frequently used modalities are acupuncture (19%–58%); massage (42%–46%); relaxation techniques, such as meditation and yoga (42%); exercise (30%); chiropractic (15%); and herbals (15%).[36]

Avoiding Triggers

One of the "seven elements of good headache management" listed by the World Health Organization is "identification of predisposing or trigger factors and their avoidance through appropriate lifestyle change."[37] Trigger avoidance is typically a part of traditional headache management, although the data supporting the efficacy of trigger avoidance have been questioned, and in 1 study graduated exposure with desensitization to triggers was found more effective than trigger avoidance.[38] Common migraine triggers include stress, negative emotions, sensory triggers (flicker, glare, eyestrain, noise, odors, and smoke), hunger, lack of sleep or excess of sleep, food and drink (chocolate, cheese, and alcohol), menstruation, and weather (cold, heat, and high humidity).[38] *As with any other complaint, PCPs should help patients identify common and individual triggers as well as modifiable risk factors. These include medication overuse, caffeine overuse, and comorbid conditions, such as obstructive sleep apnea and psychiatric comorbidities.*[38] *Anxiety and stress in particular are common comorbidities among patients with migraine and may benefit from complementary interventions.*

Mindfulness and Mind-Body Interventions: Cognitive Behavior Therapy, Biofeedback, Massage, Yoga, and Acupuncture

Psychologically mediated factors, such as problems with self-efficacy, locus of control, and various emotional states, have been found to influence the course of headache by affecting perceived pain and the overall impact of headache on disability and quality of life.[39] Of the 4% of people who consult their family doctor for headache, 28% have clinically significant levels of anxiety or depression,[40] highlighting the importance of nondrug behavioral interventions to help patients develop self-management skills and strategies to prevent and manage their headaches.

Cognitive behavior therapy and biofeedback

Cognitive behavior therapy (CBT) has been shown in systematic reviews to be effective for the treatment of chronic pain conditions.[41] The aim of CBT is to allow patients to develop preventative and acute management strategies, such as trigger identification, as well as allow for modification of maladaptive thoughts, feelings, and behaviors surrounding headache. Biofeedback can be incorporated with or without CBT as a strategy for physiologic autoregulation strategies.[42] Through biofeedback training, patients develop a degree of control over physiologic functions that contribute to the genesis of pain.[43] There have been 3 RCTs studying CBT as an adjunct to medical management, and none of these found a significant improvement in headache intensity, frequency, or number of headache days over 3 to 10 sessions of therapy.[42,44,45] Two RCTs of biofeedback also failed to show significant benefit in headache frequency or severity compared with control treatments.[43,45] In a longer study comparing biofeedback to treatment with a β-blocker, there was some suggestion that biofeedback improved headache severity and frequency at 1-year follow-up, although the primary 6-month endpoint was not significant.[46]

Massage and yoga

Techniques like massage, yoga, and acupuncture may reduce sympathetic arousal and other physiologic responses that can contribute to migraine onset.[47] In a 5-week RCT of massage therapy, a small but significant reduction in migraine frequency was seen compared with a no-intervention control group among 47 migraineurs.[47] Although this study suggests that massage therapy may be beneficial, the duration of benefit is unclear, and placebo-controlled trials are needed. Yoga has long been used to reduce the physical symptoms of chronic pain, and meditation as part of yoga may help reduce anxiety and depression associated with pain.[48,49] In a study of 72 migraineurs randomized to yoga or self-care, only the yoga group had significantly improved frequency and severity of headaches over a 3-month period.[48] Similar benefits were not seen with meditation alone.[50]

Acupuncture

A 2009 Cochrane review (24 RCTs; 14 had a sham control) concluded that there was no evidence for headache benefit with true acupuncture compared with sham; however, in the 4 studies comparing acupuncture to medications, acupuncture was more effective and was associated with significantly fewer adverse effects[51]; 7 additional RCTs have been published since that review, of which 4 were sham-controlled.[52–55] The largest of these studies included 480 migraineurs who received 20 acupuncture treatments over 4 weeks. No significant difference in the primary outcome of headache days was seen, although headache frequency and intensity did improve.[53] Foroughipour and colleagues[52] found that acupuncture add-on therapy was beneficial in reducing headache days compared with a sham control group, and Wang and colleagues[55] found that a single session of acupuncture improved pain scores within 24 hours compared with sham group. Yang and colleagues[56] compared acupuncture to treatment with topiramate and after 12 weeks found that the acupuncture group had fewer headache days and fewer adverse events (6% in the acupuncture group compared with 66% in the topiramate group). Facco and colleagues[57] showed similar benefits compared with valproic acid, although poor methodology limits the interpretation of their results.

Since the release of the 2009 Cochrane review that concluded that there was no benefit for headache with acupuncture over sham, new studies have emerged, which deserve some attention. *Acupuncture may be considered for the management of migraine, although the strength of the placebo response and duration of benefit is not clear from these studies. No conclusions can be made about massage therapy or yoga based on single limited studies. There is also insufficient evidence to support the benefit of short-term CBT or biofeedback for the management of migraine. Given the high incidence of psychiatric comorbidities among migraine patients, however, physicians should screen for anxiety and depression.*

Exercise

Headache experts have proposed that regular, moderate aerobic exercise helps reduce the frequency, severity, and duration of migraine attacks.[58,59] This may be related to the increased production of β-endorphins[60] and to changes in levels of nitric oxide[61] during aerobic exercise, which relaxes vascular smooth muscle in the systemic and cerebral circulation. There may also be a biopsychosocial role for exercise through effects on mood and quality of life. Narin and colleagues[61] studied moderate aerobic exercise in 40 migraineurs as an adjunctive to medical management and found that over 8 weeks there was significant improvement in pain that correlated with a rise in blood nitric oxide levels; this was in contrast to some case studies, which had suggested that exercise may actually precipitate migraine attacks due to excess nitric oxide production.[62] In a study comparing aerobic exercise as an adjunct to amitriptyline, significant benefit in pain frequency, intensity, and duration was seen after 12 weeks in the exercise group compared with medication alone.[63] Improvements in comorbid anxiety and depression were also greater in the exercise group. In contrast, a study comparing cycling therapy with topiramate failed to show a significant difference in pain reduction between groups after 12 weeks but did point out that adverse event rates were more common in the medication group.[64]

There is some evidence supporting a role for aerobic endurance training on the frequency and intensity of migraines; however, the method, dosage, and duration of exercise is not clear. The 2 positive RCTs both used exercise as an adjunctive to medical management with success. Also, some migraineurs (up to 22%) report exercise as a trigger factor[65]; therefore, more studies are imperative.

Nutraceuticals and Diet: Supplements, Herbals, and Foods

A deficiency of certain nutrients has been suggested to play a role in the pathophysiology of migraine through oxidative effects as well as mitochondrial dysfunction.[66,67] Riboflavin, magnesium, and CoQ10 play an important role in the production of energy in the mitochondria,[68] and studies have revealed decreased levels of these micronutrients in migraine patients.[69,70]

Magnesium

Low levels of magnesium may induce cerebral arterial vasoconstriction and increase the aggregation of platelets and thus promote serotonin release, potentiate the vasoactive action of serotonin,[71] and reduce the effect of prostacyclin-mediated relaxation of vascular smooth muscle.[72] Low levels may also enhance the sensitivity of N-methyl-D-aspartate receptors to glutamate, facilitating the development of cortical spreading depression.[73] Reduced magnesium levels were found in the serum[72] and cerebrospinal fluid[74] of migraine patients during and outside of migraine attacks. In a study of 81 migraineurs, 600 mg of magnesium daily was shown to reduce headache frequency by 41.6% over a 3-month period compared with only 15.8% in a placebo group.[74] However, 3 other RCTs using similar dosages and treatment durations did not show similar benefits.[75–77] Side effects, including diarrhea and gastric irritation, have been reported in up to 45% of patients on oral magnesium supplements.[74–76]

Riboflavin and coenzyme Q10

Two other nutrients with important roles in mitochondrial function are riboflavin and CoQ10. Sandor and colleagues[78] reported significant benefit from 300 mg of CoQ10 over placebo after 3 months of treatment. In this study, 47.6% of the 21 patients on CoQ10 compared with only 14.4% of patients on placebo had at least a 50% reduction in headache frequency. Similar benefits were found in a study of 400 mg of daily riboflavin.[79] A more recent trial of 130 migraineurs, however, randomized to combination riboflavin, CoQ10, and magnesium failed to show a significant reduction in headache frequency compared with placebo.[80]

Feverfew and butterbur

Vasoactive herbal medications have been of interest in the treatment of migraine headaches for many years. *Tanacetum parthenium* (feverfew) is an herb whose potential medical properties for headache relief were recognized even as far back as medieval times.[81] Mechanisms for its potential effect may include inhibition of prostaglandin production, interference with contractile and relaxant mechanisms in blood vessels, and release of serotonin from platelets.[81,82] Feverfew was shown to improve the frequency, severity, or number of headaches in each of 5 RCTs compared with placebo.[81–85] In the largest trial of 147 participants, 6.25 mg 3 times a day was most effective.[81] In a 48-subject RCT, 42% of subjects receiving the combination of feverfew with magnesium and riboflavin had at least a 50% reduction in migraines, but 44% of the placebo group also achieved this outcome.[86]

Petasites hybridus (butterbur) is a shrub that has been used traditionally for medicinal purposes. The antispasmodic, antiinflammatory, and vasodilatory properties of butterbur make it an attractive treatment option for migraine prevention.[87] Significant improvements in migraine frequency were shown with butterbur extract, 50 mg to 75 mg twice daily, in 3 RCTs in which it was compared with placebo.[88–90] Adverse events were limited, with gastrointestinal upset the most common (approximately 20%). Raw and unprocessed butterbur extracts contain alkaloids that are hepatotoxic and may be carcinogenic. In commercially available products in the United States, alkaloids are removed to very low levels. CYP3A4 inducers may enhance the metabolism of butterbur alkaloids to toxic metabolites, and although no specific drug interactions have been reported, concomitant administration with 3A4 inducers should be avoided.[91]

Diet

Approximately 25% of migraine patients report that their symptoms are initiated by certain foods,[92] and elimination of specific foods from a person's diet may prevent the onset of a migraine or reduce the number of symptoms experienced.[93] The most commonly reported dietary triggers are chocolate, cheese, citrus, alcohol, and coffee.[94] Some food additives, including sucralose and monosodium glutamate, may also trigger attacks.[95,96] A relationship between obesity and migraine severity has been described, potentially due to the effect of lipid-rich diets on serotonin and estrogen levels.[93,97] In a crossover study of a low-lipid compared with a normal-lipid diet, Ferrara and colleagues[98] found that obese subjects had more headache days and that a significant reduction in headache frequency was achieved with a low-lipid diet. Bunner and colleagues[99] likewise showed that 16 weeks of a low-fat vegan diet significantly improved headache pain on a visual analog scale compared with a group receiving a placebo supplement. A diet rich in omega-3 fatty acids was beneficial in improving number of headache days in 1 study,[100] and a diet incorporating 1.5 L of daily water was shown to improve quality of life ratings in another study.[101] Due to concern over food hypersensitivity (intolerance) as a trigger for migraine attacks, IgG-based elimination diets have been studied and have shown conflicting results with regard to improvement in headache days. In 1 study of 30 subjects there was headache benefit when an elimination diet was compared with a provocation diet,[102] but no significant benefit was seen over a sham diet in a larger trial of 167 subjects.[103]

Although supplementation with magnesium, riboflavin, and CoQ10 is supported by some biological plausibility, there is inconsistent and therefore insufficient data at this time to recommend for or against their use. There is some evidence supporting the efficacy of the vasoactive herbs feverfew and butterbur in the treatment of migraine, although it is not clear whether usage for longer than 4 months is safe and effective. No major adverse effects were reported in trials of feverfew, although due to the potential effects on platelet activity usage should be discussed with a health care provider, particularly in patients on blood-thinning medications or in patients with bleeding or clotting disorders. Commercially available forms of butterbur are likely safe, although it is best to avoid concomitant use with CYP3A4 inducers, and like feverfew, it has not been well studied for treatment periods of greater than 12 weeks to 16 weeks. The role of food in migraine is still controversial. There is some evidence that a low-lipid diet is beneficial, although it is not clear if this is related to specific elements of the diet or to effects on obesity. There is a need for an individualized approach to diet to relieve migraine that incorporates overall healthy lifestyle with awareness of personal triggers.

Conclusion

Although every patient requires an individual approach, some recommendations are applicable to most patients with migraine. Planning regular sleep schedules and regular meals, avoidance of high simple-carbohydrate foods or high lipid foods, adequate hydration, restriction and consistency of caffeine intake, regular aerobic exercise, and relaxation strategies are reasonable. Acupuncture is also an option for headache prevention.[104] Some patients may benefit from taking magnesium, CoQ10, riboflavin, butterbur, or feverfew, although these should be discussed with a health care provider given potential for adverse effects and lack of long-term safety data.

DEMENTIA AND DELIRIUM

Dementia is a chronic decline in cognitive abilities sufficient to result in impairment of activities of daily living. The treatment of Alzheimer dementia (the most common cause of dementia) with cholinesterase inhibitors has limited efficacy, leading many patients to seek CIM interventions. Furthermore, many patients with dementia experience neuropsychiatric symptoms and episodes of delirium.[105] Unfortunately, the pharmacologic treatment of neuropsychiatric symptoms and delirium is challenging, because available medications have drawbacks concerning the benefit-to-risk ratio. Most CIM treatments proposed for dementia and delirium are guided by 4 major principles: (1) protect or enhance cognitive reserve; (2) control vascular risk factors; (3) reduce oxidative stress; and (4) prevent delirium.

Cognitive Reserve

Studies of cognitive engagement have shown that tasks like reading, playing games, or creating art may be associated with lower risk of cognitive decline and dementia.[106] Higher levels of social engagement and physical activity have likewise been associated with less cognitive decline in observational studies.[107] Similar positive associations have been made with regard to effects on β-amyloid burden and hippocampal volumes among more cognitively engaged participants.[108] In a prospective study of 256 octogenarians, engagement in artistic activities, craft activities, and social engagement, both in midlife and late life, was associated with reduced risk of mild cognitive impairment.[109] Participation in mental activities after the onset of dementia may have an impact on quality of life. Participation in various mentally engaging activities should be encouraged based on the potential psychosocial benefit despite the unclear impact on the course of the disease.

Controlling Vascular Risk Factors

Midlife vascular risk factors (including hyperlipidemia, hypertension, obesity, and diabetes) and the metabolic syndrome have been associated with cognitive function and later-life dementia in epidemiologic studies.[110] Treatment trials for hypertension and hyperlipidemia have had mixed results in terms of the effects on dementia. On the other hand, studies of physical activity, both aerobic and resistance training, have suggested that exercise may delay cognitive decline.[111–113] Among those who already have dementia, there is some evidence that physical activity is beneficial not only for gait and balance but also for nonmotor outcomes. Although the more convincing evidence shows that exercise may be associated with improved quality of life and caregiver burden,[114] some studies have shown benefits for measures of cognition as well.[111] *Regular exercise has cardiovascular benefits and should be encouraged in all individuals as there is an association between cardiovascular health and risk of dementia. Among those with dementia, both resistance and aerobic forms of exercise have been associated with motor benefits and higher quality of life.*

Reducing Oxidative Stress

Oxidative stress may accelerate the cascade of Alzheimer disease pathologic changes that can lead to dementia and cerebrovascular disease. Although some studies have demonstrated associations between various vitamin deficiencies or antioxidants and cognitive function, most randomized trials of individual supplements have not been positive. There has been a lot of interest in vitamin B_{12} and folate as risk factors for dementia based on their relations as cofactors in the metabolism of homocysteine. Vitamin B_{12} deficiency is common in older adults[115] and is characterized by symptoms that include cognitive impairment.[116] Folate deficiency, on the other hand, is a rare occurrence in the United States due to folic acid fortification. A meta-analysis of 9 randomized trials of folic acid did not show any effect on cognitive function with up to 3 years of treatment.[117] Randomized trials of the effects of vitamin B_{12} supplementation on cognitive decline have been small and of short duration, making it difficult to interpret the results.[118] Studies of antioxidant vitamins E and C have been inconsistent, although few of the randomized trials targeted participants who are actually deficient.[118] Many of the vitamins and antioxidants of interest to researchers are dietary components that happen to be prominent in the Mediterranean diet. This is a diet high in vegetables, fruits, fish, whole grains, legumes, and monounsaturated oils and low in meats and high-fat dairy. Several prospective studies reported protective associations of adherence to the Mediterranean diet with cognitive decline[119,120] and dementias.[121] *There is no clear evidence that any vitamin or supplement is useful in the treatment or prevention of dementia; however, low intake or low vitamin status for B and E vitamins are deleterious for brain function and health and should be replaced. Few randomized clinical trials are designed to test these observed relations properly because trial participants are generally recruited without regard to nutrient intake or vitamin status.*[118]

The leaves of the ginkgo biloba tree have been made into medicinal extracts in Chinese medicine for 5000 years. Gingko contains flavonoids that have antioxidant and free radical scavenging effects and in vitro antiamyloid aggregation properties.[122] In a meta-analysis of 21 trials in which ginkgo was given to 2608 total patients with cognitive impairment, a small but inconsistent effect of 3 months to 6 months of treatment with 120 mg to 240 mg of the extract was shown on measures of cognition.[123] Two large placebo-controlled trials, 1 published in *The Lancet*[124] and 1 in *JAMA*,[125] both demonstrated lack of efficacy for gingko in reducing progression or incidence of dementia. *Based on these well-designed studies, the use of ginkgo in the treatment of dementia cannot be recommended.*

Preventing Delirium

In a review of interventions for delirium, a mean reduction in the incidence of delirium was found to be 24.7% (range of 9.7% to 31.8%) after implementation of various nonpharmacologic strategies.[126] The most common interventions associated with any clinical benefit were early mobilization, reorientation, education of nurses, and music therapy.[126] Although there is no empiric evidence that the environment alone can cause delirium, certain environmental conditions may exacerbate it. In general, attention to sensory input and provision of orientation aids are considered helpful strategies for reducing the manifestations or severity of delirium.

Aromatherapy is one of the main complementary therapies for agitation and delirium to be practiced by nurses and other health care professionals in hospital, hospice, and community settings.[127] Aromatherapy uses pure essential oils from fragrant plants (such as peppermint, marjoram, rose, and lavender) to help relieve health problems through calming effects. The claimed benefits of aromatherapy include promotion of relaxation and sleep, relief of pain, and reduction of depressive symptoms.[128] The oils used in aromatherapy are most commonly delivered through vaporizers or massaged into the skin; it has been proposed that stimulating the olfactory senses in this way triggers a psychological response to past experiences, which influence the connotation of the aroma and lead to relaxation.[128] Studies of aromatherapy in patients with dementia have all focused on agitation as the main outcome. In a 2014 Cochrane review, 7 RCTs were identified, of which only 2 were considered of high enough quality to formulate a conclusion. The results of these 2 trials with regard to improvement in agitation and behavioral symptoms were inconsistent,[129,130] and, therefore, *no conclusions could be made regarding the effectiveness of aromatherapy for the treatment of agitation related to dementia.*[128]

Conclusion

The CIM approach to managing dementia and delirium involves protecting or enhancing cognitive reserve, controlling vascular risk factors, reducing oxidative stress, and preventing delirium. With the goal of targeting multiple pathways, some investigators have begun studying multidomain interventions for dementia. In the Finnish Geriatric Intervention Study to Prevent Cognitive Impairment and Disability, a group randomized to a *2-year multidomain intervention, which included diet, exercise, cognitive training, and vascular risk monitoring, had significantly better maintenance of cognitive function on a neuropsychological test battery compared with controls.*[131]

SUMMARY

Diabetic neuropathy, migraine, and dementia, are chronic neurologic conditions frequently encountered by PCPs and for which CIM interventions are frequently used. This article reviews the evidence for some of the most frequently used or studied CIM interventions and provides some practical guidelines for each. Many studies are not of high quality, often lacking appropriate controls, having small numbers, or having short durations. There are also many fields in which positive outcomes call strongly for more studies to support preliminary evidence. The desire of patients to engage in CIM as additional therapy to more conventional treatments needs to be recognized and patients should be encouraged to discuss options with their providers. It is important that the role of self-efficacy in producing physiologic benefits not be underestimated. Health care professionals should consider evidence-informed CIM interventions when psychosocial stress is a factor, as it is in many neurologic diseases, or when patients have not responded to, tolerated, or are ineligible for conventional treatments.

REFERENCES

1. Ornstein SM, Nietert PJ, Jenkins RG, et al. The prevalence of chronic diseases and multimorbidity in primary care practice: a PPRNet report. J Am Board Fam Med 2013;26(5):518–24.

2. Erwin Wells R, Phillips RS, McCarthy EP. Patterns of mind-body therapies in adults with common neurological conditions. Neuroepidemiology 2011;36(1):46–51.

3. Boulton AJ, Vinik AI, Arezzo JC, et al. Diabetic neuropathies: a statement by the American Diabetes Association. Diabetes Care 2005;28(4):956–62.

4. Chen W, Zhang Y, Li X, et al. Chinese herbal medicine for diabetic peripheral neuropathy. Cochrane Database Syst Rev 2013;(10):CD007796.

5. Happich M, John J, Stamenitis S, et al. The quality of life and economic burden of neuropathy in diabetic patients in Germany in 2002–results from the Diabetic Microvascular Complications (DIMICO) study. Diabetes Res Clin Pract 2008; 81(2):223–30.

6. Head KA. Peripheral neuropathy: pathogenic mechanisms and alternative therapies. Altern Med Rev 2006;11(4):294–329.

7. Brunelli B, Gorson KC. The use of complementary and alternative medicines by patients with peripheral neuropathy. J Neurol Sci 2004;218(1–2):59–66.

8. Singh VP, Bali A, Singh N, et al. Advanced glycation end products and diabetic complications. Korean J Physiol Pharmacol 2014;18(1):1–14.

9. Halat KM, Dennehy CE. Botanicals and dietary supplements in diabetic peripheral neuropathy. J Am Board Fam Pract 2003;16(1):47–57.

10. Sola S, Mir MQ, Cheema FA, et al. Irbesartan and lipoic acid improve endothelial function and reduce markers of inflammation in the metabolic syndrome: results of the Irbesartan and Lipoic Acid in Endothelial Dysfunction (ISLAND) study. Circulation 2005;111(3):343–8.

11. Han T, Bai J, Liu W, et al. A systematic review and meta-analysis of alpha-lipoic acid in the treatment of diabetic peripheral neuropathy. Eur J Endocrinol 2012; 167(4):465–71.

12. Ziegler D, Hanefeld M, Ruhnau KJ, et al. Treatment of symptomatic diabetic polyneuropathy with the antioxidant alpha-lipoic acid: a 7-month multicenter randomized controlled trial (ALADIN III Study). ALADIN III Study Group. Alpha-Lipoic Acid in Diabetic Neuropathy. Diabetes Care 1999;22(8):1296–301.

13. Ametov AS, Barinov A, Dyck PJ, et al. The sensory symptoms of diabetic polyneuropathy are improved with alpha-lipoic acid: the SYDNEY trial. Diabetes Care 2003;26(3):770–6.

14. Ziegler D, Ametov A, Barinov A, et al. Oral treatment with alpha-lipoic acid improves symptomatic diabetic polyneuropathy: the SYDNEY 2 trial. Diabetes Care 2006;29(11):2365–70.

15. Rajanandh MG, Kosey S, Prathiksha G. Assessment of antioxidant supplementation on the neuropathic pain score and quality of life in diabetic neuropathy patients - a randomized controlled study. Pharmacol Rep 2014;66(1):44–8.

16. Scarpini E, Doneda P, Pizzul S, et al. L-carnitine and acetyl-L-carnitine in human nerves from normal and diabetic subjects. J Peripher Nerv Syst 1996;1(2):157–63.

17. Sima AA, Calvani M, Mehra M, et al. Acetyl-L-carnitine improves pain, nerve regeneration, and vibratory perception in patients with chronic diabetic neuropathy: an analysis of two randomized placebo-controlled trials. Diabetes Care 2005;28(1):89–94.

18. Soderstrom LH, Johnson SP, Diaz VA, et al. Association between vitamin D and diabetic neuropathy in a nationally representative sample: results from 2001-2004 NHANES. Diabet Med 2012;29(1):50–5.

19. Shehab D, Al-Jarallah K, Abdella N, et al. Prospective evaluation of the effect of short-term oral vitamin d supplementation on peripheral neuropathy in type 2 diabetes mellitus. Med Princ Pract 2015;24(3):250–6.

20. Basit A, Basit KA, Fawwad A, et al. Vitamin D for the treatment of painful diabetic neuropathy. BMJ Open Diabetes Res Care 2016;4(1):e000148.

21. Visovsky C. Acupuncture for the management of chemotherapy-induced peripheral neuropathy. J Adv Pract Oncol 2012;3(3):178–81.

22. Zhao ZQ. Neural mechanism underlying acupuncture analgesia. Prog Neurobiol 2008;85(4):355–75.

23. Chen W, Yang GY, Liu B, et al. Manual acupuncture for treatment of diabetic peripheral neuropathy: a systematic review of randomized controlled trials. PLoS One 2013;8(9):e73764.

24. Garrow AP, Xing M, Vere J, et al. Role of acupuncture in the management of diabetic painful neuropathy (DPN): a pilot RCT. Acupunct Med 2014;32(3):242–9.

25. Tong Y, Guo H, Han B. Fifteen-day acupuncture treatment relieves diabetic peripheral neuropathy. J Acupunct Meridian Stud 2010;3(2):95–103.

26. Schroder S, Liepert J, Remppis A, et al. Acupuncture treatment improves nerve conduction in peripheral neuropathy. Eur J Neurol 2007;14(3):276–81.

27. Bril V, England J, Franklin GM, et al. Evidence-based guideline: treatment of painful diabetic neuropathy: report of the American Academy of Neurology, the American Association of Neuromuscular and Electrodiagnostic Medicine, and the American Academy of Physical Medicine and Rehabilitation. Neurology 2011;76(20):1758–65.

28. Anand P, Bley K. Topical capsaicin for pain management: therapeutic potential and mechanisms of action of the new high-concentration capsaicin 8% patch. Br J Anaesth 2011;107(4):490–502.

29. Treatment of painful diabetic neuropathy with topical capsaicin. A multicenter, double-blind, vehicle-controlled study. The Capsaicin Study Group. Arch Intern Med 1991;151(11):2225–9.

30. Kulkantrakorn K, Lorsuwansiri C, Meesawatsom P. 0.025% capsaicin gel for the treatment of painful diabetic neuropathy: a randomized, double-blind, crossover, placebo-controlled trial. Pain Pract 2013;13(6):497–503.

31. Biesbroeck R, Bril V, Hollander P, et al. A double-blind comparison of topical capsaicin and oral amitriptyline in painful diabetic neuropathy. Adv Ther 1995; 12(2):111–20.

32. Ahmed F. Headache disorders: differentiating and managing the common subtypes. Br J Pain 2012;6(3):124–32.

33. Silberstein SD, Holland S, Freitag F, et al. Evidence-based guideline update: pharmacologic treatment for episodic migraine prevention in adults: report of the Quality Standards Subcommittee of the American Academy of Neurology and the American Headache Society. Neurology 2012;78(17):1337–45.

34. Adams J, Barbery G, Lui CW. Complementary and alternative medicine use for headache and migraine: a critical review of the literature. Headache 2013;53(3): 459–73.

35. Gaul C, Eismann R, Schmidt T, et al. Use of complementary and alternative medicine in patients suffering from primary headache disorders. Cephalalgia 2009;29(10):1069–78.

36. Wells RE, Bertisch SM, Buettner C, et al. Complementary and alternative medicine use among adults with migraines/severe headaches. Headache 2011; 51(7):1087–97.

37. Martin PR, Mackenzie S, Bandarian-Balooch S, et al. Enhancing cognitive-behavioural therapy for recurrent headache: design of a randomised controlled trial. BMC Neurol 2014;14:233.

38. Martin PR, Reece J, Callan M, et al. Behavioral management of the triggers of recurrent headache: a randomized controlled trial. Behav Res Ther 2014;61:1–11.

39. French DJ, Holroyd KA, Pinell C, et al. Perceived self-efficacy and headache-related disability. Headache 2000;40(8):647–56.

40. Ridsdale L, Clark LV, Dowson AJ, et al. How do patients referred to neurologists for headache differ from those managed in primary care? Br J Gen Pract 2007;57(538):388–95.

41. Williams AC, Eccleston C, Morley S. Psychological therapies for the management of chronic pain (excluding headache) in adults. Cochrane Database Syst Rev 2012;(11):CD007407.

42. Cousins S, Ridsdale L, Goldstein LH, et al. A pilot study of cognitive behavioural therapy and relaxation for migraine headache: a randomised controlled trial. J Neurol 2015;262(12):2764–72.

43. Mullally WJ, Hall K, Goldstein R. Efficacy of biofeedback in the treatment of migraine and tension type headaches. Pain Physician 2009;12(6):1005–11.

44. Harris P, Loveman E, Clegg A, et al. Systematic review of cognitive behavioural therapy for the management of headaches and migraines in adults. Br J Pain 2015;9(4):213–24.

45. Martin PR, Forsyth MR, Reece J. Cognitive-behavioral therapy versus temporal pulse amplitude biofeedback training for recurrent headache. Behav Ther 2007;38(4):350–63.

46. Kaushik R, Kaushik RM, Mahajan SK, et al. Biofeedback assisted diaphragmatic breathing and systematic relaxation versus propranolol in long term prophylaxis of migraine. Complement Ther Med 2005;13(3):165–74.

47. Lawler SP, Cameron LD. A randomized, controlled trial of massage therapy as a treatment for migraine. Ann Behav Med 2006;32(1):50–9.

48. John PJ, Sharma N, Sharma CM, et al. Effectiveness of yoga therapy in the treatment of migraine without aura: a randomized controlled trial. Headache 2007;47(5):654–61.

49. Kim D, Moon Y, Kim H. Meditation and yoga reduce emotional stress of chronic pain. Prog Neuropsychopharmacol Biol Psychiatry 2005;29:327–31.

50. Wells RE, Burch R, Paulsen RH, et al. Meditation for migraines: a pilot randomized controlled trial. Headache 2014;54(9):1484–95.

51. Linde K, Allais G, Brinkhaus B, et al. Acupuncture for migraine prophylaxis. Cochrane Database Syst Rev 2009;(1):CD001218.

52. Foroughipour M, Golchian AR, Kalhor M, et al. A sham-controlled trial of acupuncture as an adjunct in migraine prophylaxis. Acupunct Med 2014;32(1):12–6.

53. Li Y, Zheng H, Witt CM, et al. Acupuncture for migraine prophylaxis: a randomized controlled trial. CMAJ 2012;184(4):401–10.

54. Wang LP, Zhang XZ, Guo J, et al. Efficacy of acupuncture for migraine prophylaxis: a single-blinded, double-dummy, randomized controlled trial. Pain 2011;152(8):1864–71.

55. Wang LP, Zhang XZ, Guo J, et al. Efficacy of acupuncture for acute migraine attack: a multicenter single blinded, randomized controlled trial. Pain Med 2012;13(5):623–30.

56. Yang CP, Chang MH, Liu PE, et al. Acupuncture versus topiramate in chronic migraine prophylaxis: a randomized clinical trial. Cephalalgia 2011;31(15): 1510–21.

57. Facco E, Liguori A, Petti F, et al. Acupuncture versus valproic acid in the prophylaxis of migraine without aura: a prospective controlled study. Minerva Anestesiol 2013;79(6):634–42.

58. Diamond S. Managing migraines in active people. Phys Sportsmed 1996; 24(12):41–53.

59. Lockett DM, Campbell JF. The effects of aerobic exercise on migraine. Headache 1992;32(1):50–4.

60. Koseoglu E, Akboyraz A, Soyuer A, et al. Aerobic exercise and plasma beta endorphin levels in patients with migrainous headache without aura. Cephalalgia 2003;23(10):972–6.

61. Narin SO, Pinar L, Erbas D, et al. The effects of exercise and exercise-related changes in blood nitric oxide level on migraine headache. Clin Rehabil 2003; 17(6):624–30.

62. Ashina M, Bendtsen L, Jensen R, et al. Possible mechanisms of action of nitric oxide synthase inhibitors in chronic tension-type headache. Brain 1999;122(Pt 9):1629–35.

63. Santiago MD, Carvalho Dde S, Gabbai AA, et al. Amitriptyline and aerobic exercise or amitriptyline alone in the treatment of chronic migraine: a randomized comparative study. Arq Neuropsiquiatr 2014;72(11):851–5.

64. Varkey E, Cider A, Carlsson J, et al. Exercise as migraine prophylaxis: a randomized study using relaxation and topiramate as controls. Cephalalgia 2011; 31(14):1428–38.

65. Kelman L. The triggers or precipitants of the acute migraine attack. Cephalalgia 2007;27(5):394–402.

66. Lodi R, Iotti S, Cortelli P, et al. Deficient energy metabolism is associated with low free magnesium in the brains of patients with migraine and cluster headache. Brain Res Bull 2001;54(4):437–41.

67. Sparaco M, Feleppa M, Lipton RB, et al. Mitochondrial dysfunction and migraine: evidence and hypotheses. Cephalalgia 2006;26(4):361–72.

68. Bianchi A, Salomone S, Caraci F, et al. Role of magnesium, coenzyme Q10, riboflavin, and vitamin B12 in migraine prophylaxis. Vitam Horm 2004;69:297–312.

69. Hershey AD, Powers SW, Vockell AL, et al. Coenzyme Q10 deficiency and response to supplementation in pediatric and adolescent migraine. Headache 2007;47(1):73–80.

70. Mauskop A, Altura BT, Altura BM. Serum ionized magnesium levels and serum ionized calcium/ionized magnesium ratios in women with menstrual migraine. Headache 2002;42(4):242–8.

71. Altura BT, Altura BM. Withdrawal of magnesium causes vasospasm while elevated magnesium produces relaxation of tone in cerebral arteries. Neurosci Lett 1980;20(3):323–7.

72. Schoenen J, Sianard-Gainko J, Lenaerts M. Blood magnesium levels in migraine. Cephalalgia 1991;11(2):97–9.

73. Mody I, Lambert JD, Heinemann U. Low extracellular magnesium induces epileptiform activity and spreading depression in rat hippocampal slices. J Neurophysiol 1987;57(3):869–88.

74. Peikert A, Wilimzig C, Kohne-Volland R. Prophylaxis of migraine with oral magnesium: results from a prospective, multi-center, placebo-controlled and double-blind randomized study. Cephalalgia 1996;16(4):257–63.

75. Koseoglu E, Talaslioglu A, Gonul AS, et al. The effects of magnesium prophy-laxis in migraine without aura. Magnes Res 2008;21(2):101–8.

76. Pfaffenrath V, Wessely P, Meyer C, et al. Magnesium in the prophylaxis of migraine–a double-blind placebo-controlled study. Cephalalgia 1996;16(6): 436–40.

77. Tarighat Esfanjani A, Mahdavi R, Ebrahimi Mameghani M, et al. The effects of magnesium, L-carnitine, and concurrent magnesium-L-carnitine supplementa-tion in migraine prophylaxis. Biol Trace Elem Res 2012;150(1–3):42–8.

78. Sandor PS, Di Clemente L, Coppola G, et al. Efficacy of coenzyme Q10 in migraine prophylaxis: a randomized controlled trial. Neurology 2005;64(4): 713–5.

79. Schoenen J, Jacquy J, Lenaerts M. Effectiveness of high-dose riboflavin in migraine prophylaxis. A randomized controlled trial. Neurology 1998;50(2): 466–70.

80. Gaul C, Diener HC, Danesch U, et al. Improvement of migraine symptoms with a proprietary supplement containing riboflavin, magnesium and Q10: a random-ized, placebo-controlled, double-blind, multicenter trial. J Headache Pain 2015;16:516.

81. Pfaffenrath V, Diener HC, Fischer M, et al. The efficacy and safety of Tanacetum parthenium (feverfew) in migraine prophylaxis–a double-blind, multicentre, ran-domized placebo-controlled dose-response study. Cephalalgia 2002;22(7): 523–32.

82. Diener HC, Pfaffenrath V, Schnitker J, et al. Efficacy and safety of 6.25 mg t.i.d. feverfew CO2-extract (MIG-99) in migraine prevention–a randomized, double-blind, multicentre, placebo-controlled study. Cephalalgia 2005;25(11):1031–41.

83. Cady RK, Goldstein J, Nett R, et al. A double-blind placebo-controlled pilot study of sublingual feverfew and ginger (LipiGesic M) in the treatment of migraine. Headache 2011;51(7):1078–86.

84. Johnson ES, Kadam NP, Hylands DM, et al. Efficacy of feverfew as prophylactic treatment of migraine. Br Med J (Clin Res Ed) 1985;291(6495):569–73.

85. Murphy JJ, Heptinstall S, Mitchell JR. Randomised double-blind placebo-controlled trial of feverfew in migraine prevention. Lancet 1988;2(8604):189–92.

86. Maizels M, Blumenfeld A, Burchette R. A combination of riboflavin, magnesium, and feverfew for migraine prophylaxis: a randomized trial. Headache 2004; 44(9):885–90.

87. Thomet OA, Wiesmann UN, Schapowal A, et al. Role of petasin in the potential anti-inflammatory activity of a plant extract of petasites hybridus. Biochem Phar-macol 2001;61(8):1041–7.

88. Diener HC, Rahlfs VW, Danesch U. The first placebo-controlled trial of a special butterbur root extract for the prevention of migraine: reanalysis of efficacy criteria. Eur Neurol 2004;51(2):89–97.

89. Grossman W, Schmidramsl H. An extract of Petasites hybridus is effective in the prophylaxis of migraine. Altern Med Rev 2001;6(3):303–10.

90. Lipton RB, Gobel H, Einhaupl KM, et al. Petasites hybridus root (butterbur) is an effective preventive treatment for migraine. Neurology 2004;63(12):2240–4.

91. Sutherland A, Sweet BV. Butterbur: an alternative therapy for migraine preven-tion. Am J Health Syst Pharm 2010;67(9):705–11.

92. Van den Bergh V, Amery WK, Waelkens J. Trigger factors in migraine: a study conducted by the Belgian Migraine Society. Headache 1987;27(4):191–6.

93. Bic Z, Blix GG, Hopp HP, et al. The influence of a low-fat diet on incidence and severity of migraine headaches. J Womens Health Gend Based Med 1999;8(5): 623–30.
94. Fukui PT, Goncalves TR, Strabelli CG, et al. Trigger factors in migraine patients. Arq Neuropsiquiatr 2008;66(3A):494–9.
95. Bigal ME, Lipton RB. Modifiable risk factors for migraine progression. Headache 2006;46(9):1334–43.
96. Patel RM, Sarma R, Grimsley E. Popular sweetner sucralose as a migraine trigger. Headache 2006;46(8):1303–4.
97. Peterlin BL, Rosso AL, Williams MA, et al. Episodic migraine and obesity and the influence of age, race, and sex. Neurology 2013;81(15):1314–21.
98. Ferrara LA, Pacioni D, Di Fronzo V, et al. Low-lipid diet reduces frequency and severity of acute migraine attacks. Nutr Metab Cardiovasc Dis 2015;25(4): 370–5.
99. Bunner AE, Agarwal U, Gonzales JF, et al. Nutrition intervention for migraine: a randomized crossover trial. J Headache Pain 2014;15:69.
100. Ramsden CE, Faurot KR, Zamora D, et al. Targeted alteration of dietary n-3 and n-6 fatty acids for the treatment of chronic headaches: a randomized trial. Pain 2013;154(11):2441–51.
101. Spigt M, Weerkamp N, Troost J, et al. A randomized trial on the effects of regular water intake in patients with recurrent headaches. Fam Pract 2012;29(4):370–5.
102. Alpay K, Ertas M, Orhan EK, et al. Diet restriction in migraine, based on IgG against foods: a clinical double-blind, randomised, cross-over trial. Cephalalgia 2010;30(7):829–37.
103. Mitchell N, Hewitt CE, Jayakody S, et al. Randomised controlled trial of food elimination diet based on IgG antibodies for the prevention of migraine like headaches. Nutr J 2011;10:85.
104. Mauskop A. Nonmedication, alternative, and complementary treatments for migraine. Continuum (Minneap Minn) 2012;18(4):796–806.
105. Anderson D. Preventing delirium in older people. Br Med Bull 2005;73-74:25–34.
106. Treiber KA, Carlson MC, Corcoran C, et al. Cognitive stimulation and cognitive and functional decline in Alzheimer's disease: the cache county dementia progression study. J Gerontol B Psychol Sci Soc Sci 2011;66(4):416–25.
107. Crooks VC, Lubben J, Petitti DB, et al. Social network, cognitive function, and dementia incidence among elderly women. Am J Public Health 2008;98(7): 1221–7.
108. Okonkwo OC, Schultz SA, Oh JM, et al. Physical activity attenuates age-related biomarker alterations in preclinical AD. Neurology 2014;83(19):1753–60.
109. Roberts RO, Cha RH, Mielke MM, et al. Risk and protective factors for cognitive impairment in persons aged 85 years and older. Neurology 2015;84(18): 1854–61.
110. Tolppanen AM, Solomon A, Soininen H, et al. Midlife vascular risk factors and Alzheimer's disease: evidence from epidemiological studies. J Alzheimers Dis 2012;32(3):531–40.
111. Fiatarone Singh MA, Gates N, Saigal N, et al. The Study of Mental and Resistance Training (SMART) study-resistance training and/or cognitive training in mild cognitive impairment: a randomized, double-blind, double-sham controlled trial. J Am Med Dir Assoc 2014;15(12):873–80.
112. Smith PJ, Blumenthal JA, Hoffman BM, et al. Aerobic exercise and neurocognitive performance: a meta-analytic review of randomized controlled trials. Psychosom Med 2010;72(3):239–52.

113. Sofi F, Valecchi D, Bacci D, et al. Physical activity and risk of cognitive decline: a meta-analysis of prospective studies. J Intern Med 2011;269(1):107–17.
114. Littbrand H, Stenvall M, Rosendahl E. Applicability and effects of physical exercise on physical and cognitive functions and activities of daily living among people with dementia: a systematic review. Am J Phys Med Rehabil 2011;90(6): 495–518.
115. Pfeiffer CM, Schleicher RL, Johnson CL, et al. Assessing vitamin status in large population surveys by measuring biomarkers and dietary intake - two case studies: folate and vitamin D. Food Nutr Res 2012;56:1–10.
116. Briani C, Dalla Torre C, Citton V, et al. Cobalamin deficiency: clinical picture and radiological findings. Nutrients 2013;5(11):4521–39.
117. Wald DS, Kasturiratne A, Simmonds M. Effect of folic acid, with or without other B vitamins, on cognitive decline: meta-analysis of randomized trials. Am J Med 2010;123(6):522–7.e2.
118. Morris MC. Nutritional determinants of cognitive aging and dementia. Proc Nutr Soc 2012;71(1):1–13.
119. Feart C, Samieri C, Rondeau V, et al. Adherence to a Mediterranean diet, cognitive decline, and risk of dementia. JAMA 2009;302(6):638–48.
120. Scarmeas N, Stern Y, Mayeux R, et al. Mediterranean diet and mild cognitive impairment. Arch Neurol 2009;66(2):216–25.
121. Scarmeas N, Stern Y, Mayeux R, et al. Mediterranean diet, Alzheimer disease, and vascular mediation. Arch Neurol 2006;63(12):1709–17.
122. Luo Y, Smith JV, Paramasivam V, et al. Inhibition of amyloid-beta aggregation and caspase-3 activation by the Ginkgo biloba extract EGb761. Proc Natl Acad Sci U S A 2002;99(19):12197–202.
123. Yang G, Wang Y, Sun J, et al. Ginkgo biloba for mild cognitive impairment and Alzheimer's disease: a systematic review and meta-analysis of randomized controlled trials. Curr Top Med Chem 2016;16(5):520–8.
124. Vellas B, Coley N, Ousset PJ, et al. Long-term use of standardised Ginkgo biloba extract for the prevention of Alzheimer's disease (GuidAge): a randomised placebo-controlled trial. Lancet Neurol 2012;11(10):851–9.
125. DeKosky ST, Williamson JD, Fitzpatrick AL, et al. Ginkgo biloba for prevention of dementia: a randomized controlled trial. JAMA 2008;300(19):2253–62.
126. Rivosecchi RM, Smithburger PL, Svec S, et al. Nonpharmacological interventions to prevent delirium: an evidence-based systematic review. Crit Care Nurse 2015;35(1):39–50 [quiz: 1].
127. Buckle J. Aromatherapy for health professionals. Beginnings 2003;23(1):6–7.
128. Forrester LT, Maayan N, Orrell M, et al. Aromatherapy for dementia. Cochrane Database Syst Rev 2014;(2):CD003150.
129. Ballard CG, O'Brien JT, Reichelt K, et al. Aromatherapy as a safe and effective treatment for the management of agitation in severe dementia: the results of a double-blind, placebo-controlled trial with Melissa. J Clin Psychiatry 2002; 63(7):553–8.
130. Burns A, Perry E, Holmes C, et al. A double-blind placebo-controlled randomized trial of Melissa officinalis oil and donepezil for the treatment of agitation in Alzheimer's disease. Dement Geriatr Cogn Disord 2011;31(2):158–64.
131. Ngandu T, Lehtisalo J, Solomon A, et al. A 2 year multidomain intervention of diet, exercise, cognitive training, and vascular risk monitoring versus control to prevent cognitive decline in at-risk elderly people (FINGER): a randomised controlled trial. Lancet 2015;385(9984):2255–63.

Restoring Balance for People with Cancer Through Integrative Oncology

Judy A. Fulop, ND, MS[a,b,*], Ania Grimone, MS, LAc[c],
David Victorson, PhD[d,e]

KEYWORDS

- Integrative medicine • Cancer • Nutrition • Chinese medicine • Nature
- Quality of life • Ancient medicine • Mind-body medicine

KEY POINTS

- Alongside their conventional cancer therapies, patients have an opportunity to include integrative medicine to enhance their physical, emotional, mental, and spiritual well-being.
- The integrative oncology team works together with the patient's oncologist, surgeon, and radiation oncologist to provide support and augment care during and after active cancer treatment.
- Individualized integrative medicine allows patients a choice from diverse practices and treatments, including nutritional support and dietary changes, yoga, Aryuvedic medicine, traditional Chinese medicine (TCM), meditation, qigong, and other mind-body modalities.

INTRODUCTION

When faced with a life-threatening diagnosis, such as cancer, a patient's desire to focus on everything possible to support conventional medical treatments is understandable. More than 65% of individuals diagnosed with cancer in the United States report having used some form of complementary and alternative medicine (CAM) to help combat their disease, manage symptoms and treat side effects, and increase

Disclosure Statement: The authors have nothing to disclose.
[a] Naturopathic Oncology, Osher Center for Integrative Medicine, Northwestern Memorial Hospital, Northwestern Medicine, 150 East Huron Street, Suite #1100, Chicago, IL 60611, USA; [b] Adjunct Faculty, Naturopathic Medicine, National University of Health Sciences, 200 E Roosevelt Rd, Lombard, IL 60148, USA; [c] Acupuncture and Chinese Medicine, Osher Center for Integrative Medicine, Northwestern Memorial Hospital, Northwestern Medicine, 150 East Huron Street, Suite #1100, Chicago, IL 60611, USA; [d] Department of Medical Social Sciences, Northwestern University Feinberg School of Medicine, 2205 Tech Drive, Suite 2-120, Chicago, IL 60208, USA; [e] Osher Center for Integrative Medicine, Northwestern Medicine, 150 East Huron Street, Suite #1100, Chicago, IL 60611, USA
* Corresponding author. Osher Center for Integrative Medicine, Northwestern Memorial Hospital, 150 East Huron Street, Suite #1100, Chicago, IL 60611.
E-mail address: jfulop@nm.org

Prim Care Clin Office Pract 44 (2017) 323–335
http://dx.doi.org/10.1016/j.pop.2017.02.009
0095-4543/17/© 2017 Elsevier Inc. All rights reserved.

their overall well-being and quality of life.[1] Integrative oncology, or the professional discipline of integrating CAM into mainstream cancer treatments and survivorship, encompasses a diverse group of ancient traditional health and healing practices, systems, and approaches. These include such modalities as the use of nutrition, dietary and herbal supplements, acupuncture, and mind-body practices to name a few. To best understand how CAM therapies may be integrated within conventional oncology treatment it is beneficial to first rethink what constitutes disease and illness. This article presents a guiding conceptual framework from an integrative perspective, based on the concept of balance and imbalance. From this perspective, an integrative approach can be used to help restore quality of life, enhance lifestyle choices, mitigate symptoms, and support a healthy future.

WESTERN VERSUS TRADITIONAL MEDICAL APPROACHES TO UNDERSTANDING CANCER

Conventional Western medical cancer treatments focus on identifying and targeting specific cancers in different parts of the body on cellular and molecular levels, measuring tumor responses, and identifying cell signaling and growth factors.[2] Although this approach is mostly targeted to eliminate cancerous cells, the whole body is involved. Integrative medical approaches are grounded in the concept of balance and are not limited to pathology of the physical body and cellular activity. Balance occurs in the body as cells die and are replaced, as the nervous system maintains its parasympathetic and sympathetic balance, and as the immune system keeps a balance between protection from unhealthy microbes and an attack on itself as in autoimmune disease. Examples of more holistic approaches to balance are Ying and Yang of Chinese medicine[3]; Vata, Pita, Kapha doshas of Ayurvedic medicine[4]; choleric, melancholic, sanguine, and phlegmatic humors of early Hippocratic medicine[5]; and hot/cold, damp/dry characteristics of eclectic physicians.[6] Many ancient medical traditions speak of treating the root of the tree, rather than treating the branches. Treating the branches addresses the symptoms, whereas treating the roots address the cause of the imbalance, which in their ancient understanding reaches far beyond cellular function. In these traditions health is not simply the absence of physical illness, but rather a state of harmony and balance between the body, mind, and spirit and a relationship with the living environment.[7]

Traditional ancient practices of medicine (whether Chinese, Ayurvedic and Naturopathic or Native American) are unique, because they identify and address illness from a physical and energetic imbalance.[8] In these approaches it is understood that energy comprises all matter at a fundamental level, and flows within, around, and throughout the entire universe. Energy cannot be destroyed, but is changed by a variety of circumstances, which cause an imbalance. According to laws of quantum physics, energy and matter are simply two aspects of the same thing. Thus an energetic disturbance in the body on a physical or material level can also affect mind and spirit, and vice versa.

Within this context, cancer may be seen as a condition where the body is out of balance whether from a source within or from without. Becoming unbalanced at any level (physical, energetic, emotional or mental) can produce pathophysiologic changes resulting in the manifestation of disease. From a traditional medical perspective, the dynamic intersection and interaction of biochemical networks are affected by the diverse milieu in which they operate. Thus from this paradigm, cancer as an isolated entity does not exist, at least not in the way that Western conventional medicine has conceptualized it.

From an integrative medicine perspective, spirituality is just as important to health as diet, exercise, sleep, environmental exposure to elements and toxins, state of mind, and interpersonal relationships.[9] Each of these contributes to an energetic backdrop that interacts with individual components of the whole. From this understanding "everything is everything," each one of these elements has a capacity to start a chain reaction, which may contribute to health or disease by altering a unique biochemical process within the body. Any of these factors can change the energetic milieu. This in turn, can affect organs, tissues, fluids, functions, and collectively trigger further breakdown and deepen pathology. A single element may not be capable of producing disease; however, the combination of several elements over a prolonged period of time can affect this balance or homeostasis. As the body's adaptive mechanisms become strained, there is a point at which the system cannot maintain its equilibrium and the imbalance manifests itself physically.[7]

To effectively address imbalance, one must not only identify the cause and location of symptoms, but also the context from which they arise. The objective of treatment from an integrative paradigm is to identify elements that can help the body "right itself" as a whole and achieve a state of homeostasis.[10] These elements may include imbalances related to diet, such as toxic food; poor relationship with food; and negative beliefs, attitudes, and associations.[11] Other elements, such as environmental factors (ie, external factors including heat, cold, wind, damp, bacteria, viruses, mold, poisonous insects, pollution), excessive or unregulated emotions (persistent anger, sadness, fear, worry, hopelessness, and so forth),[12] and spiritual conflict (religious extremism, pressure, guilt, and so forth) may factor into this imbalance.[13] On the opposite spectrum, imbalances may be caused by a deficiency of nutrients, sleep, clean water, fresh air, exercise, loving relationships, connectedness (to people, nature, deity, or whatever is significant to the individual), meaning and purpose, fulfillment, or social support.[14]

Although current Western oncology practices are beginning to appreciate the impact of environment, lifestyle, and emotions on human biology, their primary focus at this time remains that of removing the cancer through chemotherapy, surgery, and radiation. More recent research and treatment is directed at identifying growth factors and cell signaling within the cancerous cell. An integrative treatment program advocates for the need to approach cancer treatment as a dynamic, interconnected and interdependent biomedical system that exists in a larger context and is not confined to a single tissue, organ, or body system.[15]

Integrative oncology attempts to see the forest and the trees simultaneously, understanding that for a tree to survive, all aspects of the living forest in its entirety must be addressed. Focus on treatment includes the air that the living forest breathes, the water that pulses through its veins, the soil that houses the deep living roots, the birds that migrate through the forest, and every vital connection with the rest of the planet. Within the integrative oncology paradigm, the most powerful approach to treating the whole person (and not just their symptoms or disease) is in building a vital connection between conventional and traditional medical strategies.[16] Integrative oncology approaches include supporting, nourishing, strengthening, and otherwise restoring balance; removing obstacles to the body's inert wisdom to heal and achieving balance while creating a favorable environment in which balance within the body is restored.

Many patients view cancer as a turning point, an awakening to a reality that life is finite and an opportunity to reevaluate and make positive changes in their lives,[17] including the areas of diet, exercise, job, relationships, purpose, or spirituality. As part of their journey from cancer to recovery, individuals instinctively seek to balance these areas and in doing so seek all available resources, modern and traditional, to facilitate that process.

RESTORING BALANCE THROUGH NUTRITION

Let food be your medicine and medicine be your food

—*Hippocrates*

Recommendations for nutrition and individualized approaches vary throughout the literature from nutrition having no impact on cancer to nutrition having a great impact (**Table 1**).[18,19] The general consensus is that a more plant-based living diet with a lesser amount of animal proteins is extremely beneficial for cancer prevention and treatment and for other chronic diseases.[20] Long ago naturopathic physicians believed that health and disease began in the gut. This is now gaining acceptance with the understanding of the human microbiome. The intestinal microbiome protects the tight junctions in the gut so that nutrients are absorbed while microbes, endotoxins, and other unwanted materials are screened from entering through the intestinal barrier. Because a healthy gut microbiome is required for basic nutrition, energy balance, and immune function, an imbalance here can lead to further disease through a decrease in cellular absorption no matter how healthy the diet.[21] In addition to a healthy microbiome, fiber is needed to feed the flora from a diet full of a rainbow color of vegetables, some fruits, and minimal animal protein. Because the type of foods determine which microflora live and die, an anti-inflammatory diet (avoidance of sugar, simple starches, artificial sugars, wheat/gluten, dairy, and alcohol) similar to a Mediterranean diet not only decreases inflammation throughout the body, but determines balance in the microbiome.[22]

Other options for further cancer prevention include diets low in simple carbohydrates either as a ketogenic diet, calorie-restricted diet, or a mixture of the two.[23] This perspective comes from a 22 yearlong study (N = 99) with individuals affected by Laron syndrome (genetic inability to produce growth hormone receptors, and lack of insulin-like growth factor-1) found only one cancer and zero diabetes in the population, with 20% of close blood relatives who did not have the syndrome dying of cancer.[24,25] Insulin-like growth factors have been found to be high in patients with cancer including ovarian tumors,[26] malignant biliary obstructive lesions, and early stage malignant breast cancer.[27] Close relationships exist between the insulin growth factor receptor and cell proliferation pathways.

Table 1	
Nutrition solutions for cancer-related support	
Support	**Nutrition**
Anti-oxidant	Green tea, fruits, onions, garlic, cruciferous vegetables, nuts tumeric/curcumin, peppers, tomatoes, dark leafy greens
Anti-inflammatory	Tumeric/curcumin, ginger, cardamon, fennel seeds, juniper berries, fatty fish, dark leafy greens, garlic, onions, olive oil
Anti-angiogenesis	Green tea, berries, oranges, grapefruit, lemons, apples, pineapples, cherries, red grapes, bok choy, kale
Anti-estrogenic	White button mushrooms, cruciferous veggies, pomegranates shiitake mushrooms, red grape skins, onions, garlic

Metabolic syndrome is associated with colorectal, breast, endometrial, pancreatic, and primary liver cancer.[28] For this reason addressing a metabolic syndrome and subsequent weight loss with a diet low in sugars, carbohydrates, and simple starches that are known to raise insulin-like growth factors is imperative.

A diet that reduces carbohydrate intake and uses fat as the main source of energy to induce ketosis (ketogenic diet) has been used successfully for the last 90 years in the treatment of drug-resistant refractory seizures in children with epilepsy.[29] More recently success has also been found with refractory seizures in adults.[30] In the area of cancer, research has centered on a calorie-restricted ketogenic diet to help slow glioblastoma because high ketones and low glucose starve glioblastoma cells while sparing healthy cells.[31] Studies show that fasting is safe and feasible during platinum-based chemotherapy with reduced side effects.[32]

RESTORING BALANCE DURING AND AFTER CANCER TREATMENT

Although chemotherapy, radiation, and other conventional cancer treatments are effective in killing rapidly dividing cancer cells, these treatments can stress healthy cells, leading to many debilitating side effects (eg, nausea, vomiting, fatigue, alopecia, neuropathy). Managing these side effects (**Table 2**) without affecting treatment outcomes can result in improved quality of life, avoidance or reduction in treatment dosage and delays, and improvement in compliance.

Much can and needs to be mentioned regarding the individual patient's fear of recurrence and other related anxieties that surface when treatment has finished and the individual transitions to cancer survivorship. This tremendous fear of recurrence is a leading unaddressed consequence of cancer diagnosis and treatment.[33] Referral for counseling or health coaching may be helpful. Even helping patients articulate this fear can provide great benefit.

Although more and more patients go into remission, survivors of cancer are at an increased risk for developing a second cancer.[34] Patients diagnosed with Hodgkin's lymphoma in their early years have later been diagnosed with breast cancer and other secondary neoplasms.[35] Many treatments (doxorubicin and trastuzumab) affect the mitochondria of healthy cells, especially those of the heart.[36] Restoring healthy mitochondria with a supplement, such as CoQ10 or L-carnitine, becomes of extreme importance not only in decreasing the fatigue induced by specific chemotherapy agents, but ongoing support for healthy mitochondria in cells especially heart muscle.[37]

HERBAL AND SUPPLEMENTAL SUPPORT FOR PATIENTS WITH CANCER

Integrative approaches to cancer care are individualized because of different chemotherapy treatments and the individual's own genetic polymorphisms that detoxify these treatments. However, in general there are some options that the primary care physician can suggest to their patients during treatment. These include support to manage nausea, neuropathy, fatigue, insomnia, dysgeusia, neuropathy, and imbalances of the gastrointestinal system. Care is taken to avoid any supplements and herbs that would disrupt chemotherapy and radiation treatment, that is, liver P-450 pathways or antioxidant use. **Table 2** provides common herbs, supplements, and modalities most frequently used to support patients receiving conventional cancer therapies.

Cannabinoids derived from *Cannabis sativa* and *Cannabis indica* have been used for thousands of years to help with cancer-related pain, nausea, and even on tumors. Many states now allow licensed medical marijuana dispensaries to provide

Table 2
Common herbal, supplemental, and Chinese medicine solutions for cancer-related side effects

Problem	Nutrition, Supplement, or Herbal	Chinese Medicine
Loss of taste	Nutrient deficiencies: zinc, vitamins B_3 and B_{12}	Auricular acupuncture
Nausea	Ginger, cannabidiol, medical marijuana	PC-6 pressure, sea sick bands, kidney-1 acupressure point
Diarrhea	Glutamine, probiotics	Counterclockwise abdominal massage, acupuncture, mona
Constipation	Digestive enzymes, probiotics, senna, rhubarb	Clockwise abdominal massage, black sesame seeds, ST 25 acupressure
Neuropathy	Vitamin B_6, α-lipoic acid	Low-level laser therapy, acupuncture
Insomnia	Melatonin, turkey, Tilia tomentosa, chamomile tea, kava kava	Auricular acupressure, Shenmen and T 7 acupressure, qigong, meditation
Anxiety	Magnesium, Rescue Remedy, kava kava	Ear Shenmen acupressure, Yin Tang point between eyebrows, diaphragmatic breathing, meditation
Hot flashes	Black cohosh, vitamin E at high doses	Acupuncture
Fatigue	Vitamin D (if low), eleutherococcus and other ginsengs	Astragalus
Cognitive problems	Soy lecithin, rosemary, tibetan sound meditation	

cannabinoids for specific registered medical patient populations including those with cancer.[38] Only recently has research found the endogenous endocannabinoid system in the human body.[39] These endocannabinoids have a role in memory, appetite, and the stress response. Besides the cannabis plant, cannabinoids are found in other herbals including *Echinacea* species and some mushrooms, fungi, and other lesser known herbals.

Although cannabidiol (CBD) and tetrahydrocannabinol (THC) are the most popular known cannabinoids, other cannabinoids within the whole plant also have significant therapeutic properties, including cannabigerol (antitumor, high in nonpsychoactive hemp strains), cannabichromene (analgesic, anti-inflammatory, and antibiotic), and tetrahydrocannabivarin (although psychoactive, contains antidiabetic and antiobesity properties).

C sativa and *C indica* contain at least 68 different cannabinoids, many of which hold great promise for medical use above and beyond their well-known active ingredients (CBD and THC).[40] Rather than isolating one active component and producing plants with a higher level of this component (ie, THC), use of the whole plant with all active ingredients working together is even more beneficial to the patient. This whole plant approach supports harmony and the approach to the balance within the body. Given increasing problems with the addictive and often lethal opioid epidemic in the United States, cannabinoids besides THC, such as CBD, can help with somatic, visceral, and neuropathic pain (although severe pain may require both THC and CBD). CBD alone (the nonpsychoactive cannabinoid) has been shown to reduce nausea, pain, and inhibit cancer growth on its own (eg, glioblastomas, breast, lung, prostate, and colon cancer).[41] Because CBD is derived from hemp and not the cannabis plant itself, individuals in states that do not license medical marijuana may find CBD of great benefit.

RESTORING BALANCE THROUGH HOMEOPATHY

Homeopathy has been used for hundreds of years as a holistic medical approach that uses highly diluted natural substances to relieve symptoms.[42] In the area of cancer, cell culture research show evidence of apoptosis by cell shrinkage, chromatin condensation, and DNA fragmentation. Plastic surgeons increasingly are using homeopathy with plastic surgery.[43] One study using objective measurements found that homeopathic *Arnica montana* accelerated postoperative healing with quick resolution and dramatic increase in patient satisfaction. This study showed statistical significance ($P<.05$) on two of four postoperative data points.[44] More studies are needed on therapeutic benefits of homeopathic Arnica. In addition, when conventional cancer treatment approaches have been exhausted, homeopathic remedies can help individuals transition at the end of life.[45] Whether giving patients a longer time to prepare for eventual death or helping ease pain during the process of dying, homeopathy can benefit the individual at all stages of life.

TRADITIONAL CHINESE MEDICINE TO RESTORE BALANCE

Chinese medicine has a long history of treating cancer and recognizes that its cause involves external pathogens (from outside the body), the environment, emotional maladjustment, and an improper diet with the tumor as a partial consequence of systemic disease. This approach to treatment combines partial and systemic therapy, by strengthening the body's resistance, eliminating pathogens, and regulating emotions. During radiation therapy and chemotherapy, traditional Chinese medicine (TCM) treatment can reduce toxic side effects, such as myelosupression, gastrointestinal reactions, skin and mucosal reactions, and hepatic and renal impairment. TCM with chemotherapy has shown improved efficacy with less adverse reactions.[46] For patients with advanced disease who fail conventional treatment, TCM can stabilize tumor lesions, improve symptoms, enhance quality of life, and prolong survival time. Improvement in patient's preoperative state, postoperative recovery, and decreased postoperative complications, immune function, and rehabilitation all are benefits of TCM.[47]

QIGONG TO RESTORE BALANCE

Qigong is translated from Chinese to mean "energy cultivation."[48] As an ancient healing art it involves postures, exercises, breathing techniques, and meditations that restore balance to the body. Common to all styles of qigong is the achievement of a state of tranquility, relaxation and release of tension, improved sleep, energy balance, strength and stamina, and a commitment to developing will power.[49]

In ancient China, qigong was considered a method for warding off diseases and prolonging life. Slow, deliberate movements are purported to activate circuits of energy or chi to strengthen the whole body. Randomized clinical trials have been conducted on qigong with populations of patients with cancer in which qigong had positive effects on quality of life, fatigue, and immune system functioning.[50] Women undergoing radiation therapy for 5 weekly sessions over 5 to 6 weeks were found to report less depressive symptoms over time than with women in the control group ($P<.05$). Women who reported elevated depression at the start of radiation reported less fatigue ($P<.01$) and better overall quality of life ($P<.05$).[51] Qigong also has been found to improve fragility and quality of life among patients with breast cancer receiving chemotherapy.[52]

BALANCE THROUGH EXPOSURE TO NATURE

A traditional activity called Shinrin-yoku found in China and Japan is that of forest bathing or "taking in the forest atmosphere." Compared with city environments, studies show that exposure to forest environments promote lower concentrations of cortisol, pulse rate, and blood pressure, while achieving balance through greater parasympathetic and lower sympathetic nervous system activity. Trees release phytoncides (α-pinene and β-pinene) into the forest air. Human studies (though small in subject size) showed a significant increase in natural killer cell number and activity in participants from forest fields when compared with control levels drawn one day prior to the forest trip.[53]

RESTORING BALANCE THROUGH MIND-BODY PRACTICES

Understanding of the interconnected balance between mind and body dates back several millennia, and is found in traditional Ayurvedic and Chinese Medicine, and other ancient healing traditions. The National Center for Complementary and Integrative Health defines mind-body medicine as practices that "focus on the interactions among the brain, mind, body, and behavior, with the intent to use the mind to affect physical functioning and promote health."[54] Mind-focused therapies typically include such practices as meditation, relaxation, and yoga, and are performed either stationary or in movement. Other expressive therapies (eg, music and art therapy, journaling) are sometimes included in this category. Body-focused practices typically include acupuncture, spinal manipulation, massage therapy, Feldenkrais method, and the Alexander technique.[55] Consistent with other previously mentioned ways in which imbalance can disrupt adaptive homeostatic rhythms and processes within bodily systems, the mind and body are no different.

The use of mind-body medicine tends to be higher among individuals with significant medical conditions, such as cancer, especially those who experience multiple disease and treatment-related sequelae. Important targets for mind-body therapeutic interventions have typically included symptom severity and frequency (eg, fatigue, pain, sleep), emotional and social well-being (eg, depression, anxiety, satisfaction with role participation), perceived level of health, quality of life, and functional ability. A recent systematic review on CAM use for men with prostate cancer reported that mind-body medicine use has increased over the past decade, with rates ranging between 8% and 90% (median, 30%). This trend indicated that men with more advanced disease are more likely to use mind-body medicine.[56] Many patients with late-stage breast cancer look to mind-body practices for relief of their symptoms and to enhance their emotional well-being. In addition to meditation use among women with breast cancer,[57] other mind-body practices among patients with cancer include guided imagery,[58] music therapy,[59] therapeutic touch,[60] and reflexology.[61]

Overall, mind-body practices that are tailored to individual needs of the cancer population are generally safe to use in the context of adjuvant supportive care alongside conventional cancer therapies.[55] Although mixed evidence exists regarding the efficacy of some mind-body practices, overall positive outcomes have been reported in quality of life improvement,[62] stress reduction,[63] and balance of different bodily systems and processes. These include reestablishment of normal patterns of cortisol secretion,[64] inflammation,[65] and neurotransmission.[66]

MINDFULNESS MEDITATION AND CANCER

Over the past two decades a growing body of research has shown that learning and implementing mindful awareness practices can lead to increased self-regulation and reductions in emotional distress (depression, anxiety) and pain, improvements in sleep, positive health behaviors, and overall health-related quality of life in populations of patients with cancer.[57] Mindfulness also has an important role in decreasing physiologic effects of stress on the body by reestablishing normal patterns of cortisol secretion,[67] decreasing proinflammatory cytokines, and regulating hypothalamic-pituitary-adrenal axis functioning.[68] Rooted in contemplative traditions, mindfulness enables the cultivation of nonjudgmental, moment-to-moment awareness through attentional single-mindedness.[69]

BENEFITS OF YOGA FOR SURVIVORS OF CANCER

Several studies with populations of patients with cancer report that yoga is linked to improved quality of life, including increased mental health and decreased physical symptoms.[70] Compared with control conditions, specific benefits have included improved sleep quality[71]; less mood disturbances[72]; and improved quality of life,[73] physical functioning,[72] spiritual well-being,[74] and social well-being.[75]

BRIDGING INTEGRATIVE ONCOLOGY AND PRIMARY CARE

Primary care physicians are in a unique position to support oncology care providers by entering into discussions with their patients to identify and address concerns, respond to a patient's need for information, and provide guidance without dismissing their fears. Management of side effects and end-of-life discussions also offer invaluable teachable moments for patients to consider using integrative approaches that may make the difference between deciding to receive a life-sparing treatment or a healthy life transition. Referral to a psychologist for medical hypnosis or guided imagery for fear or anxiety, a naturopathic consult to manage side effects of chemotherapy, or a laser acupuncture treatment to prevent and/or treat neuropathy can help balance a system that is in imbalance. Referrals for physical interventions, such as acupuncture, nutritional changes, homeopathy, diaphragmatic breathing exercises, yoga, and qigong, can offer a sense of ownership and ongoing support for a variety of issues. In addition, emotional support in the form of integrative psychotherapy or meditation can help alleviate some of the uncertainties and fears related to being a cancer survivor.

Practitioners of complementary modalities are often sought out by patients with cancer to respond to their fears and side effects and help regain a sense of control over what is happening to them. Together with primary care physicians, patients can be better guided and educated to form a comprehensive approach that unites oncology treatments with all possible options to complement and advance optimal healing.

ACKNOWLEDGMENTS

The authors thank Ms Stephanie Schuette for her assistance with formatting and other administrative support on this article.

REFERENCES

1. Barnes PM, Bloom B, Nahin RL. Complementary and alternative medicine use among adults and children: United States, 2007. Hyattsville (MD): US Department of Health and Human Services; Centers for Disease Control and Prevention; National Center for Health Statistics; 2008.
2. Treatments and Side Effects. Treatments and Side Effects. 2016. Available at: http://www.cancer.org/treatment/treatmentsandsideeffects/treatmenttypes/. Accessed August 3, 2016.
3. Nestler G, Dovey M. Traditional Chinese medicine. Clin Obstet Gynecol 2001; 44(4):801–13.
4. Sharma HM, Clark C. Contemporary Ayurveda: medicine and research in Maharishi Ayur-Veda. Philadelphia: Churchill Livingstone; 1998.
5. Guthrie D. A history of medicine. London: Thomas Nelson & Sons Ltd; 1945.
6. Wood M, Bégnoche FB, Light PD. Traditional Western herbalism and pulse evaluation: a conversation. Lulu. com; 2015.
7. McKee J. Holistic health and the critique of Western medicine. Soc Sci Med 1988; 26(8):775–84.
8. Qiu J. Traditional medicine: a culture in the balance. Nature 2007;448(7150): 126–8.
9. Bishop FL, Yardley L, Lewith GT. A systematic review of beliefs involved in the use of complementary and alternative medicine. J Health Psychol 2007;12(6):851–67.
10. Lu A-P, Jia H-W, Xiao C, et al. Theory of traditional Chinese medicine and therapeutic method of diseases. World J Gastroenterol 2004;10(13):1854–6.
11. Thatte UM, Dahanukar SA. Ayurveda and contemporary scientific thought. Trends Pharmacol Sci 1986;7:247–51.
12. Tseng W-S. The development of psychiatric concepts in traditional Chinese medicine. Arch Gen Psychiatry 1973;29(4):569–75.
13. Williams A. Therapeutic landscapes in holistic medicine. Soc Sci Med 1998;46(9): 1193–203.
14. Hagerty BM, Williams A. The effects of sense of belonging, social support, conflict, and loneliness on depression. Nurs Res 1999;48(4):215–9.
15. Richardson MA, Sanders T, Palmer JL, et al. Complementary/alternative medicine use in a comprehensive cancer center and the implications for oncology. J Clin Oncol 2000;18(13):2505–14.

16. Matthews T. Combining Western and alternative medicine. Haemophilia 2000; 6:40.
17. Sears SR, Stanton AL, Danoff-Burg S. The yellow brick road and the emerald city: benefit finding, positive reappraisal coping and posttraumatic growth in women with early-stage breast cancer. Health Psychol 2003;22(5):487.
18. Messina MJ, Persky V, Setchell KD, et al. Soy intake and cancer risk: a review of the in vitro and in vivo data. Nutr Cancer 1994;21(2):113–31.
19. Schmitz-Dräger BJ, Eichholzer M, Beiche B, et al. Nutrition and prostate cancer. Urol Int 2001;67(1):1–11.
20. Demark-Wahnefried W, Rogers LQ, Alfano CM, et al. Practical clinical interventions for diet, physical activity, and weight control in cancer survivors. CA Cancer J Clin 2015;65(3):167–89.
21. Hollander D. Intestinal permeability, leaky gut, and intestinal disorders. Curr Gastroenterol Rep 1999;1(5):410–6.
22. Esposito K, Marfella R, Ciotola M, et al. Effect of a Mediterranean-style diet on endothelial dysfunction and markers of vascular inflammation in the metabolic syndrome: a randomized trial. JAMA 2004;292(12):1440–6.
23. Zhou W, Mukherjee P, Kiebish MA, et al. The calorically restricted ketogenic diet, an effective alternative therapy for malignant brain cancer. Nutr Metab 2007;4(1):1.
24. Janecka A, Kołodziej-Rzepa M, Biesaga B. Clinical and molecular features of Laron syndrome, a genetic disorder protecting from cancer. In Vivo 2016;30(4):375–81.
25. Leslie M. Growth defect blocks cancer and diabetes. Science 2011;331(6019):837.
26. Gershtein E, Isaeva E, Kushlinsky D, et al. Insulin-like growth factors (IGF) and IGF-binding proteins (IGFBP) in the serum of patients with ovarian tumors. Bull Exp Biol Med 2016;160(6):814–6.
27. Karlikova M, Topolcan O, Narsanska A, et al. Circulating growth and angiogenic factors and lymph node status in early-stage breast cancer: a pilot study. Anticancer Res 2016;36(8):4209–14.
28. Uzunlulu M, Telci Caklili O, Oguz A. Association between metabolic syndrome and cancer. Ann Nutr Metab 2016;68(3):173–9.
29. Barañano KW, Hartman AL. The ketogenic diet: uses in epilepsy and other neurologic illnesses. Curr Treat Options Neurol 2008;10(6):410–9.
30. Liu YM, Wang H-S. Medium-chain triglyceride ketogenic diet, an effective treatment for drug-resistant epilepsy and a comparison with other ketogenic diets. Biomed J 2013;36(1):9.
31. Rieger J, Bähr O, Maurer GD, et al. ERGO: a pilot study of ketogenic diet in recurrent glioblastoma. Int J Oncol 2014;44(6):1843–52 [Erratum appear in Int J Oncol 2014;45(6):2605].
32. Dorff TB, Groshen S, Garcia A, et al. Safety and feasibility of fasting in combination with platinum-based chemotherapy. BMC Cancer 2016;16(1):1.
33. Lee-Jones C, Humphris G, Dixon R, et al. Fear of cancer recurrence: a literature review and proposed cognitive formulation to explain exacerbation of recurrence fears. Psychooncology 1997;6(2):95–105.
34. Kleinerman RA, Tucker MA, Tarone RE, et al. Risk of new cancers after radiotherapy in long-term survivors of retinoblastoma: an extended follow-up. J Clin Oncol 2005;23(10):2272–9.
35. Bhatia S, Robison LL, Oberlin O, et al. Breast cancer and other second neoplasms after childhood Hodgkin's disease. N Engl J Med 1996;334(12):745–51.
36. Fanous I, Dillon P. Cancer treatment-related cardiac toxicity: prevention, assessment and management. Med Oncol 2016;33(8):1–11.

37. Hockenberry MJ, Hooke MC, Gregurich M, et al. Carnitine plasma levels and fatigue in children/adolescents receiving cisplatin, ifosfamide, or doxorubicin. J Pediatr Hematol Oncol 2009;31(9):664–9.
38. Marijuana and Cancer. Marijuana and Cancer 2015. 2016. Available at: http://www.cancer.org/treatment/treatmentsandsideeffects/physicalsideeffects/chemotherapyeffects/marijuana-and-cancer. Accessed August 12, 2016.
39. Pagotto U, Marsicano G, Cota D, et al. The emerging role of the endocannabinoid system in endocrine regulation and energy balance. Endocr Rev 2006;27(1):73–100.
40. Whiting PF, Wolff RF, Deshpande S, et al. Cannabinoids for medical use: a systematic review and meta-analysis. JAMA 2015;313(24):2456–73.
41. Ramer R, Bublitz K, Freimuth N, et al. Cannabidiol inhibits lung cancer cell invasion and metastasis via intercellular adhesion molecule-1. FASEB J 2012;26(4):1535–48.
42. Ullman D. Homeopathy medicine for the 21st century. Futurist 1988;22(4):43.
43. Stevinson C, Devaraj V, Fountain-Barber A, et al. Homeopathic arnica for prevention of pain and bruising: randomized placebo-controlled trial in hand surgery. J R Soc Med 2003;96(2):60–5.
44. Chaiet SR, Marcus BC. Perioperative arnica montana for reduction of ecchymosis in rhinoplasty surgery. Ann Plast Surg 2016;76(5):477–82.
45. Miccinesi G, Bianchi E, Brunelli C, et al. End-of-life preferences in advanced cancer patients willing to discuss issues surrounding their terminal condition. Eur J Cancer Care 2012;21(5):623–33.
46. Qi F, Li A, Inagaki Y, et al. Chinese herbal medicines as adjuvant treatment during chemo-or radio-therapy for cancer. Biosci Trends 2010;4(6):297–307.
47. Li X, Yang G, Li X, et al. Traditional Chinese medicine in cancer care: a review of controlled clinical studies published in Chinese. PLoS One 2013;8(4):e60338.
48. Dorcas A, Yung P. Qigong: harmonising the breath, the body and the mind. Complement Ther Nurs Midwifery 2003;9(4):198–202.
49. Sancier KM. Therapeutic benefits of qigong exercises in combination with drugs. J Altern Complement Med 1999;5(4):383–9.
50. Soo Lee M, Chen KW, Sancier KM, et al. Qigong for cancer treatment: a systematic review of controlled clinical trials. Acta Oncol 2007;46(6):717–22.
51. Chen Z, Meng Z, Milbury K, et al. Qigong improves quality of life in women undergoing radiotherapy for breast cancer: results of a randomized controlled trial. Cancer 2013;119(9):1690–8.
52. Huang SM, Tseng LM, Chien LY, et al. Effects of non-sporting and sporting qigong on frailty and quality of life among breast cancer patients receiving chemotherapy. Eur J Oncol Nurs 2016;21:257–65.
53. Li Q, Morimoto K, Nakadai A, et al. Forest bathing enhances human natural killer activity and expression of anti-cancer proteins. International Journal of Immunopathology and Pharmacology 2007;20(2):3–8.
54. NCCAM Definition of Mind Body Medicine. 2011. Available at: https://report.nih.gov/NIHfactsheets/ViewFactSheet.aspx?csid=102.
55. Chaoul A, Milbury K, Sood AK, et al. Mind-body practices in cancer care. Curr Oncol Rep 2014;16(12):417.
56. Bishop FL, Rea A, Lewith H, et al. Complementary medicine use by men with prostate cancer: a systematic review of prevalence studies. Prostate Cancer Prostatic Dis 2011;14(1):1–13.
57. Carlson LE, Speca M, Patel KD, et al. Mindfulness-based stress reduction in relation to quality of life, mood, symptoms of stress, and immune parameters in breast and prostate cancer outpatients. Psychosom Med 2003;65(4):571–81.

58. Bedford FL. A perception theory in mind-body medicine: guided imagery and mindful meditation as cross-modal adaptation. Psychon Bull Rev 2012;19(1): 24–45.

59. Burns DS. Theoretical rationale for music selection in oncology intervention research: an integrative review. J Music Ther 2012;49(1):7–22.

60. Hart LK, Freel MI, Haylock PJ, et al. The use of healing touch in integrative oncology. Clin J Oncol Nurs 2011;15(5):519–25.

61. Wyatt G, Sikorskii A, Rahbar MH, et al. Health-related quality-of-life outcomes: a reflexology trial with patients with advanced-stage breast cancer. Oncol Nurs Forum 2012;39(6):568–77.

62. Spahn G, Choi KE, Kennemann C, et al. Can a multimodal mind-body program enhance the treatment effects of physical activity in breast cancer survivors with chronic tumor-associated fatigue? A randomized controlled trial. Integr Cancer Ther 2013;12(4):291–300.

63. Cramer H, Lauche R, Paul A, et al. Mindfulness-based stress reduction for breast cancer-a systematic review and meta-analysis. Curr Oncol 2012;19(5):e343–52.

64. Branstrom R, Kvillemo P, Akerstedt T. Effects of mindfulness training on levels of cortisol in cancer patients. Psychosomatics 2013;54(2):158–64.

65. Kiecolt-Glaser JK, Bennett JM, Andridge R, et al. Yoga's impact on inflammation, mood, and fatigue in breast cancer survivors: a randomized controlled trial. J Clin Oncol 2014;32(10):1040–9.

66. Tang YY, Holzel BK, Posner MI. The neuroscience of mindfulness meditation. Nat Rev Neurosci 2015;16(4):213–25.

67. Matousek RH, Dobkin PL, Pruessner J. Cortisol as a marker for improvement in mindfulness-based stress reduction. Complement Ther Clin Pract 2010;16(1): 13–9.

68. Carlson LE, Speca M, Patel KD, et al. Mindfulness-based stress reduction in relation to quality of life, mood, symptoms of stress and levels of cortisol, dehydroepiandrosterone sulfate (DHEAS) and melatonin in breast and prostate cancer outpatients. Psychoneuroendocrinology 2004;29(4):448–74.

69. Bishop SR, Lau M, Shapiro S, et al. Mindfulness: a proposed operational definition. Clin Psychol Sci Pract 2004;11(3):230–41.

70. Sohl SJ, Danhauer SC, Birdee GS, et al. A brief yoga intervention implemented during chemotherapy: a randomized controlled pilot study. Complement Ther Med 2016;25:139–42.

71. Cohen L, Warneke C, Fouladi RT, et al. Psychological adjustment and sleep quality in a randomized trial of the effects of a Tibetan yoga intervention in patients with lymphoma. Cancer 2004;100(10):2253–60.

72. Chandwani KD, Thornton B, Perkins GH, et al. Yoga improves quality of life and benefit finding in women undergoing radiotherapy for breast cancer. J Soc Integr Oncol 2010;8(2):43–55.

73. Rao RM, Nagendra HR, Raghuram N, et al. Influence of yoga on mood states, distress, quality of life and immune outcomes in early stage breast cancer patients undergoing surgery. Int J Yoga 2008;1(1):11–20.

74. Danhauer SC, Mihalko SL, Russell GB, et al. Restorative yoga for women with breast cancer: findings from a randomized pilot study. Psychooncology 2009; 18(4):360–8.

75. Moadel AB, Shah C, Wylie-Rosett J, et al. Randomized controlled trial of yoga among a multiethnic sample of breast cancer patients: effects on quality of life. J Clin Oncol 2007;25(28):4387–95.

Pediatric Integrative Medicine

David K. Becker, MD, MPH, MA

KEYWORDS

- Integrative medicine • Pediatric integrative medicine • Treatment planning

KEY POINTS

- Integrative pediatrics starts with the relationship with the child and family, and considers the child in the context of her or his environment.
- Treatment planning is a collaborative process, informed by evidence.
- A broad database exists to inform integrative approaches with children.

INTRODUCTION

Integrative pediatrics mirrors much of what is taught in the adult framework. For example, the breadth of modalities for the treatment of migraine or asthma can also be used when treating these conditions in school-aged children and adolescents. However, children are not simply little adults, and data evaluating treatments in adults cannot routinely be extrapolated to children without careful consideration. Fortunately, research in the use complementary modalities in children has exploded in recent years.

It is not possible in the space of this article to address all the issues that may apply to children. The focus is on several areas of interest to physicians who treat children. Additional references are provided for background on other key topics, including neurodevelopmental disorders, attention-deficit/hyperactivity disorder, and autism.

Pediatrics as a field has long advocated a biopsychosocial approach to assessment and treatment planning, recognizing that the child's family, school, and social environment affect and are affected by medical and psychological health.[1] The practice of integrative pediatrics appeals to many providers who care for children because, in addition to the integration of complementary modalities with conventional care, the holistic model actively includes the influences of social and family environments, nutrition, lifestyle choices, and psychological and spiritual health.

Osher Center for Integrative Medicine, University of California, San Francisco, 1545 Divisadero Street, 4th Floor, Box 1726, San Francisco, CA 94143-1726, USA
E-mail address: david.becker1@ucsf.edu

Prim Care Clin Office Pract 44 (2017) 337–350
http://dx.doi.org/10.1016/j.pop.2017.02.010
0095-4543/17/© 2017 Elsevier Inc. All rights reserved.

Specifically, the integrative model in pediatrics encompasses these tenets:

- The child in context (eg, family, environment, social factors, genetics)
- Relationship-based care of child and family
- Focus on wellness and prevention
- Individualized therapies
- Respectful, multidisciplinary collaboration with other providers
- Complementary approach
- Empowerment (the child heals in the context of their family, the physician does not heal him or her)
- Good medicine.

Multiple clinic visits in early infancy are used to monitor growth and development, establish a relationship with the family, and provide anticipatory guidance. Research has shown the impossible amount of time it would take to address all preventive health topics in the typical primary care visit.[2] The goal in the integrative care model should be to balance the standard preventive agenda with the specific needs of the family, while keeping in mind the potential for long-term effects of health prevention.

PRINCIPLES OF INTEGRATIVE PEDIATRICS

With the myriad of options available to families for health-related products, providers, and sources of information about them, a model for helping families make good medical decisions is essential. Factors such as evidence of effectiveness, safety, knowledge of complementary and alternative medicine providers for referrals, cost, prioritizing treatments, and behavioral counseling all must be included.

For example, when evidence of safety is high and conventional approaches have higher risks, a range of complementary approaches may reasonably be considered even when strong evidence of efficacy may be lacking. The quality of the evidence must also be balanced with the beliefs, biases, and preferences of the family, child, and the physician while attending to the obligation of being an advocate for the child in circumstances of vulnerability in the face of competing interests.

Prioritizing and Sequencing Treatments

When making referrals for therapies such as massage, acupuncture, homeopathy, yoga, or other therapies there are several important considerations:

- Provider's experience with children and/or adolescents
- Willingness of the provider to communicate openly with other caregivers
- Provider's philosophy of care: collaborative versus animosity or disdain toward conventional care
- Provider's personal knowledge of the provider (particularly in states without licensing for the given therapeutic modality)
- Cost and time involved for the family
- Potential risks and/or interferences with other treatments
- Provider's legal liability in making a specific referral
- Reasonable evidence of safety and efficacy
- Parents' willingness to continue clearly indicated conventional treatments.

Whenever possible each of these considerations is weighed and, in doing so, the least invasive, most natural treatment options are recommended, including factors that support a child's normal development. A key component to child development is the natural drive for mastery and accomplishment. Engaging this natural drive through active, participatory self-care strategies is likely to increase the success of treatment plans at least in part by engendering a sense of internal control. With sufficient time given to rapport-building and education, many children and families are open to self-regulatory skills development. For many, complex, chronic conditions (eg, headaches) may benefit from the acquisition of a mind-body skill in addition to, for example, massage or acupuncture.

Communication among all providers involved with the child is important. Exemplary integrative care involves communication with western subspecialists, as well as homeopaths, naturopaths, biofeedback practitioners, and others. This includes monitoring for herb-drug interactions, modifications of medications as symptoms change, or adjustments as other modalities become the preferred or primary treatment strategy. In addition, communication helps broaden knowledge among allopathic providers and helps the monitoring of alternative recommendations by providers with strong antipathy toward necessary allopathic treatments.

The integrative treatment plan (adapted from Ref.[3]):

- Summary of diagnosis (explained in developmentally appropriate level)
- Clarify patients and family's goals for treatment (symptom removal vs improved functioning)
- Helpful lifestyle changes (diet, exercise, sleep, schedule)
- Stress management plans (mind or body skills training)
- Parental role as coach and role model
- Vitamins, supplements, botanicals (name, best brands, dose, frequency, route, side-effects)
- Conventional treatments (pharmaceuticals, physician specialists, allied health, rehabilitation therapies, mental health)
- Preventative health recommendations
- Other recommendations: explanation of treatments, target symptoms, risks and benefits, anticipated time and cost, provider referral information if appropriate
- Educational resources (books, Web sites, articles)
- Review recommended priority and sequence of treatments
- Tracking and follow-up plan.

COMMON ACUTE AND CHRONIC PROBLEMS
Colic

Pediatric providers have recognized for decades that at about 6 weeks of age there is a tendency for a subset of infants to develop prolonged bouts of crying and fussiness. The definition of infantile colic has not evolved significantly since Wessel[4] defined it as crying more than 3 hour per day, for more than 3 days per week, for longer than 3 weeks, without an identifiable cause. Despite decades of research, no clear cause has been elucidated.[5] It has at various times been attributed to transient lactase deficiency, allergic sensitivity of the gut (eg, to dairy proteins in formula or breast milk), other abnormal gastrointestinal function, infants' difficult temperament, or ineffective maternal-infant interaction. More recently there are data suggesting that infantile colic is associated with later development of migraines.[6] No conventional treatment modalities have been shown to be effective. Several complementary modalities have shown promise but none have demonstrated effectiveness in multiple well-designed trials.

A detailed history is crucial to the assessment of a fussy infant. Classic colic is usually restricted to the late afternoon or evening hours, is self-limited, varying in intensity, and at best partially responsive to multiple soothing techniques. Symptoms of food sensitivities are usually not restricted to a consistent time of day and are frequently associated with stool changes such as mucus and/or consistently dark green stools. Gastroesophageal reflux usually presents with regurgitation associated with clear signs of pain or distress, arching of the back, or crying with the first swallows of feedings, as well as a pattern of distress that is fairly consistent through the day. Its presence should prompt evaluation for food sensitivities and possibly for issues related to parental attachment and anxiety. The use of antacids or proton pump inhibitors may provide symptomatic relief but does not address the reason for the intestinal dysfunction.

Natural health products
A few studies have looked at the use of fennel seed oil exclusively or in a blended formula. A randomized controlled trial in Russia compared 0.1% fennel seed oil emulsion to similar-appearing and tasting placebo. Compared with 24% improvement in the placebo group, the treatment group showed significant improvement in 65% of infants. Two other studies looked at blended formulas. One included fennel, chamomile, vervain, licorice, and lemon balm. The other included powdered extracts of fennel and chamomile, lemon balm, and vitamins B1, B5, and B6. Both studies found a higher response rate in the treatment compared with control groups. Evaluation of side effects was variable but none were documented. Allergic reactions to fennel and chamomile have been known to occur but are very uncommon. One trial of oral sucrose, which is frequently used for painful procedures in infants, showed short-term efficacy in colic but its effects did not last.[7]

Probiotics
Systematic reviews have been published that show the specific strain *Lactobacillus reuteri* can reduce crying time.[8] A well-designed study looked at the use of *L reuteri* (100 million CFUs once daily) compared with simethicone in breastfed infants whose mothers were put on a dairy-free diet throughout the trial. There was a marked difference in response by the first week that widened by the fourth week to 93% in the probiotic group versus only 7% in the simethicone group.[9] The same research group has also documented a quantitative and qualitative difference in the populations of healthy organisms in infants with or without colic.

Nutritional interventions
Allergic colitis in infants is usually a clinical diagnosis based on blood and/or mucus in the stool with resolution of symptoms following an elimination diet (with or without colonoscopy to rule out other diagnoses). Infant sensitivity to components of the maternal diet has been clinically recognized even without such dramatic stool changes. Cruciferous vegetables and chocolate have been associated with increased flatulence in infants. In addition, a low-allergen maternal diet (no dairy, wheat, soy, eggs, peanuts, tree nuts, and fish) has been shown to reduce colic in a study of 107 infants.[10] Also, hydrolyzed whey formula is recommended by the American Academy of Pediatrics as a treatment option for severe colic. Partially hydrolyzed formulas and casein-hydrolysate have not demonstrated efficacy in clinical trials.

Manual therapies
Chiropractic, osteopathy, and massage have been studied in the treatment of colic. Of several studies on gentle chiropractic treatment, the best-designed study showed no effect. A single unblinded osteopathic study of weekly treatments for a month showed significantly better improvement over a no-treatment control group. A Cochrane review of massage therapy for colic showed some improvement for mother-infant interaction and improved sleep but did not show improvement in colic.[7] A more recent

comprehensive Cochrane review looking at chiropractic, osteopathic, and cranial-sacral studies found statistically significant parent-reported colic symptoms.[11] However, they also noted that the studies that better limited reporting bias did not find statistically significant improvement. When considering referral for manual therapies, it is important to assess the practitioner's experience with infants and that any therapies considered are light touch, hold, and release rather than high-velocity or low-amplitude manipulation.

Summary considerations

- Ensure an accurate diagnosis by detailed history (consistent daytime symptoms suggest a different problem).
- Assess maternal-infant bond and support any family stress and infant calming techniques.

Discuss previously noted options with the family and consider an option that appeals to them, such as probiotics, chamomile tea, or gentle manipulation techniques.

Constipation

Constipation is a variably defined phenomenon that depends on stool frequency, consistency, and difficulty in passing the stool. It is among the more frequent complaints in pediatric primary care. Generally speaking, pain-free passing of the full contents of the lower colon from about 3 times a day to once in 3 days in children over the age of 1 year is expected. In all ages, stool consistency and frequency are diet-dependent, an aspect frequently neglected in conventional medical texts. This phenomenon can be observed in the first weeks of life through the different patterns commonly seen in formula-fed versus breastfed infants. Taking breastfeeding as the standard, normal stools are loose, mustardy-yellow, often with seedy or curd-like components, occasionally watery, and range in frequency from more than 12 times daily to once in 1 to 2 weeks. Formula-fed infants frequently have harder, dryer, pastier stools that occur daily. The age-related differential diagnosis of constipation is extensive and includes anatomic, neurologic, metabolic, pharmacologic, primary intestinal, and other disorders. Once these conditions are ruled out, which can usually be done with a good history and physical alone, dietary evaluation and counseling become the mainstay of assessment and management, with the occasional use of conventional agents, behavioral modifications, and/or mind-body interventions as needed. More severe cases of constipation with a longer history of stool retention and/or encopresis benefit from multimodal treatment strategies that include evacuating the colon, behavioral interventions, and diet assessment. Addressing constipation in childhood is important for adult health because about 25% of children with constipation go on to have symptoms as adults.[12] Also, when behavior problems are present, referral for behavioral health management can be helpful.[13]

Probiotics

There are relatively little data to guide the use of probiotics for constipation. Three studies have not shown efficacy.[14] However, another review of 3 adult studies and 2 pediatric studies suggests promise.[15] A clinical report in pediatrics published in 2010 did not review these studies and concluded that the use of probiotics for constipation was not supported.[16] Understanding of the microbiome and its relationship to a range of conditions remains rudimentary. However, the low risk of probiotics in healthy children make using them a reasonable strategy, particularly in infants and children who are formula fed, have restricted diets, or have been on multiple courses of antibiotics.

Nutritional and lifestyle interventions

A whole foods diet with plenty of water should generally be adequate for addressing most issues with constipation. Many, if not most, families find it difficult to maintain a whole foods diet with young children for a variety of reasons. Dietary behavioral counseling can be helpful. Food choices are only part of a plan. Toddlers in particular are dealing with the developmental drive for control that can assert itself over the natural developmental drive for self-nourishment, competency, and modeling of adults and peers. Reminding parents about what they can and cannot control is helpful. Parents should be reminded that they control which foods are available and served in the house, as well as when and in what setting they are served. However, they have little control over what a child actually puts in his or her mouth or eats (or when they defecate, for that matter). It is crucial to assist parents in efforts to let go of some battles, thereby reinforcing their ability to tolerate the inevitable frustrations of toddlers and older children when they do not get what they want. In addition to this basic guidance, ensuring adequate fiber and water is important, and trials of elimination diets may be helpful (particularly dairy). A simple guide for fiber requirements is 15 mg for every 1000 Kcal in the diet. This roughly translates to: 1 year old, 15 g; 3 year old, 20 g; 5 to 7 years, 25 g; girls older than 8 years, 25gm; and boys older than 8 years old, about 30 to 35 g.[17]

Behavioral interventions

For more difficult cases, behavioral counseling with mental health professionals may be essential. This therapy may or may not include modalities such as biofeedback and hypnosis, both of which can be helpful. For example, some children with constipation and withholding have an aversion to stooling, sometimes called defecation anxiety. These children have difficulty timing the muscular responses to the normal signals that the bowel is ready to empty. For an excellent review of a broadly integrative approach to constipation, including mind-body approaches, see Culbert and Banez.[18]

Upper Respiratory Infections

Upper respiratory and related infections (otitis, sinusitis, influenza) are among the most common reasons for office visits. Toddlers and children have on average 4 to 6 simple colds annually. Because of their frequency, the nuisance of associated symptoms, missed daycare and work, and the absence of effective conventional remedies, families frequently turn to complementary or alternative treatments. Generally speaking, when it comes to the common cold, common sense and good self-care ring true. Good sleep hygiene, regular exercise, a healthy diet, regular hand washing, and early initiation of 1 or more of these possibly effective treatments is about the best one can do.

Echinacea

A wide variety of plants and parts have been used historically and a wide variety of study results have mirrored this. Although echinacea is a safe remedy for use in children (as tolerated and if there is no allergy), Echinacea purpura does not seem effective in the treatment of upper respiratory infections (URIs) in children.[19–21]

Andrographis

Two studies have investigated the use of Andrographis in children: 1 in Russia and 1 is Chile. Although both showed positive results, the Russian study used a combination treatment regimen and both had methodological issues. Potential adverse reactions include stomach upset and hives but these rates in children are unclear. It is likely safe to use but should be done with an awareness of the absence of good evidence in favor and the potential for adverse reactions.[19]

Elderberry

In vitro evidence suggests elderberry has antiviral and immunostimulatory effects. Clinical data suggest it may be effective in reducing the length of influenza symptoms when given early. However, additional studies are necessary before clear conclusions can be drawn.[19]

Vitamin C

Vitamin C may have modest preventive and treatment effects in children at moderate doses, 250 mg to 500 mg daily during cold season or at onset of symptoms.[22] The main side effects from larger doses of vitamin C are bloating, flatulence, and diarrhea, which should abate with lower doses.

Saline irrigation

Evidence in adults suggests nasal saline irrigation may be as effective as antibiotics for acute sinusitis. Use in children depends on acceptability and whether the habit is engendered early. In infants, nasal saline drops can be very effective for improving sleep and feeding.

Zinc

Lozenges (dissolved not chewed) or syrup at approximately 15 mg per dose every couple of hours at first onset of symptoms may shorten the course. When taken for several months, zinc may reduce the number of colds in a season, missed school days, and the number of antibiotic prescriptions written. However, the potential adverse effects of taking significant doses of zinc for an extended period of time have not been well studied. In addition, nasal spray formulations should absolutely be avoided due to credible reports of permanent loss of smell.[23,24]

Honey

A single randomized controlled trial compared a teaspoon of buckwheat honey with honey-flavored dextromethorphan or no treatment. Parents reported significantly reduced cough in the buckwheat honey group and no difference in the other 2 arms. Adverse effects included hyperactivity and poor sleep.[25] A Cochrane review has now been published reviewing trials for honey for cough. Use of honey had better effectiveness than placebo and diphenhydramine, and similar efficacy as dextromethorphan.[26] Unpasteurized honey may contain botulinum toxin and should not be given to infants younger than 1 year of age.

Probiotics

There have been several studies looking at the prevention of common childhood infections, including URIs in 2 trials. In a study from Israel, the use of *Bifidobacterium lactis* or *L reuteri* significantly reduced the number of days with fever, overall episodes of fever, and antibiotic prescriptions in daycare attendees, with *L reuteri* performing better than *B lactis*; however, it had no effect on the frequency of respiratory illness specifically.[27] One well-designed study conducted in China evaluated the use of 2 probiotic preventive regimens in children 3 to 5 years of age over the winter months. Both regimens were highly effective, with the combination of *L acidophilus* and *B lactis* being particularly effective. The combination product reduced fever incidence by 73%, cough incidence by 62%, and rhinorrhea by 58% compared with controls. These results are quite remarkable and warrant repeat study. Nevertheless, they support the use of probiotics for prevention of URIs in children during the winter months.[28] Data for the treatment of URIs with probiotics are weaker but a systematic review did suggest a possible shorting of cold duration.[29]

Acute Gastroenteritis

Acute, uncomplicated gastroenteritis is another common reason for pediatric outpatient visits (not to mention the associated discomfort and foul-smelling frequent diaper changes and bathroom visits). Conventional care for uncomplicated viral gastroenteritis usually includes ensuring adequate hydration, fever control, and follow-up. Herbal remedies and supplements, particularly probiotics, offer additional therapeutic benefit. Nucleotide supplements, glutamine, and partially hydrolyzed guar gum have been advocated as treatments but have very limited data.

Chamomile

Two studies support the use of chamomile in combination with apple pectin in shortening the course of diarrhea due to viral gastroenteritis.[30]

Black tea

Black tea is an example of a plant with high tannin content. Tannins have been shown to increase colonic water and electrolyte reabsorption.[31] In addition, a mouse model showed that tannins reduced diarrhea that was then reversible with naloxone or loperamide.[32]

Homeopathy

Several studies have been conducted evaluating the use of different homeopathic remedies for acute diarrhea in children in Nicaragua, Nepal, and Honduras. The study in Honduras found no difference between placebo and a combination remedy of commonly used homeopathic remedies for acute diarrhea. The same group that conducted 3 small trials in Nicaragua and Nepal performed a meta-analysis of these studies and concluded that homeopathic treatment reduced the duration of diarrhea compared with placebo by 3.3 versus 4.1 days.[33]

Probiotics

Among natural health products for the treatment of diarrhea, probiotics are the best studied and have shown clear benefit.[34] A wide variety of strains have been studied and several systematic reviews, as well as a Cochrane review, have concluded that probiotics are effective in reducing the number of days with diarrhea and the number of stools per day. *L rhamnosus* is probably the best studied but other effective strains include *S boulardii* and *L reuteri*.[33]

Atopic Conditions

The understanding of the etiologic factors underlying the development of all types of allergic conditions is still in its infancy. There are as many theories as there are treatments for the various manifestations, including asthma, atopic dermatitis, allergic rhinitis and conjunctivitis, eosinophilic enteritis, immunoglobulin E–mediated food allergies, and others.[35] Atopic conditions have been on a rapid increase in this country for several decades. The reasons for this are unclear and several theories have also been proposed to explain this. Among the most popular theories for both underlying causes and the increasing prevalence are the hygiene hypothesis, the increase in psychological stress in modern society, and a combination model that includes genetic predispositions, environmental triggers, and nutritional triggers. A detailed discussion of these theories is beyond the scope of this article.

There are many clinical manifestations of atopic conditions. Rather than presenting different cases and the evidence base for those particular clinical scenarios, this review of treatment options presents evidence related to several treatment approaches and the evidence supporting their use.

Nutrition

The best-known primary prevention for atopic conditions is exclusive breastfeeding for at least the first 4 to 6 months. Recent evidence has intriguingly suggested a different strategy than has previously been recommended with regard to the introduction of solid foods. Traditional allergy prevention strategy has included several recommendations, including avoidance of highly allergenic foods during pregnancy and lactation, and delaying their introduction into infant or toddler diets for 1 to 3 years, as well as exclusive breast feeding for 4 to 6 months. However, it has become clear that no consistent data support these recommendations.[36] However, basic nutritional interventions may yet prove to be immensely important as primary prevention measures. Currently, evidence suggests several nutritional recommendations[36]:

- Exclusive breast feeding for 4 to 6 months.
- When formula is necessary or chosen, extensively hydrolyzed formulas have benefit over cow milk, soy, and partially hydrolyzed formulas for the prevention of atopic dermatitis.
- Early introduction (beginning by 6 months of age) of typically highly allergenic foods as complementary foods may prevent development of allergy.

Food sources rich in the omega-6 fatty acid gamma-linolenic acid have been recommended for atopic dermatitis. These include borage oil, evening primrose oil, and black currant seed. However, a meta-analysis of published studies up to 2004 did not find clinically significant evidence to support their use for this condition.[37] Interestingly, a study found that introducing fish before 9 months of age reduced the incidence of eczema in toddlers, so omega-3 fatty acids may have a role.[36] Given the wide range of health benefits of a diet rich in omega-3 fatty acids, incorporating a balance of omega-3 and omega-6 fatty acids early in the diet is well supported.

Finally, though not yet supported by good clinical data, elimination diet trials can be a consideration for children with atopic disorders. In the author's experience, specific foods can be found to be triggers in only about 25% to 30% of children with eczema and there are usually other symptoms of food intolerance, such as gastrointestinal or neurocognitive problems.

Probiotics

Probiotic use for the prevention or treatment of atopic conditions has been an active area of research. If nothing else, research to date has shown the microbiome to be an incredibly complex system with clear roles in the development of a healthy immune system. However, data guiding which strains may be helpful for which conditions, at what doses, and for how long are lacking.[38] Although the World Allergy Organization has released guidelines for the use of probiotics to prevent atopic dermatitis,[39] other global bodies have determined the evidence is lacking for a clear recommendation.[38] The population most likely to benefit are infants with a primary relative with a history of atopy. For asthma prevention, however, the data are inconclusive to date.[40] In families with a strong family history of atopic conditions, a probiotic supplement for the first 6 months of life is reasonable, as is a treatment trial for those already demonstrating evidence of atopy. However, the data supporting the latter recommendation are weaker.

Other natural health products
Many other natural health products have been studied in children and adults with atopic conditions. There are data that seem promising, such as for butterbur, Boswellia, and pcynogenol.[35] However, a recent systematic review has outlined the limitations of these data in supporting broad recommendations.[41] Two examples of thinking integratively about these approaches might be: considering butterbur for a child with an atopic condition and a history (or family history) of migraines, where there are good data supporting its use, and considering Pycnogenol for a child with both atopic disease and significant attention problems.

Mind-body
The link between stress and the function of the immune system is well established, if not specifically etiologically described. Many mind-body therapies have demonstrated efficacy in reducing the biobehavioral markers of stress. However, there are relatively few data specifically linking mind-body skills and clinical change in atopic disorders. Several studies suggest adjunctive benefit of clinical hypnosis and general relaxation techniques.[42]

Traditional Chinese medicine
There is promising early research suggesting benefits of several traditional Chinese medicine (TCM) herbal combinations for atopic dermatitis.[37,43] In a trial in adults in Beijing, a simplified 3-herb formula showed equivalent efficacy as 20 mg daily prednisone for hospitalized subjects with moderate to severe persistent asthma over 1 month. Immunologic markers were particularly interesting for an increase in interferon (IFN)-gamma levels in the herbal group, and a decrease in those levels in the steroid group. IFN-gamma is a marker of T-helper (TH)-1 activity. TH-2 markers were reduced in both groups.[44] Similarly, a mouse model of a trial of an herbal preventive and treatment remedy for anaphylaxis to peanut showed efficacy both in prevention and treatment. Potential problems with TCM herbal remedies are known risks of contamination of products imported from China and India, the strong and unpalatable tastes of many of the remedies, and out-of-pocket costs for families.

Manual therapies
Massage, particularly by parents trained in technique, can be beneficial for atopic dermatitis.[37] A New England Journal of Medicine study concluded that chiropractic manipulation for asthma is not effective.[45] Massage using certain essential oils may worsen eczema but massage with a honey mixture may be beneficial compared with massage in the same patient with a carrier emollient without the honey.[46]

Homeopathy
The data for homeopathic treatments for atopic conditions are intriguing. For example, 4 studies in adults by David Reilly and colleagues[46] have shown promise for treatment of allergic rhinitis. However, inconsistencies and the preponderance of negative trials make recommending homeopathy difficult. Referral to a traditional homeopath may be worth consideration but should be done in the context of having considered other approaches and the family's resources because it is not covered by insurance.

Other approaches
Another important point in assessing a child's atopic history is what happens if or when they travel to other parts of the country or outside the United States. Many

parents find that, for eczema in particular, there is marked improvement with travel outside their home region. Careful assessment of these environmental factors can help pinpoint triggers or alleviating factors.

Summary considerations

A recent study comparing an integrative model (nutritional manipulation, yoga, journaling, and several supplements, including fish oil and vitamin C) to standard care in adults demonstrated significant improvement in a range of behavioral and symptom markers. However, pulmonary function testing did not change.[47] Studies in pediatric populations, similar to this, are critical to demonstrate the efficacy of the integrative model, rather than individual therapies. To date, there are no such data. As always, treatment of atopic conditions in children should be based on a thorough history that will usually suggest promising directions, such as nutrition, stress management, primary preventions strategies, and identifying specific triggers. Additional therapies, as previously discussed, can be considered individually. (See discussion of vitamin D levels, in this issue.)

SUMMARY/DISCUSSION

Pediatric integrative medicine is no longer a novel approach to attending to the health of children and adolescents. This model of care is tailored to fulfill the expectations of the biopsychosocial approach to medicine. How we as child care providers approach families through developing relationship, a mindful attention to use of language, and the continued expansion of the knowledge base defines the quality of care better than labels such as conventional, allopathic, traditional, holistic, complementary, alternative, or integrative. The clinical conditions discussed here just touch the surface of available evidence and training to help address more complex issues, such as severe autoimmune disease, cancer, and complex pain syndromes. There are now pediatric residency training programs with core integrative medicine content, and clinical and research fellowships for further training. There are many doors to exploring and expanding the physician's tool set in helping children, adolescents, and their families.

REFERENCES

1. Hagan JF, Shaw JS, Duncan PM, editors. Bright futures: guidelines for health supervision of infants, children, and adolescents. 3rd edition. The American Academy of Pediatrics; 2008. p. 1–10.
2. Belamarich PF, Gandica R, Stein RE, et al. Drowning in a sea of advice: pediatricians and American Academy of Pediatrics Policy Statements. Pediatrics 2006; 118:e964–78.
3. Culbert T, Maizes V, Mendenhal T, et al. Integrative assessment & treatment planning in pediatrics. In: Culbert T, Olness K, editors. Integrative pediatrics. New York: Oxford University Press Integrative Medicine Library; 2009. p. 13–29.
4. Wessel MA, Cob JC, Jackson EB, et al. Paroxysmal fussing in infancy, sometimes call "colic." Pediatrics 1954;14(5):421–34.
5. Harb T, Matsuyama M, David M, et al. Infant colic – what works: a systematic review of interventions for breast-fed infants. J Pediatr Gastroenterol Nutr 2016;62: 668–86.
6. Qubty W, Gelfand AA. The link between infantile colic and migraine. Curr Pain Headache Rep 2016;20:31.

7. Rosen LD, Bukutu C, Le C, et al. Complementary, holistic, and integrative medicine: colic. Pediatr Rev 2007;28:381–6.

8. Xu M, Wang J, Wang N, et al. The efficacy and safety of the probiotic Bacterium Lactobacillus reuteri DSM 17938 for Infantile colic: a meta-analysis of randomized controlled trials. PLoS One 2015;10(10):e0141445.

9. Savino F, Pelle E, Palumeri E, et al. *Lactobacillus reuteri* (American type culture collection strain 55730) versus simethicone in the treatment of infantile colic: a prospective randomized study. Pediatrics 2007;119:124–30.

10. Hill DJ, Roy N, Heine RG, et al. Effect of a low-allergen maternal diet on colic among breastfed infants: a randomized, controlled trial. Pediatrics 2005;116(5): e709-15.

11. Dobson D, Lucassen PLBJ, Miller JJ, et al. Manipulative therapies for infantile colic. Cochrane Database Syst Rev 2012;(12):CD004796.

12. Bongers ME, van Wijk MP, Reitsma JB, et al. Long-term prognosis for childhood constipation: clinical outcomes in adulthood. Pediatrics 2010;126: e156–62.

13. Van Dijk M, Bongers ME, de Vries GJ, et al. Behavioral Therapy for childhood constipation: a randomized, controlled trial. Pediatrics 2008;121:e1334–41.

14. Tabbbers MM, Chmielewska A, Roseboom MG. Fermented milk containing *Bifidobacterium lactis* DN-173 010 in childhood constipation: a randomized, double-blind, controlled trial. Pediatrics 2011;127:e1392–1399.

15. Chmielewska A, Szajewska H. Systematic review of randomised controlled trials: probiotics for functional constipation. World J Gastroenterol 2010;16: 69–75.

16. Thomas DW, Greer FR. Probiotics and prebiotics in pediatrics. Pediatrics 2010; 126:1217–31.

17. Institute of Medicine. Dietary reference intakes for energy, carbohydrate. Fiber, fat, fatty acids, cholesterol, protein, and amino acids. Washington, DC: The National Academies Press; 2005. p. 386.

18. Culbert TP, Banez GA. Integrative approaches to childhood constipation and encopresis. Pediatr Clin North Am 2007;54:927–47.

19. Bukutu C, Le C, Vohra S. Complementary, holistic, and integrative medicine. Pediatr Rev 2008;12:e66–71.

20. Taylor JA, Weber W, Standish L, et al. Efficacy and safety of echinacea in treating upper respiratory tract infections in children: a randomized controlled trial. JAMA 2003;290:2824–30.

21. Turner RB, Bauer R, Woelkart K, et al. An evaluation of echinacea angustifolia in experimental rhinovirus infections. N Engl J Med 2005;353:341–8.

22. Douglas RM, Hemila H, Chalker E, et al. Vitamin C for preventing and treating the common cold. Cochrane Database Syst Rev 2007;(3):CD000980.

23. Caruso TJ, Prober CG, Gwaltney JM. Treatment of naturally acquired common colds with zinc: a structured review. Clin Infect Dis 2007;45:569–74.

24. Singh M, Das RR. Zinc for the common cold. Cochrane Database Syst Rev 2011;(2):2–59.

25. Paul IM, Beiler J, McMonagle A, et al. Effect of honey, dextromethorphan, and no treatment on nocturnal cough and sleep quality for coughing children and their parents. Arch Pediatr Adolesc Med 2007;161:1140–6.

26. Oduwole O, Meremikwu MM, Oyo-Ita A, et al. Honey for acute cough in children. Cochrane Database Syst Rev 2014;(12):CD007094.

27. Weizman Z, Asli G, Alsheikh A. Effect of a probiotic infant formula on infections in child care centers: comparison of two probiotic agents. Pediatrics 2005;115:5–9.
28. Leyer GJ, Li S, Mubasher ME, et al. Probiotic effects on cold and influenza-like symptom incidence and duration in children. Pediatrics 2009;124:e172–179.
29. King S, Glanville J, Sanders ME, et al. Effectiveness of probiotics on the duration of illness in healthy children and adults who develop common acute respiratory infectious conditions: a systematic review and meta-analysis. Br J Nutr 2014;112:41–54.
30. Gardner P. Complementary, holistic, and integrative medicine: chamomile. Pediatr Rev 2007;28:e16–8.
31. Palombo EA. Phytochemicals from traditional medicinal plants used in the treatment of diarrhoea: modes of action and effects on intestinal function. Phytother Res 2006;20:717–24.
32. Besra SE, Gomes A, Ganguly DK, et al. Antidiarrhoeal activity of hot water extract of black tea (Camellia sinensis). Phytotherapy Res 2003;17:380–4.
33. Mittra D, Bukutu C, Vohra S. Complementary, holistic, and integrative medicine: a review of therapies for diarrhea. Pediatr Rev 2008;29:349–53.
34. Guarino A, Guandalini S, Lo Vecchio A. Probiotics for prevention and treatment of diarrhea. J Clin Gastroenterol 2015;49:S37–45.
35. Rosen LD. An integrative approach to atopic disorders in children. Alt Comp Ther 2007;13:71–7.
36. Fleischer DM, Spergel JM, Assa'ad AH, et al. Primary prevention of allergic disease through nutritional interventions. J Allergy Clin Immunol 2013;1:29–35.
37. Bukutu C, Deol J, Shamseer L, et al. Complementary, holistic, and integrative medicine: atopic dermatitis. Pediatr Rev 2007;28:e87–94.
38. Bridgman SL, Kozyrskyj AL, Scott JA, et al. Gut microbiota and allergic disease in children. Ann Allergy Asthma Immunol 2016;116:99–105.
39. Fiocchi A, Pawankar R, Cuello-Garcia C, et al. World Allergy Organization-McMaster University guidelines for Allergic Disease Prevention (GLAD-P): Probiotics. World Allergy Organ J 2015;8:4.
40. Azad MB, Coneys JG, Kozyrskyj AL, et al. Probiotic supplementation during pregnancy or infancy for the prevention of asthma and wheeze: systematic review and meta-analysis. BMJ 2013;347:1–15.
41. Clark CE, Arnold E, Lasserson TJ, et al. Herbal interventions for chronic asthma in adults and children: a systematic review and meta-analysis. Prim Care Respir J 2010;19:307–14.
42. Vieira BL, Lim NR, Lohman ME. Complementary and alternative medicine for atopic dermatitis: an evidence-based review. Am J Clin Dermatol 2016;17(6):557–81.
43. Li XM. Traditional Chinese herbal remedies for asthma and food allergy. J Allergy Clin Immunol 2007;120:25–31.
44. Wen MC, Wei CH, Hu ZQ, et al. Efficacy and tolerability of anti-asthma herbal medicine intervention in adult patients with moderate-severe allergic asthma. J Allergy Clin Immunol 2005;116:517–24.
45. Balon J, Aker PD, Crowther ER, et al. A comparison of active and simulated chiropractic manipulation as adjunctive treatment for childhood asthma. N Engl J Med 1998;339:1013–20.

46. Taylor MA, Reilley D, Llewellyn-Jones RH, et al. Randomised controlled trial of homeopathy versus placebo in perennial allergic rhinitis with overview of four trial series. BMJ 2000;321:471–6.
47. Kligler B, Homel P, Blank AE, et al. Randomized trial of the effect of an integrative medicine approach to the management of asthma in adults on disease-related quality of life and pulmonary function. Altern Ther Health Med 2011; 17:10–5.

Integrative Medicine and Cardiovascular Disorders

Darshan Mehta, MD, MPH[a,b],*

KEYWORDS

- Cardiovascular disease • Integrative medicine
- Complementary and alternative medicine

KEY POINTS

- Integrative medicine (IM) use is common in patients with cardiovascular diseases (CVDs).
- The most commonly used modalities include dietary supplements/natural products, and mind-body therapies.
- Although there is an increasing body of research around the use of IM in CVD, the data, by in large, are inconclusive and more research is needed.
- Providers need to be aware of safety concerns of certain IM modalities.
- Health care providers need to continue to ask their patients about the preference around their use of IM in the management of CVD.

CARDIOVASCULAR DISORDERS

According to the World Health Organization (WHO), noncommunicable diseases (NCDs), mainly cardiovascular diseases (CVDs), cancers, chronic respiratory diseases, and diabetes, are the world's biggest killers. Of these, CVDs (disorders of the heart and blood vessels that include coronary heart disease, cerebrovascular disease, rheumatic heart disease, and other conditions) account for 17.5 million deaths: an estimated 31% of all deaths worldwide.[1] More than 75% of CVD deaths occur in low-income and middle-income countries, resulting in tremendous economic losses and millions of people trapped in poverty. In 2013, WHO led a plan to reduce the avoidable NCD burden; 2 of the 9 voluntary global targets directly focus on preventing and controlling CVDs.[2]

In the United States, the patterns are quite similar. CVDs claim more lives than all forms of cancer combined. Nearly 801,000 people died of heart disease, stroke,

[a] Osher Center for Integrative Medicine, Brigham and Women's Hospital, Harvard Medical School, 900 Commonwealth Avenue East, 3rd Floor, Boston, MA 02215, USA; [b] Benson-Henry Institute for Mind-Body Medicine, Massachusetts General Hospital, 151 Merrimac Street, 4th Floor, Boston, MA 02114, USA
* Benson-Henry Institute for Mind-Body Medicine, Massachusetts General Hospital, 151 Merrimac Street, 4th Floor, Boston, MA 02114
E-mail address: dmehta@partners.org

Prim Care Clin Office Pract 44 (2017) 351–367
http://dx.doi.org/10.1016/j.pop.2017.02.005
primarycare.theclinics.com

and other CVDs in 2013, representing one-third of all deaths.[3] Approximately 85.6 million Americans are living with some form of CVD or the after-effects of stroke. Direct and indirect costs (health expenditures and lost productivity) of CVDs and stroke total more than $316.6 billion. Although there has been a steady decline in the incidence of CVD in recent years, the prevalence of CVD risk factors (hypertension, high cholesterol, and obesity) has been increasing. Smoking, high blood pressure, high total cholesterol and low-density lipoprotein, low high-density lipoprotein, diabetes, and advanced age are the main risk factors for CVD.

Pharmacologic management continues to be the mainstay of treatment of CVD. However, increasingly numbers of individuals seek nonpharmacologic options. According to the 2002 National Health Interview Survey (NHIS) data, 36% of self-identified patients with CVD use some type of integrative medicine (IM) therapy, with this percentage increasing to 68% when including prayer.[4] Other studies have shown as many as 80% of patients with CVD use some form of IM therapy.[5] Increasing numbers of dietary supplements marketed "over the counter" claim to reduce the risks and symptoms of CVD. In addition, patients with CVD might be more likely to seek IM treatments for relaxation to decrease the psychological stress associated with this condition. Analyses from the 2002 and 2007 NHIS data found that most common categories of complementary modalities used by individuals with a self-reported diagnosis of CVD or CVD risk factors were herbal/dietary supplements and mind-body practices.[6] Given these phenomena, there has been an intentional and increased focus on understanding the role of IM therapies in management of CVD.

Cerebrovascular Disease

Epidemiology

Worldwide, WHO estimates that 15 million people suffer from a stroke each year.[1] According to the Centers for Disease Control and Prevention, stroke is responsible for nearly 130,000 American deaths each year; and every year, more than 795,000 people in the United States have a stroke. The estimated cost for stroke is approximately $34 billion each year (cost of health care services, medications to treat stroke, and missed days of work). Stroke is a leading cause of serious long-term disability.[3]

Although the etiologies of stroke are several, the phenomenon is characterized by an interruption of the blood supply to the brain, often due to a hemorrhage and/or ischemia from a burst blood vessels and clots, resulting in a decreased supply of oxygen and nutrients, causing damage to the brain tissue. The most common symptom of a stroke is sudden weakness or numbness of the face, arm, or leg, most often on one side of the body. Other symptoms include headaches, confusion, difficulty speaking or understanding speech, vision changes, balance and gait issues, loss of consciousness, and death. These effects depend on which part of the brain is injured and how severely it is affected.

Dietary supplements

There is a large body of observational and laboratory evidence suggesting that increasing plasma concentrations of total homocysteine is a causal risk factor for stroke and other vascular events.[7] By inference, reductions in total homocysteine levels have been proposed as a method to reduce the risk of stroke. Vitamin supplements, specifically vitamin E, vitamin C, beta carotene, and folic acid, have been extensively debated in the prevention and treatment of stroke. Although large observational studies initially suggested that there may some protective benefits of these antioxidants, prospective controlled studies have not shown any benefit to supplementation.[8–10] Equivocal findings are also seen in antioxidants for stroke rehabilitation; only individuals with signs of clinical malnutrition seem to benefit from intensive nutritional supplementation. Of note, data have suggested that dietary intake of magnesium, folic acid, vitamin C, and flavanones has been associated with decreased stroke risk,[11–14] suggesting that phytonutrients obtained from a diet rich in fruits and vegetables may have better long-term outcomes that may not be replicable through dietary supplements. In addition, a Mediterranean diet supplemented with extra-virgin olive oil or nuts reduced the incidence of major cardiovascular events, including stroke, in individuals with high CVD risk.[15]

More recent and ongoing research has focused on other targets using dietary supplements.[16] These include vitamin D, as low vitamin D levels have been found to be associated with increased incidence of fatal stroke.[17] Fish oil and omega-3 fatty acids have being examined as well, with current results not informing clinical guidelines one way or another.[18] One challenge in these studies has been isolating the role of the supplements from dietary fat composition, as the quantity and ratios of omega-3 fatty acids may be of significant import. Additionally, dietary calcium intake has been inversely associated with stroke risk; in particular, the attention has focused on dietary calcium obtained from dairy products.[19] Challenges in these analyses include the heterogeneity of dairy types, especially in milk and cheese consumption.

Of specific note, there have been case reports of ischemic stroke in individuals using over-the-counter dietary supplements containing ephedra.[20] Although the Food and Drug Administration has banned products containing ephedra, they are still widely available through online and foreign companies. Even "ephedra-free" products should be carefully monitored in at-risk patients.[21]

Mind-body therapies
Mind-body therapies have been found to be used more frequently among American adults with common neurologic conditions than among those without. Despite this high prevalence of use, two-thirds of adults did not discuss their mind-body practice with their health care provider.[22] Many mind-body therapies (MBTs) have been studied in the rehabilitation efforts for stroke victims. Although many initial findings revolved around case reports and pilot studies, there have been increased efforts toward systematic studies in recent years. Several challenges exist around mind-body medicine studies in stroke recovery, including methodological challenges in research (eg, bias, outcomes) and the broad heterogeneity of stroke itself (eg, etiology, manifestations, sequelae).[23]

Although several different forms of guided imagery have been described in the literature, very few have been studied prospectively. One specific form has been motor imagery, mental imagery, or mental practice: a process in which a function, a behavior, or a performance is rehearsed mentally, as if the person is actually performing it. Several small studies found improvements using these techniques for relearning of daily living tasks,[24] as well as gait function and posture.[25–29] As this process demands perception and executive function, benefits are thought to be mediated by the activation of the contralateral parietal, frontal, and prefrontal regions. Current research is examining the utilization of technology, such as brain-computer interface with imagery practices,[30] as this combination may have enhanced benefits in stroke recovery.

There has been an increase in the study of movement-based interventions in stroke recovery and rehabilitation. One recent small study found improvements in balance with yoga.[31] A meta-analyses of these small intervention studies in yoga have found meaningful improvements in health-related quality of life.[32] Tai chi also has been studied in this disease population. In one larger randomized prospective study, significant improvements were seen in physical function (balance, gait speed, lower body strength) and quality of life (perceived physical, mental health) over time; in addition, fewer falls were observed in the tai chi group compared with the controls. Several large prospective studies are under way.[33–35]

One study examined the role of transcendental meditation as a secondary prevention in black men and women with coronary heart disease; this study found a significant decrease in a composite measure of all-cause mortality, myocardial infarction, or stroke.[36] Mindfulness-based interventions have also been purported to have benefits in stroke recovery, although more prospective studies are needed.[37]

Acupuncture
There has been a growing body of evidence on the use of acupuncture in the management of stroke; particularly, stroke recovery. Acupuncture has been found to be a safe treatment option, when under the guidance of a licensed and/or experienced provider. A recent Cochrane review[38] concluded that acupuncture may have a beneficial effect on dependency (activities of daily living); global neurologic deficiency; and specific neurologic impairments, including motor function, cognitive function, depression, swallowing function, pain, and spasticity. In addition, there were no serious adverse events reported in people with stroke in the convalescent stage using acupuncture. Despite these findings, many researchers raise concerns about the risk of bias in many acupuncture studies. Large-scale multicenter trials are in process,[39] and aim to reach consensus about the most appropriate protocol of acupuncture intervention, length of treatment, and potential synergistic outcomes with other modalities in stroke rehabilitation.

Manipulative and body-based methods
There are very few studies of manipulative and manual therapies in stroke rehabilitation. Although the few published case reports have yielded positive findings, larger controlled studies are needed.

Of note, many health care professionals raise concerns about cervical manipulation as a risk factor for causing stroke, particularly due to cervical artery dissection. Surveys by neurologists have estimated the risk of cervical artery dissection or stroke following neck manipulation to be approximately 5 in 100,000 to 1 in 1 million manipulations.[40,41] Most recently, a study examining the risk of stroke in elderly patients found extremely low incidence: less than 9.8 per million chiropractic visits.[42] Although a direct cause-and-effect link has not been established between neck manipulation and the risk of stroke, the American Heart Association has put out a formal statement that health care providers should inform patients of the association before they undergo neck manipulation.[43]

Energy therapies
One controlled study was identified with the use of Reiki therapy, an energy therapy conducted by a trained practitioner typically through the gentle laying of hands on a clothed patient, in the management of stroke. It did not have any clinically useful effect on stroke recovery in subacute hospitalized patients receiving standard-of-care rehabilitation therapy.[44]

Author recommendations: cerebrovascular disease
- Acupuncture, MBT, and healthy diet may have some clinical roles in the treatment and rehabilitation of cerebrovascular disease.
- Prospective studies are under way in various IM modalities and their application in cerebrovascular disease.
- Cervical manipulation in chiropractic care deserves special mention as a risk factor for stroke.

Heart Failure

Epidemiology

Heart failure affects more than 5.8 million people in the United States and more than 37 million worldwide.[45,46] Characterized by periodic exacerbations that require treatment intensification, often in the hospital, it is the single most frequent cause of hospitalization in persons aged 65 or older. The total medical costs for patients with heart failure are expected to rise from US$20.9 billion in 2012 to $53.1 billion by 2030. As it is a complex clinical syndrome requiring the understanding of cardiac conditions, hereditary defects, and systemic diseases, assessment and management of heart failure requires the tailoring of policies to population-specific risks and understanding of individual factors. Increasingly, IM therapies have been used in the secondary and tertiary prevention of individuals with heart failure.

Dietary supplements

Heart failure is an energy-depleted state associated with low myocardial adenosine triphosphate (ATP) production, mitochondria dysfunction, abnormal calcium handling, increased reactive oxygen species generation, and endothelial dysfunction. Many of the disease-modifying therapies in heart failure act by modulation of maladaptive neuro-hormonal pathways, such as the renin-angiotensin-aldosterone axis. Coenzyme Q10 (CoQ10) has been studied as a therapeutic option to treat individuals with heart failure. Lower CoQ10 levels are seen in patients with advanced heart failure symptoms and with lower ejection fractions. A recent large prospective randomized controlled trial found there may be a mortality benefit in patients with CoQ10 supplementation (100 mg taken 3 times daily orally), with reductions in the primary 2-year end point of cardiovascular death, hospital stays for heart failure, or mechanical support or cardiac transplantation, death from cardiovascular causes, and all-cause mortality.[47] Furthermore, there does not seem to be an adverse hemodynamic profile or safety concern about CoQ10 use, although further studies and postmarketing data are needed to confirm this.

Other emerging and promising targets in the management of heart failure include addressing omega-3 fatty acids,[18] iron,[48] and vitamin D deficiencies.[49] The GISSI-HF study was one of the largest prospective randomized controlled trials conducted[50]; it found that a simple treatment of a 1-g dose of omega-3 fatty acid can provide a small beneficial advantage in terms of mortality and admission to hospital for cardiovascular reasons in patients with heart failure. A recent randomized controlled study found significant improvements in elderly patients with heart failure and vitamin D deficiency after 6 months of supplementation at 4000 IU daily.[49] Challenges in research include the preparation of these dietary supplements (food source, oral, intravenous), setting (outpatient, inpatient), heterogeneity (ie, type of omega-3 fatty acid), and paucity of trials.

Hawthorn extracts have been used as a herbal remedy for the treatment of heart failure. Several large-scale trials have examined its purported benefits,[51,52] but were unable to demonstrate benefit overall. Specific populations may still derive some benefit, as dosage and disease severity may also impact outcomes[53]; that is, a more seriously ill patient may need higher dosages (1800 mg) for significant improvements to be obtained. Shengmai, a traditional Chinese medicine, is usually used in China as a complementary and a single treatment for chronic heart failure. Considered a promising treatment option, a Cochrane review[54] found that it may exert a positive effect on heart failure; however, the studies were confounded by publication bias.

Other dietary supplements that have purported benefits based on small randomized controlled studies include probiotics (specifically, *Saccharomyces boulardii*),[55]

L-carnosine,[56] taurine,[57] and other amino acids.[58] These supplements have demonstrated benefits on physiologic (ejection fraction, blood pressure, sympathomimetic markers), functional (exercise capacity), and quality-of-life metrics. Although the results of these clinical trials are promising with regard to heart failure management, data regarding prognosis are still lacking.

Mind-body therapies
In recent years, MBTs have emerged as a mainstay in the treatment of heart failure, especially in heart failure rehabilitation programs. Heart failure is characterized by high sympathetic nerve activity with high resting sympathetic tone; MBTs often aim to reduce or suppress this sympathetic nerve activity by using practices that generate slow and deep respiration. Many of these practices have shown to improve blood pressure, ventilation, and ventilation-to-perfusion matching, as well as improve exercise tolerance, functional performance, and other patho-physiologic manifestations of heart failure. Of the various MBTs, inspiratory muscle training[59] and tai chi[60] have been studied the most extensively, and are associated with improvements in exercise capacity as well as quality of life and depression.[61] There have been several small pilot studies using yoga, biofeedback, and relaxation response therapy approaches in the management of heart failure as well.

Other integrative therapies
There has been one small study examining the use of acupuncture in the management of heart failure,[62] suggesting improvements in exercise tolerance, but much more work needs to be done. Only 2 studies examined body-based methods in the management of heart failure.[63,64] Although improvements were seen in measures of anxiety, long-term effects could not be determined.

Author recommendations: heart failure
- MBTs, especially tai chi, have emerged as a mainstay in the treatment of heart failure.
- There may some role for dietary supplements including Coenzyme q10 and hawthorn extracts.
- Further research is needed to demonstrate benefit of IM approaches in management and severity of heart failure.

Heart Valve Diseases and Cardiac Surgery (Including Coronary Artery Bypass Grafting)

Epidemiology
Worldwide, rheumatic heart disease, commonly seen in low-income countries, accounts for most of heart valve disease (HVD), with mortality estimated at 4.4 per 100,000 population.[65] In high-income countries, the greatest burden of HVD referred to hospital is due to calcific aortic valve disease, accounting for just fewer than half of deaths from all valve disease.[66] HVD requires long-term follow-up, with significant investigation and treatment costs, leading to a disproportionately large impact of HVD on health care systems. For many of these patients, long-term management will often include cardiac surgery.

Dietary supplements
Several studies have examined the incidence of postoperative atrial fibrillation and the impact of antioxidants (N-acetylcysteine, omega-3 fatty acids, vitamin C, and vitamin E). A recent meta-analysis and systemic review suggests that there may be some role for antioxidants as a prevention measure in postoperative atrial fibrillation[67]; however, other reviews have suggested no demonstrated benefit.[68,69] Specifically, as it relates

to omega-3 fatty acids, the challenges in this research stem from the heterogeneity in concentrations of the different omega-3 fatty acids.

One small prospective randomized controlled trial found that a nutritional supplement containing L-arginine, omega-3 fatty acids, and yeast RNA had improved immune biomarkers in cardiac surgery patients at high risk for infection.[70] L-arginine has been found to have benefits in exercise capacity in patients with heart transplantation,[71] as well as having improvements in insulin sensitivity and inflammatory markers in cardiac surgery patients.[72]

One small study found that the stem bark of *Terminalia arjuna*, used by the Ayurvedic physicians in India for the treatment of various CVDs, was found to have reductions in ischemic mitral regurgitation.[73]

One community-based observational study found no significant increased progression of aortic valve calcification in women taking oral calcium supplementation.[74]

One at-risk population for HVD and cardiac surgery are children born with congenital heart defects. Maternal folic acid supplementation, shown to decrease neural tube defects in the offspring, also has a positive association with decreased risk of congenital heart disease.[75]

Mind-body therapies
Studies from the 1970s and 1980s describe the use of MBT in the preoperative and postoperative care of patients undergoing cardiac surgery (often in the setting of HVD), and describe improvements in postsurgical complications and pain.[76,77] In a small controlled pilot study in children with symptomatic mitral valve prolapse, biofeedback and imagery were associated with decreased chest pain.[78] Mechanisms behind these findings are thought to be due to decreased cardiac sympathetic drive, leading to reductions in cardiovascular parameters, such as resting heart rate, blood pressure, and respiratory rate. Another large-scale prospective study demonstrated that teaching self-hypnosis preoperatively led to decreased postoperative pain medication requirement.[79]

Music therapy has been found effective in the postoperative management of cardiac surgery. Several prospective randomized studies have demonstrated benefits of music therapy (and associated relaxation activities) leading to decreases in pain and anxiety, and overall satisfaction of care.[80–84] In 1 pediatric study, the use of music was associated with significant differences intraoperative metrics, as well as pain score, sedation score, occurrence of child post-traumatic stress disorder, and occurrence of negative postoperative behavior.[85]

Several notable large-scale randomized prospective studies also looked at the role of intercessory prayer in cardiac surgery, revealing no benefit in outcomes.[81,86,87]

Given that patients with HVD and those undergoing cardiac surgery procedures, MBT may have implications in costs of care. In cardiac surgery patients, one study showed that a guided imagery program was associated with shorter average length of stay (1.5 days), a decrease in average direct pharmacy costs (~$300), and a decrease in total costs ($2000) while maintaining high overall patient satisfaction with the care and treatment provided.[88] A recent study examined the benefits of augmented MBT-based cardiac rehabilitation programs, finding lower cardiac and noncardiac hospitalization rates, offset health care costs (estimated 3-year net savings per participant up to $3500/individual), and a trend toward lower mortality.[89]

Acupuncture
Acupuncture has been used in Chinese medical practice for cardiovascular surgery.[90] Early reports described its use as anesthesia for procedures. More recently,

acupuncture treatment before cardiac surgery was found to alleviate cardiac ischemia-reperfusion injury in adult patients undergoing heart valve replacements,[91] as well as reducing intensive care unit length of stay. This type of finding has been seen in pediatric populations as well.[92] Several small randomized controlled studies have examined postoperative acupuncture, finding reductions in nausea and pain.[93,94]

Importantly, cases of endocarditis have been reported in patients who have undergone acupuncture treatments.[95,96] Although the causation and incidence of this complication is unknown, patients with HVD should be counseled accordingly.

Manipulative and body-based methods
Several small studies have examined the role of massage therapy in cardiac surgery patients. These studies have found clinically significant decreases in pain and anxiety, as well as improvements in relaxation and satisfaction.[97,98] Even simple approaches, such as foot massage, can have improvements in feelings of calm and decreased anxiety.[99,100] Osteopathic manipulative therapy also has been used in the management of cardiac surgery patients, finding immediate improvements in postsurgical functional recovery.[101]

Energy therapies
One study found that the administration of healing touch after cardiac surgery resulted in decreases in anxiety and length of stay.[102]

Author recommendations: heart valve diseases and cardiac surgery
- MBT has been found to decrease postoperative complications in cardiac surgery, often in the setting of heart disease.
- Further prospective larger-scale studies need to examine the role of IM therapies in cardiac surgery and HVD.

Peripheral Vascular Disease

Epidemiology
Peripheral vascular disease (PVD) refers to circulation disorders caused by narrowing, blockage, or spasms in vessels outside of the heart, including the arteries, veins, or lymphatic vessels. The upper and lower extremities are most commonly affected. One common form of PVD is peripheral arterial disease (PAD). PAD prevalence is sharply age-related, rising more than 10% among patients in their 60s and 70s. Although low prevalence (between 3% and 12% of the population), it seems to be higher among men than women for more severe or symptomatic disease, and there have been global increases over the past decade.[103]

Dietary supplements
Omega-3 fatty acid supplementation has been of particular interest in the management of PAD. A recent systematic review concluded that there was insufficient evidence,[104] although large prospective studies are underway.[105] In addition, flax seed (rich in alpha linoleic acid) is presently being investigated in the management of PAD, and has been found to reduce cholesterol as an adjunct to pharmacologic management.[106]

One study examined the use of standardized French maritime pine bark extract (pycnogenol) in patients with severe chronic venous insufficiency (150 mg per day for 8 weeks), and found improvements and measures of clinical symptoms.[107]

Ginkgo biloba was not found to be more effective than standard pharmacologic management of Raynaud phenomenon.[108] This was also found to be true of L-arginine in the long-term management of PAD, with suggestions that there may even be harm.[109]

Acupuncture
Small studies have looked at the use of acupuncture in the treatment of Raynaud phenomenon[110] and PAD.[111] Although these studies were small, they demonstrated the feasibility of a standardized acupuncture protocol in the treatment of these conditions.

Mind-body therapies
There has been considerable interest in the use of thermal biofeedback, in which patients use thermistors applied to the affected area and practice self-control of vasorelaxation, in the management of Raynaud phenomenon.[112] Although studies have been small, this continues to be an area of promise in the nonpharmacologic management of this condition.

Author recommendations: peripheral vascular disease
- Much research is needed in the management of PVD with IM therapies.
- There is promise in dietary supplements (omega-3 fatty acids) and acupuncture.

Rhythm Disorders

Epidemiology
The prevalence of conduction and rhythm disorders increases with age due in part to the changes in the myocardium that happen with aging. Bradyarrhythmias and tachyarrhythmias can be either asymptomatic, or cause hemodynamic changes requiring treatment.

Dietary supplements
Many medications have had their origins in herbal remedies; for example, digoxin was derived from the foxglove plant. Dietary supplements also have been linked as triggers for arrhythmias. For example, cesium consumption was found to be associated with prolonged QT interval.[113] As previously mentioned, ephedra, and even "ephedra-free," products have been associated with increased cardiac arrhythmias.[114] Other products found to have associations with cardiac arrhythmias reported in the literature include ginkgo biloba, oleander, bitter orange, horny goat weed, aconitum, and bitter melon. As such, their interactions, especially with prescribed medications, should be carefully examined.[115] Omega-3 fatty acids have been studied in the management of atrial fibrillation; although it did appear promising at one time, current data do not support its use.[116]

Mind-body therapies
As mentioned earlier, elicitation of the relaxation response elicitation during postoperative recovery,[77] found reductions in postoperative supraventricular tachycardia. These findings have been replicated with the use of clinical hypnosis. MBTs have been found to have healthy physiologic changes (increased respiratory sinus arrhythmia) in healthy subjects,[117] and in patients with coronary artery disease.[118] Most recently, a yoga-based approach was found to reduce arrhythmia burden in patients with atrial fibrillation.[119]

Acupuncture
Acupuncture has been studied in the treatment of different cardiac arrhythmias; however, these studies are limited by poor design and heterogeneity.[120] One study found acupuncture reduced the rate of arrhythmia recurrences in patients with persistent atrial fibrillation.[121]

Author recommendations: rhythm disorders
- Dietary supplements are pharmacologically active, and their interactions with other medications need to be closely monitored, especially as they pertain to rhythm disorders.
- MBTs have been shown to reduce arrhythmia burden.

Coronary Heart Disease

Epidemiology
Coronary heart disease (CHD) is the largest contributor to CVDs.[122] It is responsible for nearly one-half of cardiovascular deaths in men and more than one-third in women. Myocardial infarction, angina pectoris, and sudden coronary death are the major clinical manifestations of CHD. The initial presentation of CHD is sudden coronary death in approximately one-third of cases. Although many dietary and lifestyle factors are implicated in the development of CHD, not much is known with regard to IM in the treatment of CHD.

Natural products and dietary supplements
Garlic and garlic supplements have been of significant interest in the management of CHD, particularly in demonstration of artery plaque regression.[123] Garlic has been noted to improve risk factors associated with CHD, including hyperlipidemia.[124]

Mind-body therapies
The "stressed" or "Type A" personality has a long-held belief around its association with CHD.[125] As such, MBTs have been purported to augment treatment of CHD,[126] especially in cardiac rehabilitation efforts,[127,128] although regression of CHD has not been demonstrated in long-term studies.[129] More studies are needed in this regard.

Author recommendations: coronary heart disease
- Much research is needed in the study of IM therapies in the management of CHD.

SUMMARY

IM use among patients with CVD is common, with dietary supplements and MBTs being the most commonly used treatment modalities. More rigorous research is needed to determine the precise physiologic effects and long-term benefits on cardiovascular morbidity and mortality with IM usage. In addition, safety considerations must always be kept in mind. It is important for health care providers to ask their patients about their beliefs around IM use, and especially current or planned use of dietary supplements, when determining optimal treatment plans that minimize the risk of interactions.

REFERENCES

1. WHO. Global status report on noncommunicable diseases 2014. Geneva (Switzerland): WHO; 2014.
2. WHO. Global action plan for the prevention and control of NCDs 2013–2020. Geneva (Switzerland): WHO; 2013.
3. Mozaffarian D, Benjamin EJ, Go AS, et al. Heart disease and stroke statistics—2016 update: a report from the American Heart Association. Circulation 2016; 133(4):e38–360.
4. Yeh GY, Davis RB, Phillips RS. Use of complementary therapies in patients with cardiovascular disease. Am J Cardiol 2006;98(5):673–80.
5. Prasad K, Sharma V, Lackore K, et al. Use of complementary therapies in cardiovascular disease. Am J Cardiol 2013;111(3):339–45.

6. Anderson JG, Taylor AG. Use of complementary therapies by individuals with or at risk for cardiovascular disease: results of the 2007 national health interview survey. J Cardiovasc Nurs 2012;27(2):96–102.
7. Homocysteine Studies Collaboration. Homocysteine and risk of ischemic heart disease and stroke: a meta-analysis. JAMA 2002;288(16):2015–22.
8. Schürks M, Glynn RJ, Rist PM, et al. Effects of vitamin E on stroke subtypes: meta-analysis of randomised controlled trials. BMJ 2010;341:c5702.
9. Toole JF, Malinow M, Chambless LE, et al. Lowering homocysteine in patients with ischemic stroke to prevent recurrent stroke, myocardial infarction, and death: the vitamin intervention for stroke prevention (VISP) randomized controlled trial. JAMA 2004;291(5):565–75.
10. Törnwall ME, Virtamo J, Korhonen PA, et al. Postintervention effect of alpha tocopherol and beta carotene on different strokes: a 6-year follow-up of the alpha tocopherol, beta carotene cancer prevention study. Stroke 2004;35(8): 1908–13.
11. Cassidy A, Rimm EB, O'Reilly ÉJ, et al. Dietary flavonoids and risk of stroke in women. Stroke 2012;43(4):946–51.
12. Chen G-C, Lu D-B, Pang Z, et al. Vitamin C intake, circulating vitamin C and risk of stroke: a meta-analysis of prospective studies. J Am Heart Assoc 2013;2(6): e000329.
13. He K, Merchant A, Rimm EB, et al. Folate, vitamin B6, and B12 intakes in relation to risk of stroke among men. Stroke 2004;35(1):169–74.
14. Sluijs I, Czernichow S, Beulens JWJ, et al. Intakes of potassium, magnesium, and calcium and risk of stroke. Stroke 2014;45(4):1148–50.
15. Estruch R, Ros E, Salas-Salvadó J, et al. Primary prevention of cardiovascular disease with a Mediterranean diet. N Engl J Med 2013;368(14):1279–90.
16. Hankey GJ. Vitamin supplementation and stroke prevention. Stroke 2012; 43(10):2814–8.
17. Pilz S, Dobnig H, Fischer JE, et al. Low vitamin D levels predict stroke in patients referred to coronary angiography. Stroke 2008;39(9):2611–3.
18. Rizos EC, Ntzani EE, Bika E, et al. Association between omega-3 fatty acid supplementation and risk of major cardiovascular disease events: a systematic review and meta-analysis. JAMA 2012;308(10):1024–33.
19. de Goede J, Soedamah-Muthu SS, Pan A, et al. Dairy consumption and risk of stroke: a systematic review and updated dose–response meta-analysis of prospective cohort studies. J Am Heart Assoc 2016;5(5):e002787.
20. Chen C, Biller J, Willing SJ, et al. Ischemic stroke after using over the counter products containing ephedra. J Neurol Sci 2004;217(1):55–60.
21. Bouchard NC, Howland MAP, Greller HA, et al. Ischemic stroke associated with use of an ephedra-free dietary supplement containing synephrine. Mayo Clin Proc 2005;80(4):541–5.
22. Erwin Wells R, Phillips RS, McCarthy EP. Patterns of mind-body therapies in adults with common neurological conditions. Neuroepidemiology 2011;36(1): 46–51.
23. Louw SJ. Research in stroke rehabilitation: confounding effects of the heterogeneity of stroke, experimental bias and inappropriate outcomes measures. J Altern Complement Med 2002;8(6):691–3.
24. Liu KP, Chan CC, Lee TM, et al. Mental imagery for promoting relearning for people after stroke: a randomized controlled trial. Arch Phys Med Rehabil 2004; 85(9):1403–8.

25. Cho H, Kim J, Lee G-C. Effects of motor imagery training on balance and gait abilities in post-stroke patients: a randomized controlled trial. Clin Rehabil 2013;27(8):675–80.
26. Hosseini SA, Fallahpour M, Sayadi M, et al. The impact of mental practice on stroke patients' postural balance. J Neurol Sci 2012;322(1–2):263–7.
27. Liu H, Song L, Zhang T. Mental practice combined with physical practice to enhance hand recovery in stroke patients. Behav Neurol 2014;2014:e876416.
28. Oostra KM, Oomen A, Vanderstraeten G, et al. Influence of motor imagery training on gait rehabilitation in sub-acute stroke: a randomized controlled trial. J Rehabil Med 2015;47(3):204–9.
29. Page SJ, Levine P, Leonard A. Mental practice in chronic stroke: results of a randomized, placebo-controlled trial. Stroke 2007;38(4):1293–7.
30. Pichiorri F, Morone G, Petti M, et al. Brain–computer interface boosts motor imagery practice during stroke recovery. Ann Neurol 2015;77(5):851–65.
31. Schmid AA, Puymbroeck MV, Altenburger PA, et al. Poststroke balance improves with yoga: a pilot study. Stroke 2012;43(9):2402–7.
32. Desveaux L, Lee A, Goldstein R, et al. Yoga in the management of chronic disease: a systematic review and meta-analysis. Med Care 2015;53(7):653–61.
33. Tao J, Rao T, Lin L, et al. Evaluation of Tai Chi Yunshou exercises on community-based stroke patients with balance dysfunction: a study protocol of a cluster randomized controlled trial. BMC Complement Altern Med 2015;15(1):31.
34. Tousignant M, Corriveau H, Kairy D, et al. Tai chi-based exercise program provided via telerehabilitation compared to home visits in a post-stroke population who have returned home without intensive rehabilitation: study protocol for a randomized, non-inferiority clinical trial. Mayo Clin Proc 2014;15(1):42.
35. Zhang Y, Liu H, Zhou L, et al. Applying tai chi as a rehabilitation program for stroke patients in the recovery phase: study protocol for a randomized controlled trial. Trials 2014;15(1).
36. Schneider RH, Grim CE, Rainforth MV, et al. Stress reduction in the secondary prevention of cardiovascular disease randomized, controlled trial of transcendental meditation and health education in blacks. Circ Cardiovasc Qual Outcomes 2012;5(6):750–8.
37. Lawrence M, Booth J, Mercer S, et al. A systematic review of the benefits of mindfulness-based interventions following transient ischemic attack and stroke. Int J Stroke 2013;8(6):465–74.
38. Yang A. Acupuncture for stroke rehabilitation. Cochrane Database Syst Rev 2016;(8):CD004131.
39. Huang J, Lin Z, Wang Q, et al. The effect of a therapeutic regimen of Traditional Chinese Medicine rehabilitation for post-stroke cognitive impairment: study protocol for a randomized controlled trial. Trials 2015;16:272.
40. Gouveia LO, Castanho P, Ferreira JJ. Safety of chiropractic interventions: a systematic review. Spine 2009;34(11):E405–13.
41. Kapral MK, Bondy SJ. Cervical manipulation and risk of stroke. CMAJ 2001;165(7):907–8.
42. Whedon JM, Song Y, Mackenzie TA, et al. Risk of stroke after chiropractic spinal manipulation in medicare b beneficiaries aged 66 to 99 years with neck pain. J Manipulative Physiol Ther 2015;38(2):93–101.
43. Biller J, Sacco RL, Albuquerque FC, et al. Cervical arterial dissections and association with cervical manipulative therapy: a statement for healthcare professionals from the American Heart Association/American Stroke Association. Stroke 2014;45(10):3155–74.

44. Shiflett SC, Nayak S, Bid C, et al. Effect of Reiki treatments on functional recovery in patients in poststroke rehabilitation: a pilot study. J Altern Complement Med 2002;8(6):755–63.
45. Roger VL. Epidemiology of heart failure. Circ Res 2013;113(6):646–59.
46. Ziaeian B, Fonarow GC. Epidemiology and aetiology of heart failure. Nat Rev Cardiol 2016;13(6):368–78.
47. Mortensen SA, Rosenfeldt F, Kumar A, et al. The effect of coenzyme Q10 on morbidity and mortality in chronic heart failure. JACC Heart Fail 2014;2(6): 641–9.
48. Cohen-Solal A, Leclercq C, Deray G, et al. Iron deficiency: an emerging therapeutic target in heart failure. Heart 2014;100(18):1414–20.
49. Dalbeni A, Scaturro G, Degan M, et al. Effects of six months of vitamin D supplementation in patients with heart failure: a randomized double-blind controlled trial. Nutr Metab Cardiovasc Dis 2014;24(8):861–8.
50. Tavazzi L, Maggioni AP, Marchioli R, et al. Effect of n-3 polyunsaturated fatty acids in patients with chronic heart failure (the GISSI-HF trial): a randomised, double-blind, placebo-controlled trial. Lancet 2008;372(9645):1223–30.
51. Holubarsch CJF, Colucci WS, Meinertz T, et al, Survival and Prognosis: Investigation of Crataegus Extract WS® 1442 in CHF (SPICE) Trial Study Group. The efficacy and safety of *Crataegus* extract WS® 1442 in patients with heart failure: the SPICE trial. Eur J Heart Fail 2008;10(12):1255–63.
52. Zick SM, Vautaw BM, Gillespie B, et al. Hawthorn extract randomized blinded chronic heart failure (HERB CHF) trial. Eur J Heart Fail 2009;11(10):990–9.
53. Tassell MC, Kingston R, Gilroy D, et al. Hawthorn (*Crataegus* spp.) in the treatment of cardiovascular disease. Pharmacogn Rev 2010;4(7):32–41.
54. Zhou Q, Qin W-Z, Liu S-B, et al. Shengmai (a traditional Chinese herbal medicine) for heart failure. Cochrane Database Syst Rev 2014;(4):CD005052.
55. Costanza AC, Moscavitch SD, Faria Neto HCC, et al. Probiotic therapy with *Saccharomyces boulardii* for heart failure patients: a randomized, double-blind, placebo-controlled pilot trial. Int J Cardiol 2015;179:348–50.
56. Lombardi C, Carubelli V, Lazzarini V, et al. Effects of oral administration of orodispersible levo-carnosine on quality of life and exercise performance in patients with chronic heart failure. Nutrition 2015;31(1):72–8.
57. Beyranvand MR, Kadkhodai Khalafi M, Roshan VD, et al. Effect of taurine supplementation on exercise capacity of patients with heart failure. J Cardiol 2011; 57(3):333–7.
58. Carubelli V, Castrini AI, Lazzarini V, et al. Amino acids and derivatives, a new treatment of chronic heart failure? Heart Fail Rev 2014;20(1):39–51.
59. Cahalin LP, Arena RA. Breathing exercises and inspiratory muscle training in heart failure. Heart Fail Clin 2015;11(1):149–72.
60. Pan L, Yan J, Guo Y, et al. Effects of tai chi training on exercise capacity and quality of life in patients with chronic heart failure: a meta-analysis. Eur J Heart Fail 2013;15(3):316–23.
61. Yeh GY, McCarthy EP, Wayne PM, et al. Tai chi exercise in patients with chronic heart failure: a randomized clinical trial. Arch Intern Med 2011;171(8):750–7.
62. Kristen AV, Schuhmacher B, Strych K, et al. Acupuncture improves exercise tolerance of patients with heart failure: a placebo-controlled pilot study. Heart 2010;96(17):1396–400.
63. Chen W-L, Liu G-J, Yeh S-H, et al. Effect of back massage intervention on anxiety, comfort, and physiologic responses in patients with congestive heart failure. J Altern Complement Med 2012;19(5):464–70.

64. Jones J, Thomson P, Lauder W, et al. Reflexology has no immediate haemody-
namic effect in patients with chronic heart failure: a double blind randomised
controlled trial. Complement Ther Clin Pract 2013;19(3):133–8.

65. Coffey S, Cairns BJ, Iung B. The modern epidemiology of heart valve disease.
Heart 2016;102(1):75–85.

66. Coffey S, Cox B, Williams MJA. Lack of progress in valvular heart disease in the
pre-transcatheter aortic valve replacement era: increasing deaths and minimal
change in mortality rate over the past three decades. Am Heart J 2014;
167(4):562–7.e2.

67. Ali-Hassan-Sayegh S, Mirhosseini SJ, Rezaeisadrabadi M, et al. Antioxidant
supplementations for prevention of atrial fibrillation after cardiac surgery: an updated comprehensive systematic review and meta-analysis of 23 randomized
controlled trials. Interact Cardiovasc Thorac Surg 2014;18(5):646–54.

68. Mariani J, Doval HC, Nul D, et al. N-3 polyunsaturated fatty acids to prevent
atrial fibrillation: updated systematic review and meta-analysis of randomized
controlled trials. J Am Heart Assoc 2013;2(1):e005033.

69. Xin W, Wei W, Lin Z, et al. Fish oil and atrial fibrillation after cardiac surgery: a
meta-analysis of randomized controlled trials. PLoS One 2013;8(9):e72913.

70. Tepaske R, Velthuis H, Oudemans-van Straaten HM, et al. Effect of preoperative
oral immune-enhancing nutritional supplement on patients at high risk of infection after cardiac surgery: a randomised placebo-controlled trial. Lancet 2001;
358(9283):696–701.

71. Doutreleau S, Rouyer O, Marco PD, et al. l-Arginine supplementation improves
exercise capacity after a heart transplant. Am J Clin Nutr 2010;91(5):1261–7.

72. Lucotti P, Monti L, Setola E, et al. Oral l-arginine supplementation improves
endothelial function and ameliorates insulin sensitivity and inflammation in cardi-
opathic nondiabetic patients after an aortocoronary bypass. Metabolism 2009;
58(9):1270–6.

73. Dwivedi S, Aggarwal A, Agarwal MP, et al. Role of terminalia arjuna in ischaemic
mitral regurgitation. Int J Cardiol 2005;100(3):507–8.

74. Bhakta M, Bruce C, Messika-Zeitoun D, et al. Oral calcium supplements do not
affect the progression of aortic valve calcification or coronary artery calcification. J Am Board Fam Med 2009;22(6):610–6.

75. Feng Y, Wang S, Chen R, et al. Maternal folic acid supplementation and the risk
of congenital heart defects in offspring: a meta-analysis of epidemiological
observational studies. Sci Rep 2015;(5):8506.

76. Horowitz BFM, Fitzpatrick JJ, Flaherty GGM. Relaxation techniques for pain relief after open heart surgery. Dimens Crit Care Nurs 1984;3(6):364–71.

77. Leserman J, Stuart EM, Mamish ME, et al. The efficacy of the relaxation
response in preparing for cardiac surgery. Behav Med 1989;15(3):111–7.

78. Smith MS, Doroshow C, Womack WM, et al. Symptomatic mitral valve prolapse
in children and adolescents: catecholamines, anxiety, and biofeedback. Pediatrics 1989;84(2):290–5.

79. Whitworth JR, Burkhardt AM, Oz M. Complementary therapy and cardiac surgery. J Cardiovasc Nurs 1998;12(4):87–94.

80. Bauer BA, Cutshall SA, Anderson PG, et al. Effect of the combination of music
and nature sounds on pain and anxiety in cardiac surgical patients: a randomized study. Altern Ther Health Med 2011;17(4):16–23.

81. Krucoff MW, Crater SW, Gallup D, et al. Music, imagery, touch, and prayer as
adjuncts to interventional cardiac care: the Monitoring and Actualisation of

Noetic Trainings (MANTRA) II randomised study. Lancet Lond Eng 2005; 366(9481):211–7.

82. Nilsson U. The effect of music intervention in stress response to cardiac surgery in a randomized clinical trial. Heart Lung 2009;38(3):201–7.

83. Özer N, Karaman Özlü Z, Arslan S, et al. Effect of music on postoperative pain and physiologic parameters of patients after open heart surgery. Pain Manag Nurs 2013;14(1):20–8.

84. Voss JA, Good M, Yates B, et al. Sedative music reduces anxiety and pain during chair rest after open-heart surgery. Pain 2004;112(1):197–203.

85. Abd-Elshafy SK, Khalaf GS, Abo-Kerisha MZ, et al. Not all sounds have negative effects on children undergoing cardiac surgery. J Cardiothorac Vasc Anesth 2015;29(5):1277–84.

86. Aviles JM, Whelan SE, Hernke DAM, et al. Intercessory prayer and cardiovascular disease progression in a coronary care unit population: a randomized controlled trial. Mayo Clin Proc 2001;76(12):1192–8.

87. Benson H, Dusek JA, Sherwood JB, et al. Study of the therapeutic effects of intercessory prayer (STEP) in cardiac bypass patients: a multicenter randomized trial of uncertainty and certainty of receiving intercessory prayer. Am Heart J 2006;151(4):934–42.

88. Halpin LSM, Speir AM, CapoBianco PM, et al. Guided imagery in cardiac surgery. Outcomes Manag 2002;6(3):132–7.

89. Zeng W, Stason WB, Fournier S, et al. Benefits and costs of intensive lifestyle modification programs for symptomatic coronary disease in Medicare beneficiaries. Am Heart J 2013;165(5):785–92.

90. Cheng TO. Stamps in cardiology. Acupuncture anaesthesia for open heart surgery. Heart 2000;83(3):256.

91. Yang L, Yang J, Wang Q, et al. Cardioprotective effects of electroacupuncture pretreatment on patients undergoing heart valve replacement surgery: a randomized controlled trial. Ann Thorac Surg 2010;89(3):781–6.

92. Ni X, Xie Y, Wang Q, et al. Cardioprotective effect of transcutaneous electric acupoint stimulation in the pediatric cardiac patients: a randomized controlled clinical trial. Paediatr Anaesth 2012;22(8):805–11.

93. Coura LEF, Manoel CHU, Poffo R, et al. Randomised, controlled study of preoperative electroacupuncture for postoperative pain control after cardiac surgery. Acupunct Med 2011;29(1):16–20.

94. Korinenko Y, Vincent A, Cutshall SM, et al. Efficacy of acupuncture in prevention of postoperative nausea in cardiac surgery patients. Ann Thorac Surg 2009; 88(2):537–42.

95. Buckley DA. *Staphylococcus aureus* endocarditis as a complication of acupuncture for eczema. Br J Dermatol 2011;164(6):1405–6.

96. Stellon A. Acupuncture in patients with valvular heart disease and prosthetic valves. Acupunct Med 2003;21(3):87–91.

97. Braun LA, Stanguts C, Casanelia L, et al. Massage therapy for cardiac surgery patients—a randomized trial. J Thorac Cardiovasc Surg 2012;144(6):1453–9.e1.

98. Cutshall SM, Wentworth LJ, Engen D, et al. Effect of massage therapy on pain, anxiety, and tension in cardiac surgical patients: a pilot study. Complement Ther Clin Pract 2010;16(2):92–5.

99. Bagheri-Nesami M, Shorofi SA, Zargar N, et al. The effects of foot reflexology massage on anxiety in patients following coronary artery bypass graft surgery: a randomized controlled trial. Complement Ther Clin Pract 2014;20(1):42–7.

100. Hattan J, King L, Griffiths P. The impact of foot massage and guided relaxation following cardiac surgery: a randomized controlled trial. J Adv Nurs 2002;37(2): 199–207.
101. Noll D. The effect of OMT on postoperative medical and functional recovery of coronary artery bypass graft patients. J Am Osteopath Assoc 2013;113(8): 595–6.
102. MacIntyre B, Hamilton J, Fricke T, et al. The efficacy of healing touch in coronary artery bypass surgery recovery: a randomized clinical trial. Altern Ther Health Med 2008;14(4):24–32.
103. Criqui MH, Aboyans V. Epidemiology of peripheral artery disease. Circ Res 2015;116(9):1509–26.
104. Enns JE, Yeganeh A, Zarychanski R, et al. The impact of omega-3 polyunsaturated fatty acid supplementation on the incidence of cardiovascular events and complications in peripheral arterial disease: a systematic review and meta-analysis. BMC Cardiovasc Disord 2014;14(1).
105. Grenon SM, Owens CD, Alley H, et al. n-3 Polyunsaturated fatty acids supplementation in peripheral artery disease: the OMEGA-PAD trial. Vasc Med 2013; 18(5):263–74.
106. Edel AL, Rodriguez-Leyva D, Maddaford TG, et al. Dietary flaxseed independently lowers circulating cholesterol and lowers it beyond the effects of cholesterol-lowering medications alone in patients with peripheral artery disease. J Nutr 2015;145(4):749–57.
107. Cesarone MR, Belcaro G, Rohdewald P, et al. Improvement of signs and symptoms of chronic venous insufficiency and microangiopathy with Pycnogenol®: a prospective, controlled study. Phytomedicine 2010;17(11):835–9.
108. Choi W-S, Choi C-J, Kim K-S, et al. To compare the efficacy and safety of nifedipine sustained release with *Ginkgo biloba* extract to treat patients with primary Raynaud's phenomenon in South Korea; Korean Raynaud study (KOARA study). Clin Rheumatol 2009;28(5):553–9.
109. Wilson AM, Harada R, Nair N, et al. l-Arginine supplementation in peripheral arterial disease. Circulation 2007;116(2):188–95.
110. Appiah R, Hiller S, Caspary L, et al. Treatment of primary Raynaud's syndrome with traditional Chinese acupuncture. J Intern Med 1997;241(2):119–24.
111. Cunha RG, Rodrigues KC, Salvador M, et al. Effectiveness of laser treatment at acupuncture sites compared to traditional acupuncture in the treatment of peripheral artery disease in 2010 Annual International Conference of the IEEE Engineering in Medicine and Biology. 2010. p. 1262–5.
112. Karavidas MK, Tsai P-S, Yucha C, et al. Thermal biofeedback for primary Raynaud's phenomenon: a review of the literature. Appl Psychophysiol Biofeedback 2006;31(3):203–16.
113. Lyon AW, Mayhew WJ. Cesium toxicity: a case of self-treatment by alternate therapy gone awry. Ther Drug Monit 2003;25(1):114–6.
114. Nasir JMU, Durning SJU, Ferguson MU, et al. Exercise-induced syncope associated with QT prolongation and ephedra-free xenadrine. Mayo Clin Proc 2004; 79(8):1059–62.
115. Mashour NH, Lin GI, Frishman WH. Herbal medicine for the treatment of cardiovascular disease: clinical considerations. Arch Intern Med 1998;158(20): 2225–34.
116. Christou GA, Christou KA, Korantzopoulos P, et al. The current role of omega-3 fatty acids in the management of atrial fibrillation. Int J Mol Sci 2015;16(9): 22870–87.

117. Ditto B, Eclache M, Goldman N. Short-term autonomic and cardiovascular effects of mindfulness body scan meditation. Ann Behav Med 2006;32(3):227–34.
118. Del Pozo JM, Gevirtz RN, Scher B, et al. Biofeedback treatment increases heart rate variability in patients with known coronary artery disease. Am Heart J 2004; 147(3):545.
119. Lakkireddy D, Atkins D, Pillarisetti J, et al. Effect of yoga on arrhythmia burden, anxiety, depression, and quality of life in paroxysmal atrial fibrillation: the yoga my heart study. J Am Coll Cardiol 2013;61(11):1177–82.
120. VanWormer AM, Lindquist R, Sendelbach SE. The effects of acupuncture on cardiac arrhythmias: a literature review. Heart Lung 2008;37(6):425–31.
121. Lomuscio A, Belletti S, Battezzati PM, et al. Efficacy of acupuncture in preventing atrial fibrillation recurrences after electrical cardioversion. J Cardiovasc Electrophysiol 2011;22(3):241–7.
122. Wong ND. Epidemiological studies of CHD and the evolution of preventive cardiology. Nat Rev Cardiol 2014;11(5):276–89.
123. Koscielny J, Klüßendorf D, Latza R, et al. The antiatherosclerotic effect of *Allium sativum*. Atherosclerosis 1999;144(1):237–49.
124. Knox J, Gaster B. Dietary supplements for the prevention and treatment of coronary artery disease. J Altern Complement Med 2007;13(1):83–96.
125. Friedman M, Rosenman RH. Overt behavior pattern in coronary disease: detection of overt behavior pattern a in patients with coronary disease by a new psychophysiological procedure. JAMA 1960;173(12):1320–5.
126. Orth-Gomér K, Schneiderman N, Wang H-X, et al. Stress reduction prolongs life in women with coronary disease: the Stockholm Women's Intervention Trial for Coronary Heart Disease (SWITCHD). Circ Cardiovasc Qual Outcomes 2009; 2(1):25–32.
127. Ornish D, Scherwitz LW, Doody RS, et al. Effects of stress management training and dietary changes in treating ischemic heart disease. JAMA 1983;249(1): 54–9.
128. Paul-Labrador M, Polk D, Dwyer JH, et al. Effects of a randomized controlled trial of transcendental meditation on components of the metabolic syndrome in subjects with coronary heart disease. Arch Intern Med 2006;166(11):1218–24.
129. Lehmann N, Paul A, Moebus S, et al. Effects of lifestyle modification on coronary artery calcium progression and prognostic factors in coronary patients—3-year results of the randomized SAFE-LIFE trial. Atherosclerosis 2011;219(2):630–6.

Women's Health
Pregnancy and Conception

Judith Cuneo, MD

KEYWORDS

- Integrative medicine • Pregnancy • Prenatal care • Nutrition • Mind-body medicine
- Acupuncture • Herbs

KEY POINTS

- Preconception is an ideal time to assist women contemplating pregnancy to modify health behaviors.
- Dietary needs in pregnancy are critical and may require supplementation.
- The use of mind-body medicine in the antenatal period assists patients in childbirth preparation.
- Integrative medicine techniques can be safely and effectively used for common third-trimester obstetric complications of pregnancy.

INTRODUCTION

The focus of this article is on the care of the pregnant woman in the ambulatory setting. It reviews specific integrative medicine treatments that are recommended for low-risk obstetric patients at each stage of the prenatal period to assist primary obstetric providers to safely use integrative medicine modalities in conventional prenatal care. Integrative medicine techniques may also be safely and effectively applied to intrapartum and postpartum care; however, these topics are beyond the scope of this article.

PRECONCEPTION CARE

Addressing health behaviors during the preconception period is the ideal time to assist patients in preparing for pregnancy and institute behavioral changes that optimize their health and the health of their babies. Women contemplating pregnancy may be especially receptive to shifting behaviors that improve their health and well-being.

Using motivational interviewing techniques, the integrative clinician may facilitate and engage the patient in behavior change regarding the essential health habits that

I have no commercial or financial conflicts of interest or funding sources.
Osher Center for Integrative Medicine, University of California, San Francisco, 1545 Divisadero Street, San Francisco, CA 94115, USA
E-mail address: Judith.cuneo@ucsf.edu

Prim Care Clin Office Pract 44 (2017) 369–376
http://dx.doi.org/10.1016/j.pop.2017.02.011

are the bedrock of integrative medicine: nutrition, exercise/movement, sleep, and stress management, as needed.

Among the general pregnancy population, more than half are overweight or obese at conception. Overweight and obese women are at an increased risk of medical and obstetric complications in pregnancy, including gestational diabetes, high blood pressure, preeclampsia, preterm birth, and cesarean delivery. Infants of overweight and obese mothers are at greater risk of congenital malformation, macrosomia with potential birth injury, and childhood obesity.[1] Thus, the opportunity to work with patients in the preconception period to achieve a normal weight through diet, develop a regular exercise program, and screen for obesity-related diseases, including diabetes, must be seized.

The effects of stress in pregnancy can weaken the maternal immune system and increase the risk of premature birth, although the mechanism remains unclear. Stress may also increase risk-taking behaviors that may have a negative impact on pregnancy health.[2] An inquiry into the presence of maternal stress and implementation of stress-reducing techniques are components of integrative prenatal care.

An exploration of environmental exposures is important in preconception to bring attention to reducing chemicals in food sources and household products, including but not limited to the endocrine disruptors bisphenol A, phthalates, and glycol ethers as well as flame retardants and heavy metals.

Finally, inquiry into the stability of the partner relationship, presence of support from friends and family, and an assessment of a patient's psychosocial resources are essential factors to explore when providing holistic care to the woman contemplating pregnancy.

FIRST TRIMESTER

Dietary needs increase in the first trimester of pregnancy. Although a pregnant woman only requires an additional 300 kcal/d, attention to the quality of the calories consumed is essential, and a diet sourced from whole foods and rich with fruits, vegetables, whole grains, legumes, and lean protein sources may be ideal. Certain nutrients in the diet must be emphasized for optimal growth and development of both pregnant woman and fetus.

Folate

Folate is a B vitamin that is important for reproductive-aged women. The current US recommended dietary allowance (RDA) of folate is 600 µg for pregnant women. Supplementing with 400 µg of folic acid, the synthetic form of folate and the amount typically found in standard prenatal vitamins, before and during pregnancy helps prevent fetal neural tube defects. In addition to supplementing with folic acid, increasing dietary sources of folate, including dark leafy greens, legumes, nuts and seeds, and cruciferous vegetables, should be emphasized.

Vitamin D

Vitamin D is a fat-soluble vitamin obtained largely from consuming fortified foods or dietary supplements. It is also produced endogenously in the skin with exposure to sunlight. Vitamin D helps with absorption of calcium from the gut and allows for normal bone mineralization and growth. During pregnancy, severe maternal vitamin D deficiency has been associated with biochemical evidence of disordered skeletal homeostasis, congenital rickets, and fractures in the newborn, because newborn vitamin D levels are largely dependent on maternal vitamin D status. Recent evidence suggests that maternal vitamin D deficiency is common during pregnancy, especially among high-risk groups, including vegetarians, women with limited sun exposure, and ethnic minorities, especially those with darker skin.[3]

The serum concentration of 25-hydroxyvitamin D can be used as an indicator of nutritional vitamin D status. A serum level of at least 20 ng/mL is considered adequate.[4]

The current RDA is 600 IU for pregnant women. Most prenatal vitamins typically contain 400 IU of vitamin D per tablet. Although data on the safety of higher doses are lacking, experts agree that supplemental vitamin D is safe in dosages up to 4000 IU/d during pregnancy or lactation.[5] There are limited unprocessed food sources of vitamin D. Small amounts are present in fatty fish and egg yolks.

Omega-3 Fatty Acids

Omega-3 fatty acids are essential and can only be obtained from the diet. Omega-3 fatty acids are important in pregnancy because they serve as the building blocks of the fetal brain and retina. They may also influence the length of gestation and prevent perinatal depression.[6]

The most biologically active forms of omega-3 fatty acids are docosahexaenoic acid (DHA) and eicosapentaenoic acid (EPA), which are primarily derived from marine sources, such as seafood and algae. Confusion regarding adverse effects of environmental contaminants, including mercury, in seafood, may prevent women from consuming adequate levels of omega-3 fatty acids. For pregnant women to obtain adequate omega-3 fatty acids, a variety of sources should be consumed: walnuts, seeds (hemp, chia, and flax), 2 servings of low-mercury fish per week (mackerel, herring, salmon, sardines, or anchovies), and supplements (fish oil or algae-based DHA).[7]

Although the requirements have yet to be firmly established, it is suggested that supplemental DHA (250–350 mg/d) be taken in conjunction with EPA (400–600 mg/d) in pregnancy.[7] Fish oil supplements are essentially free from mercury, dioxins, or polychlorinated biphenyls and are the best option for supplementation. Vegetarian women can take flax seed oil (or other α-linolenic acid–rich oils) and should consider taking an algae-based source of DHA.

Iron

The RDA for iron is 30 mg/d for pregnant and women, which is found in most prenatal vitamin supplements. Patients should be encouraged to consume iron-rich foods, including dark green leafy vegetables, dried beans and peas, nuts and seeds, dried fruit, poultry, fish, and lean red meat. Iron is best absorbed when consumed with vitamin C–rich foods, such as citrus fruits and tomatoes.

Calcium

The RDA for calcium is 1200 mg/d for pregnant women over age 24 and 1200 mg/d to 1500 mg/d for pregnant women under age 24. Milk and other dairy products, such as cheese and yogurt, provide the highest sources of calcium but dark, leafy greens, calcium-fortified tofu, dried beans and peas, almonds, and seafood are good nondairy sources. Adequate vitamin D levels assist calcium absorption.

Vitamin A

Doses of 10,000 IU/d or higher of preformed vitamin A can increase the risk of birth defects, such as cleft palate and spina bifida, as well as miscarriage.[8] Pregnant women should not take more than 3000 IU/d preformed vitamin A in supplement form, generally listed on the label as vitamin A acetate or vitamin A palmitate.

SECOND TRIMESTER

Childbirth education is often pursued by pregnant women and encouraged by health care providers in the second trimester. In the United States, approximately 3.9 million women give birth each year[9] and approximately half of them attend some form of childbirth preparation course.[10] There is little evidence that childbirth education, as currently structured, is effective in producing a beneficial impact on the birth experience[11] and may instead increase a woman's fear of childbirth.[12]

The integrative medicine model can provide an alternative to conventional childbirth education. Mind-body techniques, such as yoga, mindfulness meditation, and clinical hypnosis, when taught in the context of pregnancy and birth, provide a pregnant woman and her partner skills to work with pain, fear, and stress during pregnancy, labor and birth, postpartum transition, and life with an infant. Mind-body skills induce mental relaxation, alter negative thinking related to anxiety, and change the perception of a stressful event, leading to better adapted behavior and coping skills. In addition, mind-body techniques support the normalcy of pregnancy and birth and may improve a woman's overall satisfaction with the birth experience.

A 2008 review of studies on mind-body interventions in pregnancy found that women who used mind-body interventions had infants with higher birth weights, shorter labors, fewer instrument-assisted births, and reduced maternal stress and anxiety.[13] A Cochrane review evaluated mind-body interventions during pregnancy and demonstrated their efficacy for reducing women's anxiety during pregnancy and labor and in the first 4 weeks after giving birth.[14]

Prenatal Yoga

A 2015 study examined the acute maternal and fetal effects of yoga postures, and suspected contraindicated postures, in a prospective cohort of healthy pregnant women in the third trimester. Participants assumed 26 yoga postures. Vital signs, pulse oximetry, tocometry, and continuous fetal heart rate monitoring were observed before, during, and after each posture. All 26 yoga postures (cumulative 650 poses) were well tolerated with no acute adverse maternal physiologic or fetal heart rate changes demonstrating the safety of this mind-body intervention in pregnancy.[15] Pregnant women interested in prenatal yoga should receive instruction from a trained practitioner.

Mindfulness Meditation

The Mindfulness-Based Childbirth and Parenting Program (MBCP) created by certified nurse-midwife and meditation teacher Nancy Bardacke, certified nurse midwife, is a 9-week, 38-hour, antenatal educational and experiential program for expectant women and their partners that systematically teaches mindfulness meditation in preparation for labor, birth, and the family life. The program is based on the internationally recognized mindfulness-based stress reduction program developed by Jon Kabat-Zinn, PhD, at the University of Massachusetts Medical Center. Preliminary studies demonstrate that pregnant women participants of the MBCP program report an increased ability to cope with childbirth, reduced pain in labor, reduced use of systemic opiate analgesia in labor, and lower rates of perinatal depression.[16]

For those interested in the program who live at a distance from an available course, the companion text and CD, Mindful Birthing: Training the Mind, Body, and Heart for Childbirth and Beyond, written by Bardacke[17], are widely available.

Clinical Hypnosis

Clinical hypnosis promotes an altered state of awareness, perception, or consciousness that allows for increased concentration and attention. The responsiveness of individuals to hypnotic suggestions can facilitate useful changes in perception and behavior and may change aspects of a patient's physiologic and neurologic functions. Licensed hypnotherapists use hypnosis to treat psychological or physical problems. In pregnancy, hypnosis can be used antenatally in preparation for birth; its emphasis is focusing attention on feelings of comfort and enhancing a woman's feelings of relaxation and sense of safety. Individuals can learn self-hypnosis during pregnancy for subsequent use during labor or can be guided into hypnosis by a practitioner during labor. Antenatal training is often supplemented using an audio recording of hypnotic suggestions.

A Cochrane review[18] of hypnosis for pain management in labor and birth included studies of both practitioner-guided hypnosis and self-hypnosis techniques. Seven randomized trials evaluating 1213 women received hypnosis or conventional antenatal education. There were no significant differences between women in the hypnosis group and those in the control group in terms of drug use for pain management in labor, the number of normal deliveries, or women's satisfaction with the method of pain relief. Small, single trials did report that hypnosis reduced pain intensity and shortened the length of labor.[19]

HypnoBirthing International is a United Kingdom–based, internationally recognized antenatal program that teaches hypnosis techniques to expectant women. Trained practitioners are available in 46 countries, but for those without access to a practitioner, the textbook and companion CD *Hypnobirthing, The Mongan Method*, written by counselor, hypnotherapist, and program founder, Marie F. Mongan, MEd, are widely available.[20]

THIRD TRIMESTER
Breech Presentation and Moxibustion

Breech presentation at 37 weeks of gestation and beyond complicates approximately 4% of pregnancies, and more than 85% of pregnant women with a persistent breech presentation are delivered by cesarean.[21] In a recent study, the rate of attempted external cephalic version (ECV) was 46%; thus, ECV for fetal malpresentation is likely underused.[22] Considering that most patients with a successful ECV give birth vaginally, the procedure should be offered to all patients when clinically appropriate. When contraindications to ECV are present, patients decline ECV, or if ECV has failed, however, integrative medicine modalities may be useful.

Moxibustion used simultaneously with acupuncture has been studied for its effects at correcting breech presentation. Moxibustion is a traditional Chinese medicine therapy using moxa from dried mugwort that is burned near a patient's skin to stimulate the BL 67 acupoint. The treatment is typically applied several times per week over the course of the treatment period, although which kind of moxibustion method works best to correct fetal malpresentation (timing during pregnancy, number of sessions, and length of sessions) is unknown.

A Cochrane review[23] evaluated evidence to support the use of moxibustion for correcting breech presentation. Six studies with 1087 subjects compared moxibustion to observation or postural methods and reported a rate of cephalic version among the moxibustion group of 72.5% versus 53.2% in the control group. In terms of safety, no significant differences were found in the comparison of moxibustion with other techniques. The review concluded that moxibustion combined with acupuncture may result in fewer births by cesarean section and, when combined with postural management techniques, may reduce the number of noncephalic presentations at birth.[23]

Post-term Pregnancy and Integrative Medicine Techniques

Post-term pregnancy refers to a pregnancy that has reached or extended beyond 42 0/7 weeks of gestation from the last menstrual period. Late-term pregnancy is defined as one that has reached between 41 0/7 weeks and 41 6/7 weeks of gestation.[24] In 2011, the overall incidence of post-term pregnancy in the United States was 5.5%.[25] Integrative medicine modalities may be useful in preventing post-term pregnancy, labor induction, and potential complications.

Partus Preparators

Partus prepatators are herbs historically used during the last weeks of pregnancy to tone and prepare the uterus and to hasten the onset of labor.

Red raspberry leaf

Red raspberry leaf can be found in many popular pregnancy teas. It is often promoted to prevent miscarriage, ease morning sickness, and ensure a quick birth.

A survey of 172 certified nurse midwives found that 63% of midwives using herbal preparations recommended red raspberry leaf.[26] A double-blind, placebo-controlled study randomized 192 low-risk, nulliparous women to receive raspberry leaf tablets or placebo, from 32 weeks' gestation until delivery. Raspberry leaf was not associated with any adverse effects in mother or baby but did not shorten the first stage of labor. One clinically significant finding was a shortening of the second stage of labor (mean difference, 9.59 minutes).[27] A retrospective study of women taking raspberry leaf from 30 weeks to 35 weeks onward failed to find any significant adverse outcomes in mother or infant compared with controls.[28] Further studies are needed to evaluate safety and efficacy.

Evening primrose oil

Evening primrose oil has historically been used to hasten cervical ripening in an effort to shorten labor and decrease the incidence of post-term pregnancies. Evening primrose oil is used orally and/or applied to the cervix for these purposes. Findings suggest that the oral administration of evening primrose oil from the 37th gestational week until birth does not shorten gestation or decrease the overall length of labor. It may also be associated with an increase in the incidence of prolonged rupture of membranes, oxytocin augmentation, arrest of descent, and vacuum extraction.[29] Current evidence does not support its use for this indication at this time.

Blue cohosh (Caulophyllum thalictroides) and black cohosh (Actaea racemosa)

Blue cohosh (*Caulophyllum thalictroides*) and black cohosh (*Actaea racemosa*) are 2 herbs often used in combination as partus preparators. There have been a small number of case reports implicating blue cohosh, used in combination with black cohosh, with neonatal myocardial infarction, multiorgan failure, congestive heart failure, and perinatal stroke in infants born to mothers taking the herbs several weeks before birth.[30–33] Women should be strongly cautioned against the use of these herbs in pregnancy.

Post-term Pregnancy and Labor Induction with Acupuncture

To determine the efficacy and safety of acupuncture for third-trimester cervical ripening or induction of labor, a Cochrane review[34] included 14 trials with data reporting on 2220 women. The trials reported on 3 primary outcomes—caesarean section, serious neonatal morbidity, and maternal mortality—and concluded that acupuncture for induction of labor seems safe, has no known adverse effects to the fetus, and may be effective. There is a need for more well-designed randomized controlled trials to evaluate the role of acupuncture to induce labor and for these trials to assess clinically meaningful outcomes.[34]

Probiotics and Maternal Group B Streptococcus Rectovaginal Colonization

There is considerable interest in the relationship between probiotic use and group B streptococcus (GBS) rectovaginal colonization in pregnant women in the third trimester. At this time there is no evidence to support the use of probiotics to prevent or treat GBS colonization in the pregnant woman; however, a clinical trial is under way to determine if oral probiotic supplementation during the second half of pregnancy decreases maternal GBS rectovaginal colonization at 35 weeks' to 37 weeks' gestational age, thereby decreasing need for maternal antibiotic administration at time of labor. The importance of this study is that it may offer a safer alternative to intrapartum antibiotic treatment of GBS colonized pregnant women.[35]

REFERENCES

1. American College of Obstetricians and Gynecologists. ACOG committee opinion No. 549: obesity in pregnancy. Obstet Gynecol 2013;121:213–7.
2. Woods S, Melville J, Guo Y, et al. Psychosocial stress during pregnancy. Am J Obstet Gynecol 2010;202(1):61.e1-7.
3. American College of Obstetricians and Gynecologists. ACOG committee opinion. Vitamin D screening and supplementation during pregnancy. Washington, DC: American College of Obstetricians and Gynecologists; 2015.
4. Holick MF. Vitamin D deficiency. N Engl J Med 2007;357:266–81.
5. Institute of Medicine of the National Academies (US). Dietary reference intakes for calcium and vitamin D. Washington, DC: National Academy Press; 2010.
6. Coletta J, Bell S, Roman A, et al. Omega 3 fatty acids and pregnancy. Rev Obstet Gynecol 2010;3(4):163–71.
7. Greenberg JA, Bell SJ, Ausdal WV. Omega-3 fatty acid supplementation during pregnancy. Rev Obstet Gynecol 2008;1(4):162–9.
8. Oakley GP, Erickson JD. Vitamin A and birth defects. N Engl J Med 1995;333(21): 1414–5.
9. Hamilton BE, Martin JA, Ventura SJ, et al. Births: preliminary data for 2012. National vital statistics reports. Hyattsville (MD): National Center for Health Statistics; 2013.
10. Declercq ER, Sakala C, Corry MP, et al. Listening to mothers iii: pregnancy and birth. New York: Childbirth Connection; 2013.
11. Gagnon AJ, Sandall J. Individual or group antenatal education for childbirth or parenthood, or both. Cochrane Database Syst Rev 2007;(3):CD002869.
12. Sorenson DL. Uncertainty in pregnancy. NAACOGS Clin Issu Perinat Womens Health Nurs 1990;1(3):289–96.
13. Beddoe AE, Lee KA. Mind-body interventions during pregnancy. J Obstet Gynecol Neonatal Nurs 2008;37(2):165–75.
14. Marc I, Toureche N, Ernst E, et al. Mind-body interventions during pregnancy for preventing or treating women's anxiety. Cochrane Database Syst Rev 2011;(7):CD007559.
15. Pollis R, Gussman D, Kuo YH. Yoga in pregnancy: an examination of maternal and fetal responses to 26 yoga postures. Obstet Gynecol 2015;126(6):1237–41.

16. Duncan L, Cohn M, Chao M, et al. Mind in labor: effects of mind/body training on childbirth appraisals and pain medication use during labor [abstract]. J Altern Complement Med 2014;20(5):A17.

17. Bardacke N. Mindful Birthing: Training the mind, body and heart for childbirth and beyond. New York: HarperCollins; 2012.

18. Madden K, Middleton P, Cyna AM, et al. Hypnosis for pain management during labour and childbirth. Cochrane Database Syst Rev 2016;(5):CD009356.

19. Madden K, Middleton P, Cyna A, et al. Hypnosis for pain management during labor and childbirth. Cochrane Database Syst Rev 2012;(11):CD009356.

20. Mongan M. Hypnobirthing: The Mongan Method: A Natural Approach to a safe, easier, morecomfortable birthing. Deerfield Beach (FL): Health Communications, Inc; 2015.

21. Lee HC, El-Sayed YY, Gould JB. Population trends in cesarean delivery for breech presentation in the United States, 1997-2003. Am J Obstet Gynecol 2008;199:59.e1-8.

22. Clock C, Kurtzman J, White J, et al. Cesarean risk after successful external cephalic version: a matched, retrospective analysis. J Perinatol 2009;29:96–100.

23. Coyle ME, Smith CA, Peat B. Cephalic version by moxibustion for breech presentation. Cochrane Database Syst Rev 2012;(15):CD003928.

24. Spong CY. Defining "term" pregnancy: recommendations from the defining "term" pregnancy workgroup. JAMA 2013;309:2445–6.

25. Martin JA, Hamilton BE, Osterman MJ, et al. Births: final data for 2012. Natl Vital Stat Rep 2013;62(9):1–27.

26. McFarlin BL, Gibson MH, O'Rear J, et al. A national survey of herbal preparation use by nurse-midwives for labor stimulation. Review of the literature and recommendations for practice. J Nurse Midwifery 1999;44(3):205–16.

27. Simpson M, Parsons M, Greenwood J, et al. Raspberry leaf in pregnancy: its safety and efficacy in labor. J Midwifery Womens Health 2001;46(2):51–9.

28. Parsons M, Simpson M, Ponton T. Raspberry leaf and its effect on labour: safety and efficacy. Aust Coll Midwives Inc J 1999;12(3):20–5.

29. Dove D, Johnson P. Oral evening primrose oil: its effect on length of pregnancy and selected intrapartum outcomes in low-risk nulliparous women. J Nurse Midwifery 1999;44(3):320–4.

30. Wright I. Neonatal effects of maternal consumption of blue cohosh. J Pediatr 1999;134(3):384–5.

31. Jones TK, Lawson BM. Profound neonatal congestive heart failure caused by maternal consumption of blue cohosh herbal medication. J Pediatr 1998;132(3 Pt 1):550–2.

32. Gunn TR, Wright IM. The use of black and blue cohosh in labour. N Z Med J 1996; 109(1032):410–1.

33. Finkel RS, Zarlengo KM. Blue cohosh and perinatal stroke. NEJM 2004;351(3): 302–3.

34. Smith CA, Crowther CA, Grant SJ. Acupuncture for induction of labour. Cochrane Database Syst Rev 2013;(8):CD002962.

35. Oral Probiotic Supplementation and Group B Streptococcus Rectovaginal Colonization in Pregnant Women: a Randomized Double-blind Placebo-controlled Trial. ClinicalTrials.gov Identifier: NCT01479478.

Women's Health

Polycystic Ovarian Syndrome, Menopause, and Osteoporosis

Melinda Ring, MD, ABOIM[a,b,]*

KEYWORDS

- Integrative medicine • Women's health • Polycystic ovarian syndrome • Menopause
- Osteoporosis • Dietary supplements • Bioidentical hormones • Nutrition

KEY POINTS

- A total of 54.5% of women report use of at least one complementary and integrative medicine approach specifically for obstetric or gynecologic problems, with dietary supplements and mind-body approaches topping the list.
- Integrative approaches may help women with polycystic ovarian syndrome address the underlying insulin resistance, menstrual irregularities, and hyperandrogen symptoms.
- Women in perimenopause and menopause struggle with an array of issues that impact their quality of life. Understanding the issues around menopause hormone therapy, such as bioidentical hormones and the use of compounded hormones, is critical. Acupuncture, mind-body therapies, and some dietary supplements can be helpful in symptom management.
- Primary care providers need to understand the importance of choosing dietary supplements, such as calcium, magnesium, and vitamin D, as well as other marketed options, when counseling women on the prevention and treatment of osteoporosis.

INTRODUCTION

Women account for 57% of expenses in doctors' offices and make approximately 80% of decisions for their families.[1] Surveys consistently show that a significantly higher percentage of women with chronic medical conditions report use of complementary and integrative medicine (CIM) approaches compared with men (51.5% vs 44.3%).[2] A total of 54.5% of women report use of at least one CIM approach specifically for obstetric or gynecologic problems, with dietary supplements and mind-body approaches topping the list.[3] Most physicians providing women's health care in this

The author has no commercial or financial conflicts of interest or funding sources.
[a] Osher Center for Integrative Medicine at Northwestern University, 150 East Huron Avenue, Suite 1100, Chicago, IL 60611, USA; [b] Departments of Medicine and Medical Social Sciences, Northwestern University Feinberg School of Medicine, Chicago, IL, USA
* Osher Center for Integrative Medicine at Northwestern University, 150 East Huron Avenue, Suite 1100, Chicago, IL 60611.
E-mail address: mring@nm.org

study express supportive attitudes, with nearly three-quarters agreeing that clinical care should integrate the best conventional and CIM practices; however, primary care providers remain an underutilized resource by patients for guidance in the safe and appropriate use of integrative therapies. This article provides a practical overview of the most appropriate integrative therapies to consider in the management of commonly seen women's health conditions: polycystic ovarian syndrome (PCOS), menopause, and osteoporosis.

POLYCYSTIC OVARIAN SYNDROME

PCOS impacts 5% to 50% of women of reproductive age, affecting as many as 5 million women in the United States.[4,5] PCOS most often manifests with oligomenorrhea or amenorrhea due to ovulatory dysfunction present in 70% of women, accompanied by signs of androgen excess, such as acne and hirsutism (the latter found in 70% of women).[6] The third variable of classic polycystic ovarian morphology is found to a variable degree and may be present in women without the other classic metabolic features of PCOS. PCOS may be diagnosed as early as puberty or discovered during an evaluation for anovulatory infertility. Often times it is overlooked because of the heterogeneity in levels of expression. The current understanding of the pathophysiology, diagnostic approach, and conventional treatment is available through recent reviews.[7] Once PCOS is confirmed, an integrative approach to PCOS should address the obvious symptoms, the emotional impact, and a proactive strategy for metabolic sequelae, including increased risks for insulin resistance and cardiovascular disease.[8,9]

Nutrition/Lifestyle

Although not included in any of the diagnostic criteria, central weight gain, visceral fat accumulation, and insulin resistance are common features of PCOS. Impaired glucose tolerance is found in one-third of women with PCOS and type 2 diabetes in 8% to 10%.[10] Weight management plays a central role in the expression of symptoms and long-term consequences in women with PCOS. Fifty percent to 70% of women with PCOS are obese and should be informed that even 5% to 10% weight loss of body mass is associated with significant improvement in the clinical metabolic and hormonal markers.[11–13] The underlying insulin resistance can make weight loss challenging, so addressing this issue along with other barriers to weight loss can help patients succeed. A multifaceted approach through nutrition, physical activity, and supplements may be beneficial.

Physical activity

Physical activity provides diverse benefits in PCOS, such as improved insulin sensitivity, preservation of lean body mass, and positive impact on mood. A 2010 systematic review of exercise therapy in PCOS identified 8 studies (5 randomized controlled and 3 cohort) involving moderate-intensity physical activity (aerobic and/or resistance) for 12 to 24 weeks' duration.[14] Physical activity was noted to result in improved ovulation, reduced insulin resistance (9%–30%), and weight loss (4.5%–10%). In a comparative study between exercise versus a low-calorie diet in 40 women with PCOS, the exercise cohort had higher ovulation rates, better insulin sensitivity, and greater reduction in waist measurements despite less absolute weight loss.[15] The inclusion of high-intensity interval training (HIIT) may have an extra benefit in terms of insulin sensitivity compared with cardio forms of exercise.[16] Recommendations about physical activity should be individualized, following currently understood principles of optimal intensity and duration of exercise. The Institute of Lifestyle Medicine provides excellent resources for counseling patients on physical activity.

Nutrition

Although several studies comparing low-carbohydrate versus low-protein diet showed no significant difference in weight loss, androgens, glucose metabolism, and leptin, 2 studies on low-carbohydrate diets were associated with improved depression scores and lower fasting insulin.[17–19] In 2010 the first study examining impact of glycemic index (GI) rather than just total carbohydrate/protein content in PCOS (n = 96) showed that an ad libitum low-GI diet led to greater improvements in insulin resistance (P = .03) and menstrual cyclicity (95% compared with 63%; P = .03) when compared with a macronutrient-matched healthy diet.[20] Intermittent fasting or fasting-mimicking diets, in which intake is restricted to a certain number of hours a day or low-calorie intake days are interspersed with moderate-calorie intake days, has been shown to improve insulin sensitivity and decrease weight, though it has not been studied specifically in PCOS.[21,22] At this point it is reasonable for nondiabetic patients with PCOS to consider either a lower-carbohydrate diet with inclusion of low-GI, high-fiber carbohydrates or a trial of a monitored intermittent fasting approach, based on patients' starting point and interests.

Dietary soy

Soy contains phytoestrogens, or plant-based compounds with weak estrogenic effects, raising questions of its relative harm versus benefit in PCOS. One study explored the intake of 36 g of soy daily for 6 months in 12 obese women with PCOS and demonstrated decreases in low-density lipoprotein cholesterol but no hormonal impact.[23] A review of 7 soy intervention studies done on women using 32 to 200 mg/d of isoflavones showed increased menstrual cycle length.[24] Currently the evidence does not imply that soy prevents ovulation but may delay it. At present it is appropriate to counsel women with PCOS who struggle with infertility to avoid or limit soy products. Otherwise, intake of a serving daily of whole soy (eg, edamame, soy milk, or tofu) can be part of a healthy diet.

Supplements

Omega-3 fatty acids

In comparison with control subjects, patients with PCOS have decreased fibrinolytic activity, higher levels of plasminogen activator inhibitor-1, and increased C-reactive protein levels (in both obese and nonobese women), all of which are markers for inflammation.[25,26] Several recent studies point to the beneficial effect of omega-3 fatty acids (eicosapentaenoic acid and docosahexaenoic acid totaling 1200–1500 mg daily); after 6 months improvements included lower body mass index, androgen levels, and insulin resistance.[27,28]

Inositol family

The compound d-chiro-inositol (DCI) is a mediator of insulin action that forms naturally in the human body from the metabolism of dietary pinitol and myo-inositol.[29] The use of DCI supplements in studies suggests improved insulin sensitivity, triglyceride and testosterone levels, blood pressure, ovulation, and weight loss.[30,31] In one study 44 obese women received either DCI 1200 mg daily or placebo for 6 weeks; active treatment resulted in an improvement in insulin resistance (P = .07), a 55% reduction in the mean serum-free testosterone concentration (P = .006), and an increase from 27% to 86% ovulation compared with placebo (P <.001). In another study, 25 women received inositol for 6 months. Twenty-two out of the 25 (88%) patients had one spontaneous menstrual cycle during treatment, of whom 18 (72%) maintained normal ovulatory activity. A total of 10 pregnancies (40% of patients) were obtained. Although no interactions with herbs and supplements are known, there is concern that high consumption of inositol might exacerbate bipolar disorder. The dosage is as follows: DCI 600 mg daily if less than 60 kg, 1200 mg daily if heavier; pinitol 600 mg twice daily.

Chromium

Chromium is an essential trace mineral that enhances the action of insulin; the supplement chromium picolinate may help improve glucose tolerance in women with PCOS, according to several studies.[32,33] Although chromium did not seem to alter hormones in earlier studies, a 2015 study in adolescents over 6 months showed improved menstrual cycles and lower free testosterone, though no changes in acne or hirsutism were noted.[34] The adequate intake of chromium is 25 mcg daily; in humans short-term use of chromium at 1000 mcg daily is safe; these doses are not recommended in pregnancy or renal insufficiency. The dosage is as follows: chromium picolinate 600 to 1000 mcg daily.

Vitamin D

Observational studies correlate vitamin D deficiency with insulin resistance, menstrual and ovulatory irregularities, lower pregnancy success, hirsutism, and obesity.[35] In a small trial of 13 women with PCOS and vitamin D deficiency, normal menstrual cycles resumed within 2 months in 7 of the 9 women who had irregular menstrual cycles when vitamin D with calcium was replenished.[36] Another uncontrolled pilot study also observed improvements, with 50% (23 of 46) of oligomenorrhea or amenorrheic women reporting improvements in menstrual frequency after 24 weeks of vitamin D replacement.[37] Although studies are small, at the minimum, identifying and correcting vitamin D deficiency is recommended.

N-acetyl cysteine

N-acetyl cysteine (NAC) has multiple actions, including increasing the antioxidant glutathione; lowering inflammatory markers, such as tumor necrosis factor alpha; and improving insulin sensitivity.[38,39] Three studies using NAC as adjuvant therapy to clomiphene showed improved ovulation and pregnancy rates, with no adverse effects or ovarian hyperstimulation[40,41] It also has been shown to improve insulin sensitivity in PCOS and diabetes.[39,42] The dosage is as follows: NAC 1200 to 1800 mg/d in divided doses.

Botanicals

Cinnamomum cassia has been studied in vitro and in humans with studies showing a positive impact on glycemic control in diabetic patients.[43] A pilot study published in the July 2007 issue of *Fertility and Sterility* showed that 0.25 to 0.5 teaspoon (tsp) of cinnamon powder reduced insulin resistance in 15 women with PCOS. A 2015 randomized controlled study compared intake of cinnamon capsules 1500 mg versus placebo.[44] Menstrual cyclicity improved in the cinnamon but not the placebo group at 6 months (0.75 vs 0.25, $P = .0085$); surprisingly, insulin resistance was not shown to be impacted. Although additional studies are warranted, at the minimum inclusion of *Cinnamomum cassia* in dietary form is reasonable (0.25–1.0 tsp; 1 tsp = 4.75 g).

Chaste tree berry

Chaste tree berry *(Vitex agnus-castus)* has multiple endocrine effects, including improving estrogen/progesterone balance through increased luteinizing hormone and mild inhibition of follicle-stimulating hormone secretion and reduction of prolactin secretion. Most studies on chasteberry for infertility or PCOS have used a blend of herbs, making it difficult to determine the role of a solitary component. Examples of reported findings include increased pregnancy rate, cycle length, and progesterone levels.[45–47] These studies are difficult to extrapolate given the proprietary nature of the supplements; however, the trends toward improvement with no side effects warrant further consideration. Several small studies in the German literature also reported a benefit of *Vitex* for acne with self-reports of improvement of up to 70%.[48] However, it is important to note that because of its hormonal effect, *Vitex* may interfere with oral contraceptives and should not be used concurrently. *Vitex* products are available in many different forms. The dosage is as follows: Typical daily intake is 20 to 40 mg of dried herb.

Other herbs

Many other herbs are commonly used by Western and traditional Chinese medicine (TCM) herbalists in PCOS, though use is based on historical use or small studies.[49–51] Examples include *Paeonia lactiflora* (white peony), *Gymnema sylvestre*, *Tribulus terrestris*, *Glycyrrhiza glabra* or *Glycyrrhiza uralensis* (licorice root), *Cimicifuga racemosa* (black cohosh), *Camellia sinensis* (green tea), *Mentha spicata labiatae* (spearmint tea) and *Saw palmetto*. Small studies on single or combination herbal formulas have reported benefits ranging from decreased hirsutism and hyperandrogenism (spearmint, saw palmetto, peony, Chinese licorice) to improved ovulation and fertility (black cohosh, TCM formulas). Although phytotherapy may have a potential role in addressing hormonal imbalances in PCOS, the limited data on dosing and preparations as well as drug-herb interactions limit their use (Please see Charles Falzon and Anna Balabanova article, "Phytotherapy: An Introduction to Herbal Medicine," in this issue). It is best to work closely with a practitioner well versed in the use of herbal medicine for women who express an interest in including them in their regimen.

Complementary Healing Approaches

Acupuncture

Acupuncture has the potential to impact on PCOS via its effects on the sympathetic nervous system, the endocrine system, and the neuroendocrine system.[52,53] A 2016 Cochrane Review included 5 randomized controlled trials (RCTs) with 413 women, though the studies were considered overall low quality.[54] Two studies reported improved menstrual frequency; 2 of 3 studies reported improved ovulation. Acupuncture may be considered as adjunctive therapy, though women should be advised data on fertility are limited.

Mind-body therapies

Women with PCOS have significantly increased prevalence of depression and anxiety.[55] Mood disorders may be directly related to biochemical imbalances (androgens, insulin resistance) and also exacerbated by stress related to body image issues and infertility. Addressing concerns through mind-body approaches, self-care, and cognitive behavioral therapy should be encouraged for all women (Please see Mary Talen and colleagues article, "Integrative Medicine and Mood, Mental Health and Emotional Health," in this issue).

Therapeutic Checklist

Next is a summary of integrative therapeutic options for PCOS. Many women with PCOS do well with attention to diet, exercise, supplement, and acupuncture. Some women will benefit from medications when symptoms or sequelae are more advanced.

- Minimize exposure to hormone-disrupting chemicals.
- Consider weight loss to achieve ideal body weight. Consider a low-carbohydrate, low-glycemic/high-fiber diet or intermittent fasting protocols.
- For women with infertility, consider limiting soy intake, otherwise favor 1 to 2 servings (1 oz is approximately 25 g) soy-rich foods daily.

- For physical activity, aim for 150 minutes per week and consider including HIIT.
- Consider the following supplements:
  - Vitamin D based on levels or 1000 to 2000 IU daily
  - Omega 3 fatty acids 1200 to 1500 mg daily
  - Chromium picolinate 600 to 1000 mcg daily
  - DCI/pinitol 600 mg to 1200 mg daily based on weight
  - *Cinnamon cassia* 0.25–1.0 tsp (1 tsp = approximately 4.5 g)
  - *Vitex agnus-castus* extract 20 to 40 mg
- Consider consultation with an integrative medicine physician, naturopathic doctor, or TCM provider with expertise in phytotherapy.
- Consider acupuncture for oligomenorrhea and mood benefits.
- Mind-body therapies can help women cope with stress, depression, and anxiety related to PCOS.

MENOPAUSE

Compared with 100 years ago when life expectancy and the age of menopause were closely aligned, today women in the United States live on average one-third of their life after menopause.[56] A systematic review of 9 surveys concluded that 50.5% of women reported using integrative medicine therapies specifically for menopausal symptoms, though 55% did not disclose use to their health care professional.[57]

Natural menopause, confirmed after a woman has no menstrual cycles for 12 consecutive months, occurs on average at 51 years of age. Although most women experience menopause between 45 and 55 years of age, menopause is only considered premature at 40 years of age or younger. Induced menopause from gynecologic surgery, medications, or other interventions results in all the same symptoms but often times with a more dramatic presentation due to the abrupt onset.

Symptoms and physical changes often start 4 to 8 years before menopause as hormones start to shift (**Table 1**). This perimenopause transition time manifests with more frequent cycles, night sweats, insomnia, and mood swings and often begins when a woman is in her late 30s to mid 40s. A primary care provider is ideally situated to help a woman understand that changes she is experiencing are natural and normal, elicit her goals for the menopausal transition and beyond, and share current understanding about risks and benefits for varied therapeutic approaches. In addition to counseling, many online videos and resources are available to educate patients.

Table 1
Common symptoms in perimenopause and menopause

Vasomotor symptoms (hot flush, night sweats)	Dizziness
Palpitations	Dyspareunia (painful intercourse)
Vaginal atrophy	Urine incontinence, frequency, or infections
Paresthesias	Hair thinning (scalp) or increased growth (facial)
Fatigue	Mood changes
Insomnia	Low libido
Irregular or more frequent menses (perimenopause)	Headaches/migraines
Memory issues/fogginess	Musculoskeletal aches
Central weight gain	Decreased muscle mass

Hormone Therapy: Bioidentical Hormones

For decades the use of menopausal hormones was the standard of care for any menopausal woman, regardless of time since her last menses. The premature halt of the combined estrogen/progestin arm of the Women's Health Initiative (WHI) in 2002 due to increased risk of heart disease and breast cancer led to a dramatic reversal of this practice. Women, confused and seeking a solution for their menopausal symptoms, turned to physicians who could prescribe bioidentical hormones from compounding pharmacies, touted by celebrities and prescribing practitioners as a safer effective alternative. Since then reanalysis of WHI, new evidence, and increased options have clarified risks and benefits, leading to recommendations by major organizations that now support use of hormone therapy (HT) in women without contraindications if they are within 10 years of menopause and younger than 60 years, using HT in general at the lowest dose for the shortest duration needed to manage menopause symptoms.[58,59] A growing recognition of the chronicity of symptoms in a significant portion of women, along with increased data on cancer and cardiovascular risks, versus benefits on mortality rate and health conditions, led to a call for a more individualized approach to HT that takes into consideration a woman's preferences, symptoms and quality of life, and personal risks.[60]

Hormone Therapy: Terminology

Although a full guide to prescribing menopausal HT is beyond the scope of this article, it is important to have an understanding of the spectrum of formulations available.

Natural versus bioidentical versus synthetic

The term natural hormones is generally not relevant and should be discouraged, since it implies that hormones are derived from a naturally occurring source but tells nothing about the actual content. A more important distinction is whether hormones are bioidentical, meaning that their molecular structure is identical to the hormones women make in their bodies, versus synthetic, or of a chemical structure not formulated in humans. Bioidentical estrogens are 17 beta-estradiol, estrone, and estriol; the only bioidentical progestogen is progesterone. Conjugated equine estrogens are examples of synthetic estrogen, and medroxyprogesterone acetate is a synthetic progestogen. Bioidentical HT (BHT) was previously only available to women prescribed through compounding pharmacies. However, over the past decade numerous pharmaceutical versions are available. Proponents of bioidentical hormones point to studies of the differential effects of bioidentical hormones versus synthetic progestogens on lipids, glucose regulation, sleep, mood, fluid-electrolyte balance, breast tenderness, and breast cancer risk.[61-64] Given the widespread availability of bioidentical hormones, efficacy in addressing the symptoms of menopause, and possible preferential risk and side-effect profile, the use of bioidentical versions is reasonable and appropriate for any woman seeking HT.

Compounded versus pharmaceutical

A 2015 survey developed by the North American Menopause Society showed that 31% of women who had ever used HT reported use of compounded formulations, 35% of current HT users, and 41% of ever-users aged 40 to 49 years.[65,66] Major societies have urged caution in use of compounded hormones stating concerns about the lack of oversight by the US Food and Drug Administration (FDA), lack of adequate scientific evidence of safety and efficacy, and potential harm.[67] However, compounded hormones do play an important role in providing options for women who cannot take standard forms or doses of pharmaceutical BHT or who might benefit from hormones not available through FDA-approved medications (eg, transdermal testosterone for female sexual desire disorder).[68] When prescribing HT through a compounding pharmacy, it is important to verify it is an accredited pharmacy that applies the current Good Manufacturing Practice and US Pharmacopoeia tenets (**Table 2**).

Dietary Supplements and Nutrition Strategies

Many dietary herbal supplements are considered useful in menopause; often time combinations are incorporated into one formula to address different symptoms (eg, vasomotor symptoms, mood, insomnia). Although good-quality data are lacking in general for dietary supplements, the following show the greatest promise in menopause.

Phytoestrogens

Phytoestrogens are compounds found in plants that have a phenolic ring that allows them to bind to estrogen receptors. Phytoestrogens are 100 to 100,000 times weaker than the endogenous hormone and act similarly to selective estrogen receptor modulators in that their activity in different tissues may be antiestrogenic or proestrogenic. The most potent and common type of phytoestrogen in supplements is called isoflavones. A 2016 review in the *Journal of the American Medical Association* included 21 RCTs in a meta-analysis that examined a composite of all soy (*Glycine max*) isoflavones (dietary, supplements, and extracts) (12 studies), dietary soy isoflavones alone (4 studies), supplements and extracts of soy isoflavones alone (8 studies), and red clover isoflavones (7 studies).[69] The report concludes that composite and specific phytoestrogen supplementations are associated with modest reductions in the frequency of hot flashes and vaginal dryness but not night sweats.

Sage

Sage *(Salvia officinalis)* has been used in traditional herbal medicine for excessive sweating and hot flushes. It may have some estrogenic activity due to its constituent geraniol as well as neuromodulatory activity. In 71 women with at least 5 hot flushes daily, a 280-mg thujone-free sage spissum extract, equivalent to 3.4-g tincture of fresh sage leaves, led to a significant decrease in the total score of the mean number of

Table 2 Examples of bioidentical hormone options	
Estrogens	
Compounded	Biest cream (estradiol E2 and estriol E3), often prescribed as 20:80, meaning, 20% E2/80% E3; 1.25 mg–5.0 mg once to twice daily E2 and/or E3 in creams for topical or vaginal application; sublingual drops
Pharmaceutical	Estradiol patch (eg, Vivelle-Dot 0.025, 0.0375, 0.05, 0.075, 0.1 mg twice weekly) Estradiol gel (eg, EstroGel 0.06% 1.25 g pump daily) Estradiol ring (eg, Femring 0.05 or 0.1 mg daily) Estradiol spray (eg, Evamist 1.53 mg spray 1–3 daily)
Progestogens	
Compounded	Progesterone capsule continuous: 50 mg twice daily or 100 mg once to twice daily; cyclic: 200–400 mg daily for 12 d Progesterone cream, sublingual drops, or topical oil
Pharmaceutical	Progesterone capsule (eg, Prometrium 100 or 200 mg capsules) continuous: 100 mg daily; cyclic: 200 mg last 12–14 d of estrogen treatment each cycle

intensity-rated hot flashes by 50% within 4 weeks and by 64% within 8 weeks (P <.0001).[70] Additional studies are warranted to explore the potential role of sage in the treatment of vasomotor symptoms.

Black cohosh

Black cohosh (*Cimicifuga racemosa*) is one of the most popular herbs used for menopause in the United States. It is unclear whether black cohosh has estrogenic effects, though it does not directly bind estrogen receptors or stimulate the growth of estrogen-dependent tumors.[71,72]

The most consistent evidence is for a specific extract called Remifemin, which has been shown in multiple studies to significantly reduce menopausal symptom indices and hot flash frequency compared with placebo.[73,74] However, other studies and systematic reviews on black cohosh have been inconclusive.[75,76] Some issues of safety, in particular with regard to hepatotoxicity, have been raised, although in general long-term use has been shown to be very safe.[77,78] Overall, black cohosh seems to have the potential to provide relief for some women. Based on studies, typical doses are as follows: black cohosh standardized to contain 1 mg of 27-deoxyactein, 20 mg twice daily.

OTHER HERBALS

Flaxseed, chasteberry, kudzu, alfalfa, hops, licorice, evening primrose oil, *Panax ginseng*, wild yam, and vitamin E have all been promoted for menopausal symptoms relief; but studies are either lacking or conflicting on potential benefits.

Mind and Body Approaches

Acupuncture

A 2015 meta-analysis of 12 studies that met inclusion criteria evaluated the effect of acupuncture treatments occurring once to twice weekly over 5 to 12 weeks in a total of 869 participants.[79] The conclusion was that acupuncture

- Significantly reduced the frequency and severity of hot flashes, with effects lasting up to 3 months
- Significantly decreased psychological, somatic, and urogenital subscale scores on the Menopause Rating Scale
- Improved the vasomotor subscale score on the Menopause-Specific Quality of Life Questionnaire

Given the relative safety of acupuncture and its growing availability through trained practitioners of well-established schools of TCM, referral to or support of acupuncture as part of a menopause symptom strategy is warranted. Primary care providers do not need to prescribe a certain amount of treatments or specific acupuncture goals; the acupuncturist will conduct a full history, typically including pulse and tongue evaluation, to formulate a TCM diagnosis and individualized plan of care. The primary care provider can then support patients by monitoring the impact of treatment in follow-up visits.

Mind-body medicine

A 2010 systematic review of mind-body therapies explored interventions, such as yoga, meditation-based programs, tai chi, and other relaxation practices, including muscle relaxation and breath-based techniques, relaxation response training, and low-frequency sound-wave therapy.[80] Although the quality of the studies was variable, the conclusions suggest that inclusion of a form of mind-body medicine in a woman's management plan should be a priority. Eight of the 9 studies of yoga, tai chi, and meditation-based programs reported improvement in overall menopausal and vasomotor symptoms.

- Yoga programs improved sleep and mood in 6 of 7 trials.
- Nine trials suggest that breath-based and other relaxation therapies show promise for reducing symptoms, including vasomotor complaints.

A 2014 review examined how mind-body therapies could impact not just isolated symptoms but also clusters of symptoms, whereby hot flashes co-occurred with sleep, cognitive function, mood, or pain.[81] Mindfulness-based stress-reduction training improved sleep and mood symptoms along with hot flushes. The single yoga trial included significantly reduced hot flushes and improved cognitive symptoms, sleep, and pain symptoms.

OSTEOPOROSIS

Osteoporosis is a major health concern in women, especially after menopause, as lower estrogen levels lead to accelerated bone mass, microarchitecture disruption and decreased bone strength, and the associated increased risk of fractures. Current guidelines for initial management of osteoporosis when found on a bone density screening are guided by calculation of fracture risk using the World Health Organization's Fracture Risk Assessment tool, and typically include lifestyle recommendations and the first-line pharmaceutical option of an oral bisphosphonate.[82] Many patients seek additional advice for nonpharmaceutical integrative approaches to clarify questions about supplement needs, support their efforts to maintain bone health while on treatment, or as an alternative option due to side effects or contraindications to medications.

Supplements

Calcium
Calcium is a mineral necessary for building and maintaining bone health. Sufficient calcium intake may range from approximately 500 mg to approximately 1500 mg per day, depending on age, sex, and dietary factors.[83] Although high calcium intake does not ensure strong bones and low calcium intake does not necessarily result in weaker bones,[84] calcium remains an essential nutrient in inhibiting bone resorption. When determining calcium supplement doses, it is best to first calculate dietary intake to avoid excessive supplementation. The International Osteoporosis Foundation provides one example of a convenient online calculator that includes both dairy and plant-based foods.

Calcium supplements may be obtained as tablets, capsules, powders, and liquids. Doses more than 500 mg should be given in divided doses to maximize absorption (**Table 3**).

Concerns have been raised in recent years regarding the risk-benefit assessment of calcium supplements. The small reduction in fractures may be outweighed by potential risks ranging from cardiovascular events to gastrointestinal symptoms.[85–88] Currently the author's recommendation is to recommend calcium supplements when dietary intake is insufficient, with the caveat that supplementation should be complemented by adequate vitamin D, magnesium, vitamin K2, and other bone-building nutrients.[89]

Vitamin D
Vitamin D plays an important role in calcium absorption and working with vitamin K to stimulate bone mineralization. Low vitamin D has also been associated with an

Table 3
Forms of calcium supplementation

Calcium Form (Author Recommendation)	Dose Equivalence for 500 mg Elemental Calcium	Comments
Calcium carbonate (*acceptable*)	1250 mg	It is more commonly available and less expensive than calcium citrate. It provides 40% elemental calcium and consequently requires fewer tablets. It is generally well absorbed when taken with a meal.
Calcium phosphate (*not recommended*)	1282 mg	Calcium phosphate is in cow's milk, nuts, seeds, beans, broccoli, dark leafy greens, black-eyed peas, figs, oranges, tofu, and salmon or sardine. It contains 39% elemental calcium. However, supplement forms of this type of calcium, found as tricalcium phosphate, are not bioavailable. It is best to get this form from whole food.
Calcium citrate (*recommended*)	2350 mg	Calcium citrate is recommended for individuals with suspected achlorhydria, inflammatory bowel disease, or absorption disorders. It provides 24% elemental calcium. This form is well absorbed with or without a meal.
Calcium lactate (*not recommended*)	3846 mg	Calcium lactate is found in food sources like aged cheese and baking powder. It contains 9%–13% elemental calcium and is not a good choice for people who are lactose intolerant.
Calcium gluconate (*not recommended*)	5556 mg	Calcium gluconate has very low levels of elemental calcium, about 9%–15%. Large amounts would need to be taken to have an impact on bone health, and its bioavailability is unknown because of contradicting studies.
MCHC (*recommended*)	2500 mg	MCHC is a concentrate of whole bone. As such, MCHC contains calcium, phosphorus, zinc, copper, bone matrix proteins, amino acids, and glycosaminoglycans. This compound offers approximately 20%–24% elemental calcium in a form promoted as more bioavailable, though studies question that claim. MCHC has proven to be effective in preventing bone loss in patients with autoimmune chronic active hepatitis on corticosteroid therapy.[129]
OHC (*recommended*)	1250 mg	OHC is a protein-mineral complex shown to produce a higher osteogenic effect than calcium carbonate after oral administration.[129] OHC is made up of approximately 40% elemental calcium as well as phosphorus and bone metabolism proteins. This supplement may have a greater effect on bone metabolism than calcium carbonate for women with osteoporosis.[129]

Abbreviations: MCHC, microcrystalline hydroxyapatite compound; OHC, ossein-hydroxyapatite complex.

Data from Cornuz J, Feskanich D, Willett WC, et al. Smoking, smoking cessation, and risk of hip fracture in women. Am J Med 1999;106(3):311–4.

increased risk of falls.[90] Despite revisions to recommended intake levels from the Institute of Medicine (IOM) and the Endocrine Society, vitamin D deficiency remains prevalent.[91] A 2006 epidemiologic study found that 64% of postmenopausal women with osteoporosis were deficient in vitamin D.[92] Levels of 25-hydroxyvitamin D of 20 ng/mL or greater is considered sufficient to maintain proper bone mineral density by the IOM. However, some studies have shown this level is inadequate. Both population-based studies and meta-analyses suggest levels of at least 40 ng/mL are optimal for bone health.[93–95]

Vitamin D can be obtained through exposure to sunlight, various food sources, and supplements. Fatty fish, such as salmon, mackerel, and whitefish, are naturally rich in vitamin D. Fortified foods include some brands of orange juice, yogurts, and milk. Health care professionals need to keep in mind that in general, 100 IU of vitamin D per day may increase the vitamin D blood test only 1 ng/mL (2.5 nmol/L) after 2 to 3 months. Therefore, typical over-the-counter doses of 400 IU are inadequate to support a patient who has low levels; specific recommendations may range from 5000 to more than 10,000 IU daily in the case of true deficiency.

- A dosage of 400 IU per day increases vitamin D blood levels 4 ng/mL.
- A dosage of 800 IU per day increases vitamin D blood levels 8 ng/mL.
- A dosage 1000 IU per day increases vitamin D blood levels 10 ng/mL.

For patients who do not have access to testing, a general safe recommendation is vitamin D3 1000 to 2000 IU per day.[96]

Vitamin K2

Menaquinones (the K2 family) are one of 2 naturally occurring forms of vitamin K, synthesized by gut microflora. Vitamin K and vitamin D work synergistically to promote bone mineralization for the prevention and treatment of osteoporosis.[97] For postmenopausal Asian women, K2 supplementation resulted in improvement of vertebral bone mineral density and prevention of fractures, and some results show an additive effect when used with a bisphosphonate.[98,99] However, other studies in Europeans and older Americans did not find a difference in bone mineral density after 1 year of use.[100,101]

Daily recommended vitamin K intake for adult women is 90 mcg, but higher doses may be needed for optimal bone health; studies have used 45 mg of menaquinone (MK)-4.[102] Vitamin K2 is found in animal products, such as cheese, egg yolk, chicken, beef, and natto, a fermented soybean. For supplementation, the MK-7 form of vitamin K2 is preferred because of bioavailability and efficacy in increasing vitamin K serum levels.[103] Although vitamin K does not increase hypercoagulability, it should not be used along with anticoagulants, such as warfarin.

Magnesium

Magnesium, the second most abundant cation in intracellular spaces, plays an essential role in the synthesis and metabolism of vitamin D. Intake of this micronutrient is strongly associated with bone density, and epidemiologic studies have shown that dietary magnesium restriction promotes osteoporosis.[104] According to the National Health and Nutrition Examination Survey almost half (48%) of the US population consumed less than the required amount of magnesium (320 mg) from food in 2005 to 2006.[105] Magnesium levels can be measured in serum or urine (24 hours), though some prefer red blood cell magnesium levels as it indicates more of the intracellular level.[106] Magnesium deficiency can be addressed through diet, though supplements are often indicated. Common dietary sources include green vegetables, seeds, nuts, some legumes, and whole grains. In the absence of deficiency, magnesium is often prescribed in a 2:1 ratio with calcium (eg, calcium 500 mg/magnesium 250 mg). Patients with deficiency may require doses ranging from 250 to 1000 mg of elemental magnesium. Using sustained-release and divided doses can minimize the laxative effect. Magnesium comes as different chelates (magnesium oxide, citrate, glycinate, malate, and so forth), magnesium citrate, and magnesium hydroxide (**Table 4**).

Strontium
Ninety-nine percent of strontium in the body is in bone. Strontium ranelate has been shown in therapeutic doses to stimulate bone formation and reduce resorption, associated with improved density and decreased vertebral fractures when used up to 56 months.[107–109] At excessive doses, strontium, however, can adversely impact bone by impairing mineralization and interfering with calcium absorption and vitamin D synthesis. For osteoporosis, strontium ranelate at 2 g/d, providing 680 mg elemental strontium, has been used; it is available in the United States as a dietary supplement and as an approved prescription medication in Europe. Strontium chloride has not been well studied; a 2016 case report described positive increases in density after 2.5 years use of strontium chloride 680 mg daily.[110] Patients with renal insufficiency or thromboembolic disorders should not use strontium.

Additional supplements
The herb horsetail (*Equisetum arvense*) contains a high amount of silicon; it has been suggested as a possible natural support for bone density. One small study showed that 270 mg orally for 2-month intervals separated by 2 weeks of no treatment for up to 1 year significantly increased bone density compared with no treatment in post-menopausal women with osteoporosis.[111,112]

Manganese, zinc, boron, and copper may impact on bone health through varied mechanisms, including osteoblast/osteoclast activity and vitamin metabolism. Data are limited, and encouraging intake at recommended daily levels is appropriate at this time. There is currently no scientific evidence to support the use of black cohosh, dong quai, wild yam, chondroitin sulfate, or shark cartilage for osteoporosis, though they are often promoted for this indication.

Hormones

Menopause hormone therapy
The use of estrogen is widely considered effective and appropriate for preventing osteoporosis-related fracture in at-risk women younger than 60 years or within

Table 4 Magnesium chelates	
Magnesium oxide	Tends to be less expensive but less absorbed and greater laxative effect
Magnesium citrate	Better absorption; may have some laxative effect
Magnesium chloride, gluconate, diglycinate, aspartate, lactate, orotate	Better absorption; less likely to have a laxative effect, so recommended when higher doses are needed
Magnesium malate, taurate, hydroxide	Promoted for other health conditions; not typically used for magnesium deficiency (malate: fibromyalgia; taurate migraine; hydroxide: antacid)

10 years of menopause.[113] Estrogen replacement is covered in the menopause section.

Androgens

Like estrogen, androgens (testosterone and dehydroepiandrosterone [DHEA]) impact on bone remodeling. Testosterone has been shown in men to possibly improve bone density but is not currently recommended for this use in women.[114,115] The prohormone DHEA is produced in the adrenal glands and metabolized to androgens or estrogens. In a low-estrogen environment, such as postmenopause, DHEA tends to have more estrogenic effects. Some studies do support the use of DHEA orally to improve bone mineral density in older women with osteoporosis or osteopenia, though results have been contradictory.[116,117] The dosage used in studies was DHEA 50 mg daily, though it may be beneficial to start with lower doses of 5 to 10 mg to monitor for side effects (signs of estrogen or testosterone excess). Serum levels can be monitored by checking DHEA sulfate. DHEA should be avoided in women with hormone-sensitive conditions.

Lifestyle Factors

Diet

Key additional points in counseling patients on the impact of diet and bone health are as follows:

- Salt intake: Excessive sodium can increase urinary calcium excretion; stay within the recommended daily intake of less than 2400 mg.[118]
- Protein intake: Protein intake is important for bone health, but excess animal protein seems to have a negative impact. Acid-forming diets, those with high animal protein intake, significantly increases urinary calcium excretion versus diets rich in plants that create a more alkaline diet. Encourage appropriate amounts of protein, preferably plant based.[119,120]
- Omega-3s: Fish oil containing omega-3 fatty acids may have beneficial effects on calcium absorption and bone mineralization.[121,122]
- Caffeine: Caffeine increases calcium excretion, though studies on development of osteoporosis are mixed.[123,124] Recommend moderation in caffeine intake (<300 mg caffeine/day)

Physical activity

Weight-bearing exercise is a standard recommendation in the prevention of osteoporosis. Mechanical loading of the bone through physical activity, whether weight lifting or low-impact or high-impact aerobic exercise, can enhance bone mass. The optimal duration and timing are unclear; however, the relation of a sedentary lifestyle to fracture risk is certain.[125]

Tobacco use

Smoking is related to decreased bone loss and increased fracture rates.[126] Even exposure to second-hand smoke either during childhood or as an adult predisposes to later bone loss.[127] Smoking cessations seems to reduce the risk of low bone mass and fractures, with positive changes noted even within the first year of quitting.[128,129]

WOMEN'S HEALTH SUMMARY

Women face unique challenges whether during pregnancy, reproductive years, or through the menopausal transition. The partnership with a health professional who listens to women's individualized goals, needs, and preferences and is willing to explore an integrative model of care can provide immense support to patients while also creating a rewarding practice of medicine.

REFERENCES

1. Fact sheet: general facts on women and job based health. 2006. Available at: https://www.dol.gov/ebsa/newsroom/fshlth5.html. Accessed July 22, 2016.
2. Alwhaibi M, Sambamoorthi U. Sex differences in the use of complementary and alternative medicine among adults with multiple chronic conditions. Evid Based Complement Alternat Med 2016;2016:2067095.
3. Furlow ML, Patel DA, Sen A, et al. Physician and patient attitudes towards complementary and alternative medicine in obstetrics and gynecology. BMC Complement Altern Med 2008;8(1):1.
4. Azziz R, Woods KS, Reyna R, et al. The prevalence and features of the polycystic ovary syndrome in an unselected population. J Clin Endocrinol Metab 2004; 89:2745–9.
5. Hart R, Hickey M, Franks S. Definitions, prevalence and symptoms of polycystic ovaries and polycystic ovary syndrome. Best Pract Res Clin Obstet Gynaecol 2004;18:671–83.
6. Amsterdam ESHRE/ASRM-Sponsored 3rd PCOS Consensus Workshop Group. Consensus on women's health aspects of polycystic ovary syndrome (PCOS). Hum Reprod 2012;27(1):14–24.
7. McCartney CR, Marshall JC. Polycystic ovary syndrome. N Engl J Med 2016; 375(1):54–64.
8. Goodman NF, Cobin RH, Futterweit W, et al. American association of clinical endocrinologists, american college of endocrinology, and androgen excess and pcos society disease state clinical review: guide to the best practices in the evaluation and treatment of polycystic ovary syndrome–part 1. Endocr Pract 2015;21(11):1291–300.
9. Wild RA, Carmina E, Diamanti-Kandarakis E, et al. Assessment of cardiovascular risk and prevention of cardiovascular disease in women with the polycystic ovary syndrome: a consensus statement by the Androgen Excess and Polycystic Ovary Syndrome (AE-PCOS) Society. J Clin Endocrinol Metab 2010;95(5):2038–49.
10. Legro RS, Kunselman AR, Dodson WC, et al. Prevalence and predictors of risk for type 2 diabetes mellitus and impaired glucose tolerance in polycystic ovary syndrome: a prospective, controlled study in 254 affected women 1. J Clin Endocrinol Metab 1999;84(1):165–9.
11. Huber-Buchholz MM, Carey DG, Norman RJ. Restoration of reproductive potential by lifestyle modification in obese polycystic ovary syndrome: role of insulin sensitivity and luteinizing hormone. J Clin Endocrinol Metab 1999;84:1470–4.
12. Kiddy DS, Hamilton-Fairley D, Bush A, et al. Improvement in endocrine and ovarian function during dietary treatment of obese women with polycystic ovary syndrome. Clin Endocrinol (Oxf) 1992;36:105–11.
13. Pasquali R, Casimirri F, Vicennati V. Weight control and its beneficial effect on fertility in women with obesity and polycystic ovary syndrome. Hum Reprod 1997;12(Suppl 1):82–7.
14. Harrison CL, Lombard CB, Moran LJ, et al. Exercise therapy in polycystic ovary syndrome: a systematic review. Hum Reprod Update 2011;17(2):171–83.
15. Palomba S, Giallauria F, Falbo A, et al. Structured exercise training programme versus hypocaloric hyperproteinic diet in obese polycystic ovary syndrome

patients with anovulatory infertility: a 24-week pilot study. Hum Reprod 2008; 23(3):642–50.

16. Trapp EG, Chisholm DJ, Freund J, et al. The effects of high-intensity intermittent exercise training on fat loss and fasting insulin levels of young women. Int J Obes (Lond) 2008;32(4):684–91.

17. Ravn P, Haugen AG, Glintborg D. Overweight in polycystic ovary syndrome. An update on evidence based advice on diet, exercise and metformin use for weight loss. Minerva Endocrinol 2013;38(1):59–76.

18. Douglas CC, Gower BA, Darnell BE, et al. Role of diet in the treatment of poly-cystic ovary syndrome. Fertil Steril 2006;85:679–88.

19. Galletly C, Moran L, Noakes M, et al. Psychological benefits of a high-protein, low-carbohydrate diet in obese women with polycystic ovary syndrome – a pilot study. Appetite 2007;49:590–3.

20. Mehrabani HH, Salehpour S, Amiri Z, et al. Beneficial effects of a high-protein, low-glycemic-load hypocaloric diet in overweight and obese women with poly-cystic ovary syndrome: a randomized controlled intervention study. J Am Coll Nutr 2012;31(2):117–25.

21. Longo VD, Mattson MP. Fasting: molecular mechanisms and clinical applica-tions. Cell Metab 2014;19(2):181–92.

22. Halberg N, Henriksen M, Söderhamn N, et al. Effect of intermittent fasting and refeeding on insulin action in healthy men. J Appl Physiol (1985) 2005;99(6): 2128–36.

23. Romualdi D, Costantini B, Campagna G. Is there a role for soy isoflavones in the therapeutic approach to polycystic ovary syndrome? Results from a pilot study. Fertil Steril 2007;90(5):1826–33.

24. Kurzer MS. Hormonal effects of soy in premenopausal women and men. J Nutr 2002;132:570S–3S.

25. Kelly CC, Lyall H, Petrie JR, et al. Low grade chronic inflammation in women with polycystic ovarian syndrome. J Clin Endocrinol Metab 2001;86:2453–5.

26. Boulman N, Levy Y, Leiba R, et al. Increased C-reactive protein levels in the polycystic ovary syndrome: a marker of cardiovascular disease. J Clin Endocri-nol Metab 2004;89:2160–5.

27. Oner G, Muderris II. Efficacy of omega-3 in the treatment of polycystic ovary syndrome. J Obstet Gynaecol 2013;33(3):289–91.

28. Rafraf M, Mohammadi E, Asghari-Jafarabadi M, et al. Omega-3 fatty acids improve glucose metabolism without effects on obesity values and serum visfatin levels in women with polycystic ovary syndrome. J Am Coll Nutr 2012;31(5):361–8.

29. Davis A, Christiansen M, Horowitz JF, et al. Effect of pinitol treatment on insulin action in subjects with insulin resistance. Diabetes Care 2000;23:1000–5.

30. Nestler JE, Jakubowicz DJ, Reamer P, et al. Ovulatory and metabolic effects of D-chiro-inositol in the polycystic ovary syndrome. N Engl J Med 1999;340(17): 1314–20.

31. Iuorno MJ, Jakubowicz DJ, Baillargeon JP, et al. Effects of d-chiro-inositol in lean women with the polycystic ovary syndrome. Endocr Pract 2002;8(6):417–23.

32. Lydic ML, McNurlan M, Bembo S, et al. Chromium picolinate improves insulin sensitivity in obese subjects with polycystic ovary syndrome. Fertil Steril 2006; 86(1):243–6.

33. Lucidi RS, Thyer AC, Easton CA, et al. Effect of chromium supplementation on insulin resistance and ovarian and menstrual cyclicity in women with polycystic ovary syndrome. Fertil Steril 2005;84(6):1755–7.

34. Amr N, Abdel-Rahim HE. The effect of chromium supplementation on polycystic ovary syndrome in adolescents. J Pediatr Adolesc Gynecol 2015;28(2):114–8.
35. Thomson RL, Spedding S, Buckley JD. Vitamin D in the aetiology and management of polycystic ovary syndrome. Clin Endocrinol 2012;77(3):343–50.
36. Thys-Jacobs S, Donovan D, Papadopoulos A, et al. Vitamin D and calcium dysregulation in the polycystic ovarian syndrome. Steroids 1999;64(6):430–5.
37. Muscogiuri G, Policola C, Prioletta A, et al. Low levels of 25 (OH) D and insulin-resistance: 2 unrelated features or a cause-effect in PCOS? Clin Nutr 2012; 31(4):476–80.
38. Kilic-Okman T, Kucuk M. N-acetylcysteine treatment for PCOS. Int J Gynaecol Obstet 2004;85(3):296–7.
39. Fulghesu AM, Ciampelli M, Muzj G, et al. N-acetylcysteine treatment improved insulin sensitivity in women with polycystic ovary syndrome. Fertil Steril 2002; 77(6):1128–35.
40. Rizk AY, Bedaiwy MA, Al-Inany HG. N-acetyl cysteine is a novel adjuvant to clomiphene citrate in clomiphene- resistant patients with PCOS. Fertil Steril 2005;83(2):367–70.
41. Salehpour S, Sene AA, Saharkhiz N, et al. N-acetylcysteine as an adjuvant to clomiphene citrate for successful induction of ovulation in infertile patients with polycystic ovary syndrome. J Obstet Gynaecol Res 2012;38(9):1182–6.
42. Millea PJ. N-acetylcysteine: multiple clinical applications. Am Fam Physician 2009;80(3):265–9.
43. Akilen R, Tsiami A, Devendra D, et al. Cinnamon in glycaemic control: systematic review and meta analysis. Clin Nutr 2012;31(5):609–15.
44. Kort DH, Lobo RA. Preliminary evidence that cinnamon improves menstrual cyclicity in women with polycystic ovary syndrome: a randomized controlled trial. Obstet Gynecol Surv 2015;70(2):94–5.
45. Milewicz A, Gejdel E, Sworen H, et al. Vitex agnus castus extract in the treatment of luteal phase defects due to latent hyperprolactinemia. Results of a randomized placebo-controlled double-blind study. Arzneimittelforschung 1993;43: 752–6 [in German].
46. Westphal LM, Polan ML, Trant AS, et al. A nutritional supplement for improving fertility in women: a pilot study. J Reprod Med 2004;49:289–93.
47. Westphal LM, Polan ML, Trant AS. Double-blind, placebo-controlled study of Fertilityblend: a nutritional supplement for improving fertility in women. Clin Exp Obstet Gynecol 2006;33(4):205–8.
48. Giss G, Rothenburg W. Phytotherapeutic treatment of acne. Z Haut Geschlechtskr 1968;43:645 [in German].
49. Hywood A. Phytotherapy for polycystic ovarian syndrome (PCOS). Townsend Lett Doctors Patients 2004;256:28–34.
50. Zhang J, Li T, Zhou L, et al. Chinese herbal medicine for subfertile women with polycystic ovarian syndrome. Cochrane Database Syst Rev 2010;(9):CD007535.
51. Arentz S, Abbott JA, Smith CA, et al. Herbal medicine for the management of polycystic ovary syndrome (PCOS) and associated oligo/amenorrhoea and hyperandrogenism; a review of the laboratory evidence for effects with corroborative clinical findings. BMC Complement Altern Med 2014;14(1):511.
52. Lim CE, Wong WS. Current evidence of acupuncture on polycystic ovarian syndrome. Gynecol Endocrinol 2010;26(6):473–8.
53. Stener-Victorin E, Jedel E, Janson PO, et al. Low-frequency electroacupuncture and physical exercise decrease high muscle sympathetic nerve activity in polycystic ovary syndrome. Am J Physiol Regul Integr Comp Physiol 2009;297:R387–95.

54. Lim CED, Ng RWC, Xu K, et al. Acupuncture for polycystic ovarian syndrome. Cochrane Database Syst Rev 2016;(5):CD007689.

55. Barry JA, Kuczmierczyk AR, Hardiman PJ. Anxiety and depression in polycystic ovary syndrome: a systematic review and meta-analysis. Hum Reprod 2011; 26(9):2442–51.

56. Health, United States, 2015-Centers for Disease Control and Prevention 2016. Available at: http://www.cdc.gov/nchs/data/hus/hus15.pdf. Accessed July 22, 2016.

57. Posadzki P, Lee MS, Moon TW, et al. Prevalence of complementary and alternative medicine (CAM) use by menopausal women: a systematic review of surveys. Maturitas 2013;75(1):34–43.

58. North American Menopause Society. The 2012 hormone therapy position statement of: the North American Menopause Society. Menopause 2012;19:257–71.

59. Stuenkel CA, Davis SR, Gompel A, et al. Treatment of symptoms of the menopause: an Endocrine Society clinical practice guideline. J Clin Endocrinol Metab 2015;100(11):3975–4011.

60. Lipold LD, Batur P, Kagan R. Is there a time limit for systemic menopausal hormone therapy? Cleve Clin J Med 2016;83(8):605.

61. Bakken K, Fournier A, Lund E, et al. Menopausal hormone therapy and breast cancer risk: impact of different treatments. The European Prospective Investigation into Cancer and Nutrition. Int J Cancer 2011;128(1):144–56.

62. Cummings JA, Brizendine L. Comparison of physical and emotional side effects of progesterone or medroxyprogesterone in early postmenopausal women. Menopause 2002;9(4):253–63.

63. de Lignières B. Oral micronized progesterone. Clin Ther 1999;21(1):41–60.

64. Fournier A, Alban F, Sylvie M, et al. Use of different postmenopausal hormone therapies and risk of histology-and hormone receptor–defined invasive breast cancer. J Clin Oncol 2008;26(8):1260–8.

65. Gass ML, Stuenkel CA, Utian WH, et al. Use of compounded hormone therapy in the United States: report of the North American Menopause Society survey. Menopause 2015;22(12):1276–85.

66. Pinkerton JV, Santoro N. Compounded bioidentical hormone therapy: identifying use trends and knowledge gaps among US women. Menopause 2015; 22(9):926.

67. Davis R, Batur P, Thacker HL. Risks and effectiveness of compounded bioidentical hormone therapy: a case series. J Womens Health (Larchmt) 2014; 23(8):642–8.

68. Sood R, Shuster L, Smith R, et al. Counseling postmenopausal women about bioidentical hormones: ten discussion points for practicing physicians. J Am Board Fam Med 2011;24(2):202–10.

69. Franco OH, Chowdhury R, Troup J, et al. Use of plant-based therapies and menopausal symptoms: a systematic review and meta-analysis. JAMA 2016; 315(23):2554–63.

70. Bommer S, Klein P, Suter A. First time proof of sage's tolerability and efficacy in menopausal women with hot flushes. Adv Ther 2011;28(6):490–500.

71. Liske E, Hänggi W, Henneicke-von Zepelin HH, et al. Physiological investigation of a unique extract of black cohosh (Cimicifugae racemosae rhizoma): a 6-month clinical study demonstrates no systemic estrogenic effect. J Womens Health Gend Based Med 2002;11(2):163–74.

72. Jacobson JS, Troxel AB, Evans J, et al. Randomized trial of black cohosh for the treatment of hot flashes among women with a history of breast cancer. J Clin Oncol 2001;19(10):2739–45.

73. Vermes G, Bánhidy F, Acs N. The effects of Remifemin® on subjective symptoms of menopause. Adv Ther 2005;22(2):148–54.

74. Ross SM. Menopause: a standardized isopropanolic black cohosh extract (remifemin) is found to be safe and effective for menopausal symptoms. Holist Nurs Pract 2012;26(1):58–61.

75. Newton KM, Reed SD, LaCroix AZ, et al. Treatment of vasomotor symptoms of menopause with black cohosh, multibotanicals, soy, hormone therapy, or placebo: a randomized trial. Ann Intern Med 2006;145(12):869–79.

76. Borrelli F, Ernst E. Black cohosh (Cimicifuga racemosa) for menopausal symptoms: a systematic review of its efficacy. Pharm Res 2008;58(1):8–14.

77. Huntley A, Ernst E. A systematic review of the safety of black cohosh. Menopause 2003;10(1):58–64.

78. Low Dog T, Powell KL, Weisman SM. Critical evaluation of the safety of Cimicifuga racemosa in menopause symptom relief. Menopause 2003;10(4):299–313.

79. Chiu HY, Pan CH, Shyu YK, et al. Effects of acupuncture on menopause-related symptoms and quality of life in women in natural menopause: a meta-analysis of randomized controlled trials. Menopause 2015;22(2):234–44.

80. Innes KE, Selfe TK, Vishnu A. Mind-body therapies for menopausal symptoms: a systematic review. Maturitas 2010;66(2):135–49.

81. Woods NF, Mitchell ES, Schnall JG, et al. Effects of mind–body therapies on symptom clusters during the menopausal transition. Climacteric 2014;17(1):10–22.

82. Crandall CJ, Newberry SJ, Diamant A, et al. Comparative effectiveness of pharmacologic treatments to prevent fractures: an updated systematic review. Ann Intern Med 2014;161(10):711–23.

83. Ross AC, Taylor CL, Yaktine AL, et al. Dietary reference intakes for calcium and vitamin D. Washington, DC: National Academies Press; 2011.

84. Feskanich D, Willett WC, Colditz GA. Calcium, vitamin D, milk consumption, and hip fractures: a prospective study among postmenopausal women. Am J Clin Nutr 2003;77(2):504–11.

85. Jackson RD, LaCroix AZ, Gass M, et al. Calcium plus vitamin D supplementation and the risk of fractures. N Engl J Med 2006;354(7):669–83.

86. Bolland MJ, Barber PA, Doughty RN, et al. Vascular events in healthy older women receiving calcium supplementation: randomised controlled trial. BMJ 2008;336(7638):262–6.

87. Bolland MJ, Avenell A, Baron JA, et al. Effect of calcium supplements on risk of myocardial infarction and cardiovascular events: meta-analysis. BMJ 2010;341:c3691.

88. Lewis JR, Zhu K, Prince RL. Adverse events from calcium supplementation: relationship to errors in myocardial infarction self-reporting in randomized controlled trials of calcium supplementation. J Bone Miner Res 2012;27(3):719–22.

89. Boonen S, Lips P, Bouillon R, et al. Need for additional calcium to reduce the risk of hip fracture with vitamin D supplementation: evidence from a comparative meta-analysis of randomized controlled trials. J Clin Endocrinol Metab 2007;92(4):1415–23.

90. Murad MH, Elamin KB, Abu Elnour NO, et al. The effect of vitamin D on falls: a systematic review and meta-analysis. J Clin Endocrinol Metab 2011;96(10): 2997–3006.
91. Ross AC, Manson JE, Abrams SA, et al. The 2011 report on dietary reference intakes for calcium and vitamin D from the Institute of Medicine: what clinicians need to know. J Clin Endocrinol Metab 2011;96(1):53–8.
92. Lips P, Hosking D, Lippuner K, et al. The prevalence of vitamin D inadequacy amongst women with osteoporosis: an international epidemiological investigation. J Intern Med 2006;260(3):245–54.
93. Bischoff-Ferrari HA, Dietrich T, Orav EJ, et al. Positive association between 25-hydroxyvitamin D levels and bone mineral density: a population-based study of younger and older adults. Am J Med 2004;116(9):634–9.
94. Bischoff-Ferrari HA. The 25-hydroxyvitamin D threshold for better health. J Steroid Biochem Mol Biol 2007;103(3):614–9.
95. Moyad MA. Vitamin D: a rapid review. Dermatol Nurs 2009;21(1):25.
96. Schild A, Herter-Aeberli I, Fattinger K, et al. Oral vitamin D supplements increase serum 25-hydroxyvitamin D in postmenopausal women and reduce bone calcium flux measured by 41Ca skeletal labeling. J Nutr 2015;145(10):2333–40.
97. Flore R, Ponziani FR, Di Rienzo TA, et al. Something more to say about calcium homeostasis: the role of vitamin K2 in vascular calcification and osteoporosis. Eur Rev Med Pharmacol Sci 2013;17(18):2433–40.
98. Huang ZB, Wan SL, Lu YJ, et al. Does vitamin K2 play a role in the prevention and treatment of osteoporosis for postmenopausal women: a meta-analysis of randomized controlled trials. Osteoporos Int 2015;26(3):1175–86.
99. Suzuki K, Tsuji S, Fukushima Y, et al. Clinical results of alendronate monotherapy and combined therapy with menatetrenone (VitK2) in postmenopausal RA patients. Mod Rheumatol 2013;23(3):450–5.
100. Emaus N, Gjesdal CG, Almås B, et al. Vitamin K2 supplementation does not influence bone loss in early menopausal women: a randomised double-blind placebo-controlled trial. Osteoporos Int 2010;21(10):1731–40.
101. Cockayne S, Adamson J, Lanham-New S, et al. Vitamin K and the prevention of fractures: systematic review and meta-analysis of randomized controlled trials. Arch Intern Med 2006;166(12):1256–61.
102. Pearson DA. Bone health and osteoporosis: the role of vitamin K and potential antagonism by anticoagulants. Nutr Clin Pract 2007;22(5):517–44.
103. Sato T, Schurgers LJ, Uenishi K. Comparison of menaquinone-4 and menaquinone-7 bioavailability in healthy women. Nutr J 2012;11(1):1.
104. Rude RK, Singer FR, Gruber HE. Skeletal and hormonal effects of magnesium deficiency. J Am Coll Nutr 2009;28(2):131–41.
105. Moshfegh A, Goldman J, Ahuja J, et al. What we eat in America, NHANES 2005-2006: usual nutrient intakes from food and water compared to 1997 dietary reference intakes for vitamin D, calcium, phosphorus, and magnesium. US Department of Agriculture, Agricultural Research Service; 2009.
106. Witkowski M, Hubert J, Mazur A. Methods of assessment of magnesium status in humans: a systematic review. Magnes Res 2012;24(4):163–80.
107. Reginster JY, Kaufman JM, Goemaere S, et al. Maintenance of antifracture efficacy over 10 years with strontium ranelate in postmenopausal osteoporosis. Osteoporos Int 2012;23(3):1115–22.
108. Roux C, Fechtenbaum J, Kolta S, et al. Strontium ranelate reduces the risk of vertebral fracture in young postmenopausal women with severe osteoporosis. Ann Rheum Dis 2008;67(12):1736–8.

109. O'Donnell S, Cranney A, Wells GA, et al. Strontium ranelate for preventing and treating postmenopausal osteoporosis. Cochrane Database Syst Rev 2006;(3):CD005326.
110. Westberg SM. Use of strontium chloride for the treatment of osteoporosis: a case report. Altern Ther Health Med 2016;22(3):66–70.
111. Corletto F. Female climacteric osteoporosis therapy with titrated horsetail (Equisetum arvense) extract plus calcium (osteosil calcium): randomized double blind study. Miner Ortoped Traumatol 1999;50(5):201–6.
112. Badole S, Kotwal S. Equisetum arvense: ethanopharmacological and phytochemical review with reference to osteoporosis. Intern J Pharm Sci Health Care 2014;1(4):131–41.
113. Lobo RA, Davis SR, De Villiers TJ, et al. Prevention of diseases after menopause. Climacteric 2014;17(5):540–56.
114. Ebeling PR. Osteoporosis in men. N Engl J Med 2008;358(14):1474–82.
115. Elraiyah T, Sonbol MB, Wang Z, et al. Clinical review: the benefits and harms of systemic testosterone therapy in postmenopausal women with normal adrenal function: a systematic review and meta-analysis. J Clin Endocrinol Metab 2014;99(10):3543–50.
116. Villareal DT, Holloszy JO, Kohrt WM. Effects of DHEA replacement on bone mineral density and body composition in elderly women and men. Obstet Gynecol Surv 2001;56(4):221–2.
117. Elraiyah T, Sonbol MB, Wang Z, et al. The benefits and harms of systemic dehydroepiandrosterone (DHEA) in postmenopausal women with normal adrenal function: a systematic review and meta-analysis. J Clin Endocrinol Metab 2014;99(10):3536–42.
118. Sabto J, Powell MJ, Breidahl MJ, et al. Influence of urinary sodium on calcium excretion in normal individuals. A redefinition of hypercalciuria. Med J Aust 1984;140(6):354–6.
119. Hannan MT, Tucker KL, Dawson-Hughes B, et al. Effect of dietary protein on bone loss in elderly men and women: the Framingham Osteoporosis Study. J Bone Miner Res 2000;15(12):2504–12.
120. Sellmeyer DE, Stone KL, Sebastian A, et al. A high ratio of dietary animal to vegetable protein increases the rate of bone loss and the risk of fracture in postmenopausal women. Am J Clin Nutr 2001;73(1):118–22.
121. Maggio M, Artoni A, Lauretani F, et al. The impact of omega-3 fatty acids on osteoporosis. Curr Pharm Des 2009;15(36):4157–64.
122. Tartibian B, Hajizadeh MB, Kanaley J, et al. Long-term aerobic exercise and omega-3 supplementation modulate osteoporosis through inflammatory mechanisms in post-menopausal women: a randomized, repeated measures study. Nutr Metab (Lond) 2011;8(1):1.
123. Kiel DP, Felson DT, Hannan MT, et al. Caffeine and the risk of hip fracture: the Framingham Study. Am J Epidemiol 1990;132(4):675–84.
124. Conlisk AJ, Galuska DA. Is caffeine associated with bone mineral density in young adult women? Prev Med 2000;31(5):562–8.
125. Todd JA, Robinson RJ. Osteoporosis and exercise. Postgrad Med J 2003; 79(932):320–3.
126. Kanis JA, Johnell O, Oden A, et al. Smoking and fracture risk: a meta-analysis. Osteoporos Int 2005;16(2):155–62.
127. Kim KH, Lee CM, Park SM, et al. Secondhand smoke exposure and osteoporosis in never-smoking postmenopausal women: the Fourth Korea

National Health and Nutrition Examination Survey. Osteoporos Int 2013; 24(2):523–32.

128. Oncken C, Prestwood K, Kleppinger A, et al. Impact of smoking cessation on bone mineral density in postmenopausal women. J Womens Health (Larchmt) 2006;15(10):1141–50.

129. Cornuz J, Feskanich D, Willett WC, et al. Smoking, smoking cessation, and risk of hip fracture in women. Am J Med 1999;106(3):311–4.

Moving?

Make sure your subscription moves with you!

To notify us of your new address, find your **Clinics Account Number** (located on your mailing label above your name), and contact customer service at:

Email: journalscustomerservice-usa@elsevier.com

800-654-2452 (subscribers in the U.S. & Canada)
314-447-8871 (subscribers outside of the U.S. & Canada)

Fax number: 314-447-8029

Elsevier Health Sciences Division
Subscription Customer Service
3251 Riverport Lane
Maryland Heights, MO 63043

*To ensure uninterrupted delivery of your subscription, please notify us at least 4 weeks in advance of move.

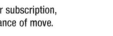

Printed and bound by CPI Group (UK) Ltd, Croydon, CR0 4YY

12/10/2024

01773487-0002